HEALTHY BOATING & SAILING

Optimize your
HEALTH & PERFORMANCE
on the water

Michael Martin Cohen, M.D.

Nautical Health Publishing, LLC

Copyright © 2019 by Michael Martin Cohen, MD

All rights reserved. No part of this publication may be reproduced, distributed, or transmitted in any form or by any means, including photocopying, recording, or other electronic or mechanical methods, without the prior written permission of the publisher, except in the case of brief quotations embodied in critical reviews and certain other noncommercial uses permitted by copyright law.

Editor: Natalie L. Silver, Silver Scribe Editorial Services

Publisher: Nautical Health Publishing, LLC

Book Design: Andrea Reider Books   andreareider@gmail.com

Healthy Boating & Sailing/ Michael Martin Cohen, MD

ISBN print 978-1-7343543-2-4
ISBN ebook: 978-1-7343543-5-5

Contents

Chapter 1	Seasickness	1
Chapter 2	Sound, Smell, and Navigation	29
Chapter 3	Cold Weather Sailing	53
Chapter 4	Heat and Dehydration	77
Chapter 5	Sailor's Skin	101
Chapter 6	Hazardous Marine Life	123
Chapter 7	Voyaging and the "Sea Diseases"	157
Chapter 8	Sailing Vision	173
Chapter 9	Sailing Nutrition	199
Chapter 10	Exercise	227
Chapter 11	Accidents and Injuries	253
Chapter 12	Sleep	279
Chapter 13	Sailing Psychology 1	303
Chapter 14	Sailing Psychology 2	319

Appendix 341

A. Motion Questionnaire & Behavioral Countermeasures 341
B. Drugs That Interfere with Sweating 345
C. Calculating Sweat 346
D. Fitness Docs 348
E. Sleep & Insomnia 352
F. Goals 359
G. Metric & English Conversion Tables 362

Index 367

Preface (2019)

A great deal has changed since the prior edition was published in 1983. For one thing, marine engines have become more reliable, and for another, the reference to celestial navigation—in this age of GPS—seems somewhat quaint. However, the human body's ability to function on the water remains something of a riddle. For that matter, how human beings function *on dry land* remains largely a mystery too! And therein lies the conundrum… Even though the amount of information on the physiology of sailing has grown exponentially, the dissemination of that information has been haphazard. There have been articles about it in many boating magazines, but not always in-depth enough to really understand the issues, or with enough substance to affect decision-making. But at least there is interest out there for learning more.

In order to provide some real understanding of the challenges faced by boaters and sailors, I have tried to go much deeper into the subject matter. But of course, that means that the narrative occasionally becomes a bit dense, so I have tried to simplify as much as possible. If there are chapters that are not of interest, feel free to skip them and perhaps come back to them later. Despite the radical change in the title (previously *Dr. Cohen's Healthy Sailor Book*) the pattern of chapters roughly follows the 1983 edition. The title change also reflects an attempt to address boaters in general, not just sailors. Except for a very few sections, most of the information is equally pertinent to powerboaters, fishermen, and even windsurfers.

I have also tried to inject some nautical history into the text. Nautical history is wonderfully instructive and, until the twentieth century, most historical culture clashes were defined, at least in part, by maritime "adventures."

Although there are some specific recommendations for the treatment of common ailments, this is not a first-aid book. The recommendations contained herein are for educational purposes only. All medication decisions must be left to you, and your personal physician or health care provider.

There are a number of quality, maritime first-aid books available, and before you set off on the water, you will need one (or perhaps more than one) along with a nautical first-aid kit. There are plenty of first-aid kits available with a completeness and sophistication commensurate with the kind of boating you will be doing: lake, bay, coastal, or blue water.

I wish you happy and healthy boating and sailing. May you always have fair winds and following seas!

Michael Martin Cohen, M.D.

for Elisse, Jordan, and Bradley,
Sam and Trudy,
Kandy and Charles

"The price of anything is the amount of life you exchange for it."
—*Henry David Thoreau*

Introduction

Healthy Boating & Sailing—the title is relatively straightforward. The subtitle—*Optimize* Your *Health and Performance on the Water*—*e*xpresses the importance of *performance* as well as health. Unless we are sitting at home thinking about our next adventure, we are always performing something (i.e., fishing, boating, cruising, or racing).

I wanted to include the term *biohacking* in the subtitle of this book to discuss performance on the water, but I resisted for fear it might scare some people away from reading an essential manual for life on the water. Even though the term is now absent from the cover of the book, biohacking is at the heart of this volume. But—what does that term even mean? And what is its relationship to health and performance?

The term *hacking* originated in the 1950s at MIT, and by the 1970s there were already a number of definitions, but one of the original (and the one that most applies to us) is the following:

> "A person who enjoys exploring the details of programmable systems and how to stretch their capabilities, as opposed to most users, who prefer to learn only the minimum necessary."[1]

So, the original usage was not pejorative and only later did the term become associated with malicious deeds such as hacking into private databases. We are using the term in the nonmalicious sense as in the definition above. The only substitution needed is "your body" for "programmable system"—and if you think about it, our body is a programmable system; we're just learning how to program it!

Biohacking is a relatively new term with the first known usage in the 1990s. It was originally used to describe biologic self-experimentation (often by implanting chips or magnets under the skin or, more recently, by attempting gene self-editing—yes, there are people out there who are attempting to use off-the-shelf science to edit their own genes). This type of physical alteration of the human body is most certainly *not* what we are talking about. Rather, at the other end of the spectrum is the more "natural" self-experimentation in order to make our body *perform* better. In a very real sense, we are experimenting on ourselves all the time. Instead of relying on a large randomized placebo controlled double-blind study, we often rely on our own personal trials. We try different things and judge which ones work better for us.

But rather than just trying x, y, and then z to see which one works better *for us,* biohacking takes a more scientific approach. It exploits the explosion of scientific information—data that has traditionally resided in some laboratory or your doctor's office—to better understand your body so that it can function optimally. The data (information) is there, or you can get it; you just need patience and inquisitiveness to acquire it.

It is not a quest of knowledge for knowledge's sake. It is a quest for knowledge that produces a change in action, a change in behavior. If the information doesn't lead somewhere, then it is just an interesting exercise.

So, in our context biohacking simply means knowing as much as possible about the human body—your body—as it deals with the stresses of the nautical environment, making whatever changes are needed to stay healthy and perform at peak efficiency. I will share a few examples to make this even clearer.

Let's assume you are a racing sailor who is often dehydrated at the end of a race. This has important implications, as even mild dehydration will reduce performance and can be the difference between medaling or not. You could consult texts and see the recommendations for the *average person* in your situation. Certainly, that is useful. But imagine how much more useful it would be if you could drill down deeper and learn how to measure *your* dehydration in order to better prepare so that you are not dehydrated for the next race.

Here's another scenario. Consider the problem of sleep and what you do to manage it or fight fatigue. There are lists of tips on how to get a good night's sleep (and they are included in Chapter 12), but again these are based on the average person (and who of us is average, anyway). For example, unless you hack into your own sleep pattern and discover what the problem is, you may never be able to get off the daily use of sleeping pills—which were never developed for daily use. And if fatigue in competition is an issue, you may need to hack into your cardiorespiratory system and determine your VO_2 max or your lactate threshold. And do you need those nutritional supplements? Almost certainly not. With few exceptions, they produce no positive effect on your health or performance, and actually many can be harmful.

There *is* a great deal of information currently available on biohacking, but most of this information has never made it to the boaters and sailors who could really use it. Definitely bits and pieces have made it into boating magazines and more recently online. But much of it remains unavailable to the average sailor, sequestered in scientific journals. My hope is that this book will provide this data so that you can improve both your health and your performance on the water.

The first chapters deal with issues that involve the way the body functions on the water. One could consider these initial chapters "Biohacking the Body." This would include chapters such as "Seasickness," "Cold Weather Sailing," "Heat and Dehydration,"

Introduction

and "Sailor's Skin." These chapters help you keep your body performing well despite what the nautical environment can throw at you.

The middle chapters—including "Hazardous Marine Life" and "Voyaging and the Sea Diseases"—involve "Biohacking the Environment" to stay safe among maritime predators, both large (sharks) and small (mosquitoes), understanding how to avoid the former and prepare for the latter.

The remainder of the book involves "Biohacking the Brain." They involve understanding those most basic human needs, such as nutrition, exercise, sleep, vision, and the mind itself, to allow the boater to perform at his or her best. These chapters detail what you should eat in this nautical environment, how you obtain the best sleep with a limited crew, and what you can do to improve your nautical mind.

As you drill down, you will find that some of the information you discover applies equally to your existence on land and sea, whereas other information is specific to our nautical environment. The only thing that matters is that you keep on hacking.

Note

1. MIT Jargon File, 1975, as cited in Ben Yagoda, "A Short History of 'Hack,'" *New Yorker*, March 6, 2014.

Chapter 1

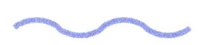

Seasickness

"And I'm never, never sick at sea!
What, never?
No, never!
What, never?
Well, hardly ever!
He's hardly ever sick at sea!
Then give three cheers, and one cheer more
For the hardy Captain of the Pinafore!"

—*W. S. Gilbert,* HMS Pinafore

"The misery I endured from sea-sickness is far
far beyond what I ever guessed at. If it was not for
sea-sickness, the whole world would be sailors."

—*Charles Darwin, letter to his father*

According to an English sailor's proverb, "The only cure for seasickness is to sit on the shady side of an old brick church in the country." Despite its obvious facetiousness, this proverb highlights the fact that seasickness is a disorder we inflict upon ourselves. Seasickness did not exist until our ancestors relinquished the relative security of land for the uncertainty of a raft or canoe. Written accounts of its challenges date back at least as far as the ancient Greeks. Hippocrates wrote, "Sailing on the sea proves that motion disturbs the body," a statement that contains more insight and less misconjecture than most of what was written during the next two thousand years. In fact, our English word *nausea* is derived from the Greek word *naus*, which means ship.

Because of our long familiarity with seasickness, numerous misconceptions and old wives' tales surround the illness. Nevertheless, we have made major advances in our understanding of both its cause and treatment. The first advance (in the nineteenth century) was the awareness that motion is the cause of motion sickness and that seasickness is simply one form of motion sickness (essentially Hippocrates's discovery). Riding in cars, trains, airplanes, spacecraft, and even on elephants and camels produces the same symptoms. Lawrence of Arabia, for example, suffered from "camel sickness"—a doubly appropriate term since camels have been referred to as the "ships of the desert." More recently, about 30 percent of the astronauts and cosmonauts who have flown in space have experienced motion sickness, or "spacecraft sickness." If you include those who suffered from mild symptoms—and many of the early astronauts *denied* they were sick to avoid being kept off future flights—the percentage affected is much higher. Additionally, people have experienced simulator sickness and virtual reality sickness.[1]

When humans depended solely on active locomotion—their own two feet—to get around, there was no problem. Running, jumping, somersaulting, and other such activities do not usually cause motion sickness. Only with the advent of passive locomotion (initially sailing and the riding of some domesticated animals) did motion sickness appear. We may find some consolation in noting that most other animal species are also liable to experience motion sickness when subjected to passive locomotion, including birds, dogs, horses, sheep, pigs, and even fish.[2]

The next advance was the recognition that motion sickness is a disorder of the brain and not of the stomach. Previous studies were mainly concerned with the stomach, which explains the variety of diets that had been proposed for the embarking passenger as well as for those already in the throes of seasickness. A popular theory in the nineteenth century attributed seasickness to the shifting of the stomach and intestines.[3]

How important are the effects of seasickness on world history? One could make a case that the world would be a very different place today without the debilitating symptoms that seasickness produces. If it were not for seasickness, the British Empire might have been quite a bit smaller and I might be speaking French, Dutch, or even from the point of view of a Native American. Why? In 1588, the Spanish Armada was launched to defeat Elizabethan England and restore Catholicism. Unfortunately for the Armada forces, the weather was very poor in the channel, and the Spanish ships were manned by soldiers (rather than sailors) who were not used to being on the sea. Many of the soldiers were seasick. The man in charge of the Armada was Don Alonso Pérez de Guzmán. He had no experience with naval battles and was frequently seasick himself. So, the Spanish Admiral and much of his crew were battling not only the English but the storm and seasickness. Thus began English dominance of the sea. This dominance was once again threatened two centuries later by Napoleon, who launched a Franco-Spanish force of thirty-three ships against the English. In one of the most decisive naval battles in history, the British fleet under Admiral Lord Nelson defeated the French and Spanish at the Battle of Trafalgar, off the coast of Spain. Nelson, one of the greatest nautical heroes in history was *constantly* seasick: and he was indeed seasick on the way to Cape Trafalgar.

Even this brief historical review allows a glimpse into the real challenges that human beings face when they take to the water. But let's turn now to a discussion of seasickness itself by looking at the vestibular (balance) system. Why look at this first? Because people who do not have a functioning vestibular balance system do not experience motion sickness, including seasickness. Ever.

The Vestibular Balance System

There are three parts to the inner ear: the cochlea or hearing apparatus (which we will address in Chapter 2), the semicircular canals, and the utricle and saccule (aka U&S; Figure 1.1). Since these structures are embedded in the skull, they move with movements of the head; that is, if the head is moved up or down or to the right or left, these structures move the same amount. The implication of this will soon become clear.

The U&S developed first in evolutionary terms, and their major task is relatively straightforward: to determine the direction of gravity (i.e., sensing up from down). Both consist of an array of *hair cells* upon which is balanced a solid mass of calcium carbonate crystals embedded in a gelatinous matrix (Figure 1.2A). The entire structure is bathed in a watery fluid called *endolymph*. Since the crystalline-gelatinous matrix is three times as dense as the endolymph, when the head is tilted away from the vertical position, gravity attracts the matrix (Figure 1.2B). As the matrix shifts, the hair cells are bent, producing a change in the number of nerve impulses relayed to the brain. The U&S function identically, except that in the utricle the hair cells are oriented horizontally whereas in the saccule, they are oriented vertically.

(Note: For those of you thinking that this is getting somewhat esoteric, please—bear with me. Unless you understand the vestibular system, you will never be able to properly exercise your judgment about some of the nonsensical approaches to motion sickness. Plus, the next time you or a relative are told by some health care professional that the cause of your dizziness and vertigo is those "crystals" in your inner ear, you will understand. In fact, what happens is that a few of the crystals (see Figure 1.2) become dislodged and end up in the semicircular canals, a condition which we will examine shortly.)

Although the U&S developed as gravity detectors, they also register linear acceleration: i.e., movement forward or backward, right or left, and up or down. Gravity is a form of linear acceleration with a constant value of 32 feet per second squared and a constant direction of being, perpendicular to the earth. The key to understanding this dual function of gravity orientation and linear acceleration is our knowledge of inertia. The law of inertia[4] states that *any mass at rest tends to remain at rest and any mass in motion tends to remain in motion unless acted upon by an outside force.* Let us look at what happens during a common experience—forward acceleration in a car. As the car accelerates, the U&S also accelerate forward—however the crystalline-gelatinous matrix that lies upon the hair cells does not. Because of inertia, the matrix is temporarily "left behind." Again, the hair cells are bent, this time signaling forward linear acceleration (Figure 1.2C). Usually there is no confusion as to whether we are experiencing head tilt or forward acceleration. After all, we can feel our body being thrust backward (inertia again), and we can see that we are moving forward. In other words, *we place the information in context aided*

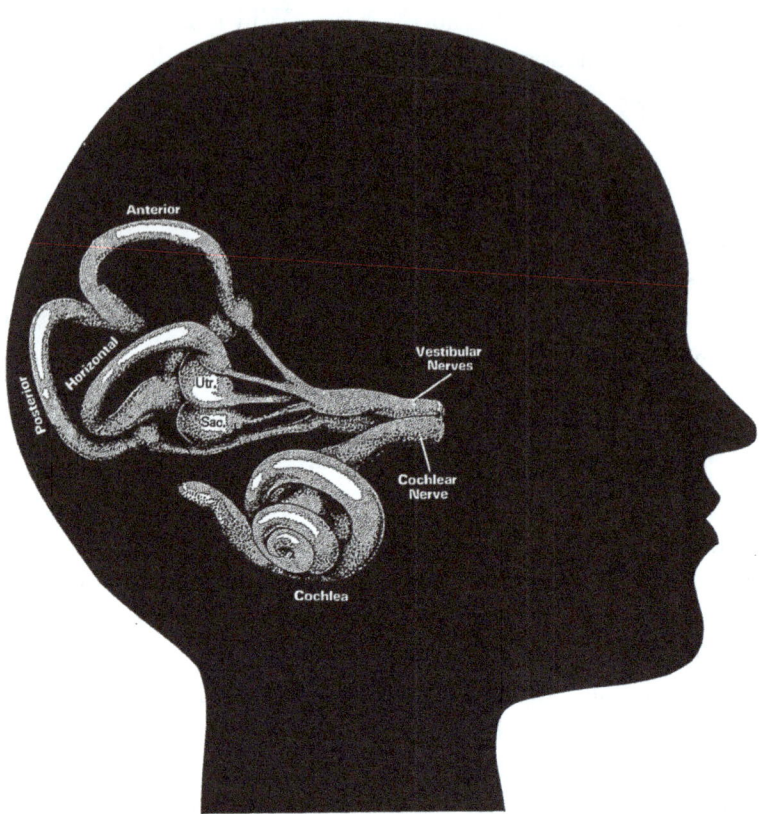

Figure 1.1 The vestibular (balance) system (not to scale). Notice the cochlea or hearing apparatus. This will be discussed in Chapter 2. Our concern now is with the vestibular system consisting of the three semicircular canals (anterior, posterior, and horizontal) and the smaller utricle and saccule (referred to as U&S). Nerve impulses from this system are carried to the brain along the vestibular nerve.

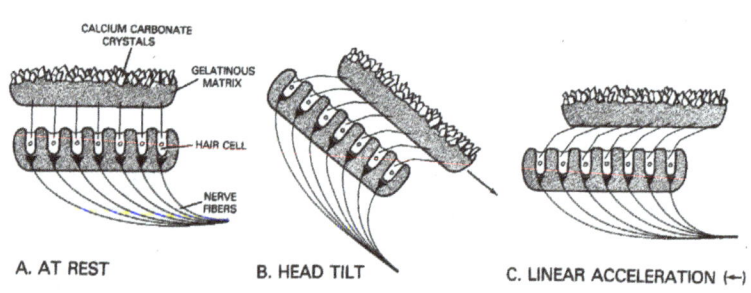

Figure 1.2 The utricle and saccule (U&S)

by the information from our other senses. When we are deprived of our other senses, especially vision, it may be impossible to tell the difference. This presents a continual hazard for pilots who fly without instruments during periods of reduced visibility. Deprived of visual cues, the pilot may misinterpret rapid forward acceleration as backward head tilt (compare Figure 1.2B and C); backward head tilt is, after all, more common. Because the pilot has the illusion that he or she has been gaining altitude (when in fact he or she has not) he or she may "level off" the plane prematurely, producing a nosedive with disastrous consequences.

The U&S function well up to a point, but to allow a greater degree of movement, a more sophisticated device is needed: the semicircular canals, which measure rotatory acceleration. There are three semicircular canals on each side of the head: the horizontal, the anterior, and the posterior (Figure 1.1).

The canals are perpendicular to one another so that all three dimensions of space can be analyzed without gaps in the coverage. Each canal is a small, circular, unbroken tube filled with endolymph. At one point in each canal, there is a swelling that contains the *cupula*, a jellylike, elastic structure (Figure 1.3A). The cupula protrudes into the tube much like a swinging door. And like a swinging door, it can bend to either side, but at rest, it tends to remain in a neutral position. The cupula has no independent motion. Rather, it is passively displaced by the endolymph in the canal. To ensure that the canals *do not* respond to gravity, nature employed a cunning stratagem by reducing the density of the cupula until it was exactly the same as the surrounding endolymph. If the cupula were either lighter or heavier, it would bend with head tilting. Since it is the same density, head tilting has no effect.

Embedded in the base of the cupula are numerous hair cells (just like the ones in the U&S). If the moving endolymph displaces the cupula in one direction, the hair cells are stimulated; if in the opposite direction, they are inhibited.

What happens when we rotate our head to the left? Since the movement is restricted to the horizontal plane, only the horizontal canals are involved. The left horizontal canal is rotated to the left by the same amount, say 20 degrees, since it is embedded in the skull. But the endolymph tends to remain at rest because of inertia. Thus, *relative to the canal*, the endolymph is moving in the opposite direction, to the right (Figure 1.3B). This relative motion of the endolymph bends the cupula, which stimulates the hair and nerve cells. Each canal is paired with one on the opposite side with which it works in tandem. If one canal is stimulated, its mate is inhibited. During a leftward head rotation, for example, the right horizontal canal is inhibited. These same concepts apply to non-horizontal head movements, except that more than one set of canals is involved. Various combinations of canals provide the brain with very precise information regarding rotation of the head and body.

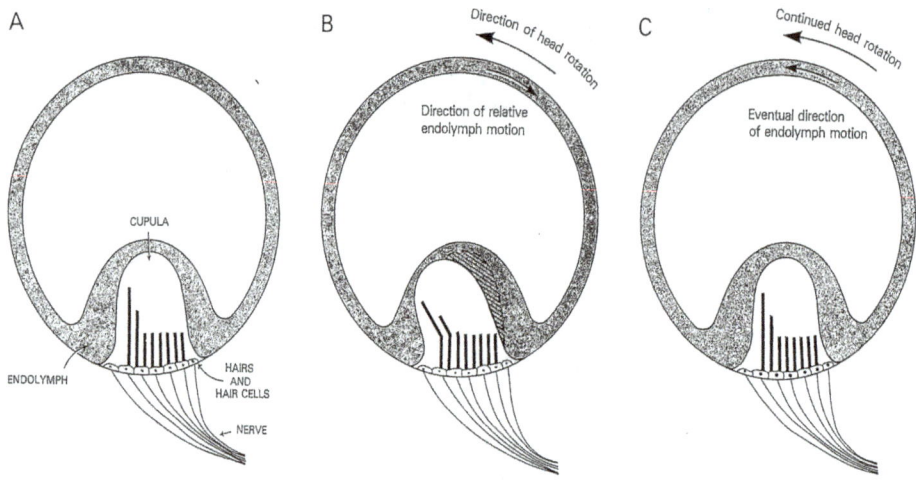

Figure 1.3 Function of the semicircular canals

The Current Theory of Motion Sickness

Sensory Conflict in the Brain

OK, that topic may have been challenging, but here is a different kind of challenge—a philosophical challenge: what is the purpose of a brain, any brain? The simple answer is to solve problems—in this case, the problem of balance in an unstable environment. To solve this problem, the brain gathers all the information it can get, from as many systems as it can access, and attempts to meld that information into a meaningful reality. We have already discussed one of the systems—the *vestibular system*. It is the most important system in terms of detecting instability and without it (because of disease or birth defect), a person will not suffer from motion sickness of any kind, including seasickness.

The second vital system is *vision*. Visual information supplements the information that the vestibular system provides. If we trip over a curbstone and fall forward, not only does our vestibular system signal the fall, but also we see that upcoming face-plant. On occasion, the visual system can "override" the information that the vestibular system gives us. Ice skaters, for example, use visual cues to help prevent dizziness when spinning. They learn to rely on the visual signals and suppress the unwanted vestibular signals.

The third system consists of *position sensors* in the joints and tendons of the neck, which signal movement of the head on the body.

All this information is precisely integrated and analyzed in the hindbrain in a structure we can call the motion analyzer (Figure 1.4). The motion analyzer is composed of nerve cells that respond to signals from all three systems. It processes the data and rapidly arrives at a meaningful response—the brain as a living computer, if you will.

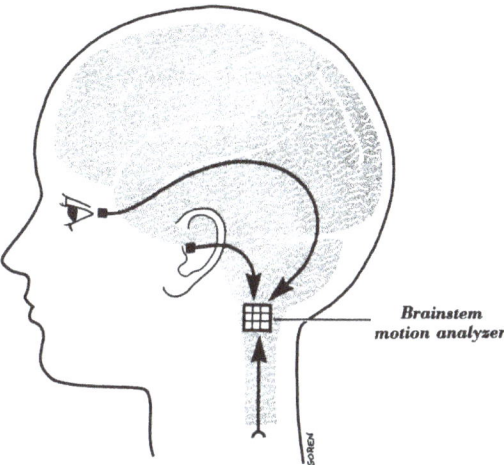

Figure 1.4 The motion analyzer

Normally, the three systems provide consistent information. In health, having three systems working together is a blessing, because they provide more sources of information, allowing smooth, coordinated movement and therefore better predictions to manage balance issues. And even if disease should affect one of the systems (e.g., visual loss), the other two can take up most of the slack. Redundancy becomes a curse, however, when the three systems are at variance with one another. *A conflict in the information that these three sources provide the brain is the cause of motion sickness.*[5]

This conflict explains why seasickness frequently occurs or is exacerbated by going below decks. Let us suppose that a crew member is seated at the navigation table facing forward during a rolling motion to starboard. The vestibular system senses this movement and informs the brain. However, since the hull of the boat has rolled to starboard by the same amount as the navigator, there is no significant change in what the navigator sees (Figure 1.5).

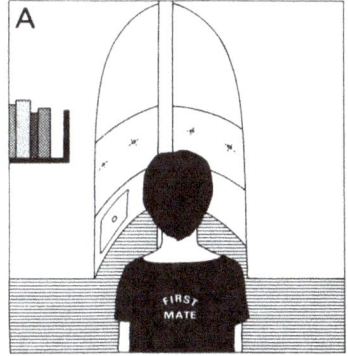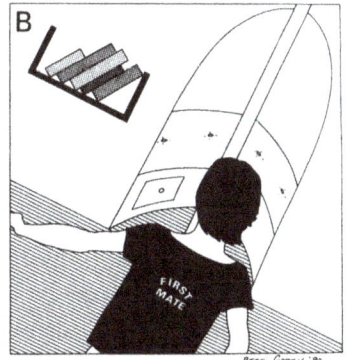

Figure 1.5 Rolling motion to starboard with visual-vestibular conflict

The visual system informs the brain that nothing has changed; however, the brain's motion analyzer has clearly received two sets of conflicting information. If, in addition, the head should jerk forward-backward or side-to-side on the body, a third set of erroneous information is provided. Actually, these extra, involuntary head movements seem to be very important in producing seasickness. As we will see, reducing them by stabilizing the head tends to ameliorate the seasickness.[6]

As if this is not enough, the brain must deal with yet another set of conflicting information arising from within the vestibular system itself. Normally, the semicircular canals and U&S act as complementary systems, which they have been doing since they first appeared in fish over a million years ago. However, in a rough sea, the vestibular system is stimulated in a chaotic fashion. In response to waves, a boat (as well as its crew) is subjected to six different motions: three rotatory (roll, pitch, and yaw), which primarily stimulate the canals, and three linear (surge, heave, and sway), which primarily stimulate the U&S (Figure 1.6).

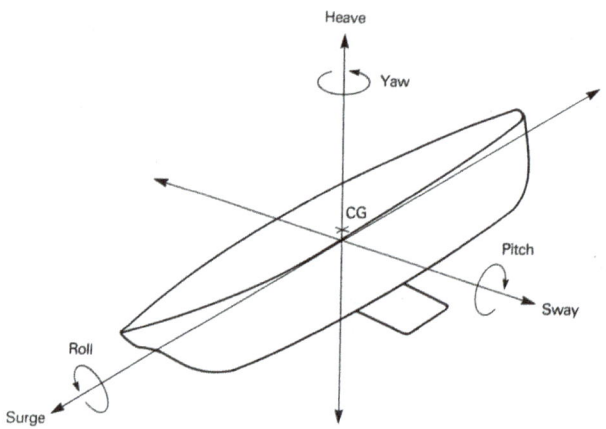

Figure 1.6 The six motions of a boat: three rotational (roll, pitch, and jaw) and three linear (surge, heave, and sway)

Combined rotatory and linear motions (such as pitching plus heaving or rolling plus surging) or rotations about two or more axes simultaneously (such as rolling plus pitching or pitching plus yawing) are very effective in producing seasickness. These complex motions trigger the release of conflicting and irreconcilable sensory information from within the semicircular canals and the U&S.[7]

Any theory of seasickness (and the other forms of motion sickness) should explain the three phases of the disorder. The first phase is seasickness caused by the sensory mismatch. Following prolonged stimulation during the first phase, the brain's motion analyzer eventually learns that this is "the new normal" and the symptoms decline and disappear. The second stage is adaptation, which can take up to three days or more in severe cases. The third phase is weird but makes sense if we realize that the brain has learned to accept the new environment with its new rules. This phase has been termed *mal de debarquement*, referring to the seasickness symptoms the sailor experiences when stepping ashore after recovering from a bout of seasickness (*mal de mer*). If the term *sea legs* connotes the ability to walk around the boat without experiencing sickness or disequilibrium, then perhaps *land legs* would be an appropriate term for the ability to adjust quickly back to life on land.[8] For a recent excellent review of the physiology and treatment of motion sickness see F. Schmal's "Neuronal Mechanisms and the Treatment of Motion Sickness."[9]

Symptoms and Signs

With all this conflicting information, it may seem surprising that the brain does not rebel more often. Well, it probably does! Many cases go unrecognized and we *undoubtedly underestimate* the incidence of seasickness by concentrating on the nausea, vomiting, and "dry heaves." We tend to neglect the "head" symptoms and signs, such as skin pallor, cold sweating, headache, malaise, and dizziness (Table 1.1). These symptoms are frequently attributed to such things as fatigue, anxiety, or dietary indiscretions.

HEAD SYMPTOMS

Skin Pallor
Cold Swelling
Headache
Malaise
Dizziness
Drowsiness
Yawning and sighing
Hyperventilation
Increased salivation or dry mouth

GUT SYMPTOMS

Disinclination to eat
Stomach awareness
Queasiness
Nausea
Vomiting or
Dry Heaves

Table 1.1 Common symptoms and signs of seasickness

The most consistent early sign of seasickness is skin pallor. It invariably precedes other symptoms and signs but may be easily overlooked. Cold sweating is next to appear but is a less reliable symptom. Headache is common during the early stage. It tends to be mild, usually a dull aching over the eyes or a bandlike constriction around the head. *Performance is often impaired even at this early stage.* By this time, the boater may feel somewhat drowsy and begin to lose interest in his or her surroundings and in food. Although he or she may not have nausea or stomach pain, he or she may become increasingly aware of the stomach region. This heightened stomach awareness then blends imperceptibly into queasiness and nausea.

Up to this point, if the abnormal motion ceases, the seasickness may abate, and the sailor rapidly recovers a sense of well-being. If the stimulus continues, the major manifestations of nausea and vomiting usually occur. The Rubicon has been crossed. The syndrome now takes on a life of its own and, even if the stimulus moderates, the symptoms may endure for an appreciable period of time.

Nausea and vomiting are not invariably linked to one another; some people vomit without premonitory nausea, whereas others experience intense nausea but never vomit. Many individuals find some relief after a bout of vomiting, that is, until a fresh wave of nausea and vomiting occurs.

Because intense nausea and vomiting (or the dry heaves) are so conspicuous, there is a tendency to equate them with every case of seasickness: not so. Some individuals have little or no nausea or vomiting but are nonetheless more uncomfortable than their mates draped over the leeward rail. Those with predominantly "head" symptoms mope about the deck preferring to be left alone. When this torpid state becomes extreme, it resembles a severe depression, and its sufferers occasionally beg to be thrown overboard, as life has lost all its charm. Performance of duty may be more hampered in these individuals than in crew members who are vomiting intermittently.

Whether or not a person develops seasickness, and whether the person has primarily head symptoms or gut symptoms, depends for the most part on three factors:

(1) the sea conditions
(2) individual susceptibility
(3) prior experience

If the sea conditions are severe enough, even the most iron-gutted sailor may become sick (if he or she has a functioning vestibular system). Some evidence suggests that heading directly into the wave system is the point of sailing most likely to cause seasickness. In this situation it is impossible to avoid the combination of multiple rotatory and linear motions described earlier in this chapter. Prior experience does seem to offer some protection but is by no means foolproof.[10]

The experience of K. Adlard Coles is worth examining. In his classic text *Heavy Weather Sailing*, he refers to numerous encounters with gale-force and near-gale-force conditions, but only twice does he give explicit descriptions of seasickness. One episode occurred while crossing the English Channel during a race. A second episode took place during a race across the Bay of Biscay, a notoriously "retched" body of water.[11]

The Coles accounts certainly support the sensory conflict theory of seasickness. No other theory can explain the occurrence of seasickness after awakening and feeling "well and refreshed." This phenomenon is not uncommon. Seasickness may first rear its ugly head after the sailor awakens, or the sailor may lie down because of seasickness and awake feeling much better, only to have the symptoms recur as soon as he or she gets up.

Individual Variability and Sensitivity

These two episodes also highlight the difficulty of predicting when seasickness will occur in those of us who are generally immune (and Coles would seem to be in the "hardly ever" category). After all, the people at each end of the spectrum present no challenge. Some fortunate individuals have yet to experience their own "moment of truth"—although if their vestibular systems are intact, there is no reason to suppose that they are *totally* immune. At the opposite end of the spectrum are those people who are extremely susceptible. They tend to be weeded out early and avoid water travel at all costs.

Most sailors fall between these extremes. It would be helpful if we could identify the unique factors that induce seasickness in each person. Possibly some people are more susceptible to the vestibular, visual, and neck-position conflict, whereas others possess less tolerance for the canal-U&S conflict. So far, however, this is merely speculation. Until researchers study this topic in more detail, all we can do is to try to eliminate each of the known precipitating factors.

The effect of the *size of the vessel* on seasickness has received little analysis. Nevertheless, it is well known that some people tend to be more susceptible to seasickness on either small or large boats. In fact, the sensory rearrangement that occurs in the motion analyzer is quite specific. For example, adaptation to the motion of an ocean liner by no means guarantees protection in a 100-foot yacht or small sailboat (and vice versa). Each situation presents the motion analyzer with a new learning experience. See also Appendix A.

In any given sea, *individual variation* determines who becomes sick, as well as the severity and duration of the symptoms. We can make a few generalizations, however. Genetic variability accounts for more than 50 percent of the risk. People who suffer from migraines, especially those with well-defined visual aura, are particularly susceptible. Women tend to be more susceptible than men to all forms of motion sickness, including seasickness—of course they are also more susceptible to migraines. Women are at even higher risk during menstruation and pregnancy, suggesting that hormonal changes play some, as yet unexplained, role. There are also age-related differences in susceptibility. Children below the age of two are almost totally immune. The risk then increases throughout childhood until adolescence, when it begins to decline *slowly*. The elderly are fairly immune. Adults prone to migraines and those with a history of Meniere's disease (an inner ear disorder) are more susceptible. Anyone actively playing video games, watching high definition movies, scrolling on tablets or smart phones, or engaging in virtual reality is also at increased risk. Most likely the specific brain wiring of a person's vestibular connections (motion analyzer) plays a role—see endnote 5 for more on this.

Regardless of these general trends, there is much individual variation in seasickness, and this depends on two factors: susceptibility and adaptation. If the motion is weak (a mild sea swell), the most susceptible are usually the first to develop head symptoms (such as skin pallor, cold sweating, and dizziness), which may be followed by gut symptoms. Resistant crew members may develop only head symptoms or nothing at all. With a severe stimulus (for example, when a boat leaves a protected harbor and heads directly into a rough sea), the more sensitive people tend to develop nausea and vomiting right away. The head symptoms may be overshadowed completely.

Since roughly one in three people are moderately or highly susceptible to motion sickness, it was only a matter of time until researchers began to examine genetic factors.[12] In one genome-wide association study of more than eighty thousand individuals (from the 23andMe database) who self-identified as having motion sickness, researchers found thirty-five gene variations associated with motion sickness. With thirty-five gene associations, there is still a long way to go to identify which genes or combination of genes increase the risk of motion sickness, but it's a start. These variations were interestingly near genes associated with the development of our three key systems—vision, balance, and position sense.

There is some evidence that adaptation and habituation do occur—although some people never habituate. The ability to adapt, as well as the rapidity with which adaptation takes place, is an individual trait. The motion analyzer is usually able to reconcile the chaos within about seventy-two hours, but a minority remains seasick for an entire journey. Fortunately, this occurs in less than 5 percent of the population. One study showed that regular seafarers seem to do better than non-seafarers on a nautical platform.[13]

In general, people exhibit these traits in four varying combinations, from worst to best: (1) high susceptibility/slow adaptation, the worst combination; (2) high susceptibility/fast adaptation, which yields an initially severe reaction that diminishes rapidly; (3) low susceptibility/slow adaptation, which produces prolonged head symptoms sometimes intermittently punctuated by nausea and vomiting; and (4) low susceptibility/fast adaptation, the ideal combination. See also Appendix A.

On the Wrong Tack

Since motion sickness is due to sensory conflict, several myths can now be jettisoned. Because the stomach is an "innocent bystander," dietary prescriptions and proscriptions are not necessary. There is no evidence that diet has any effect on seasickness whatsoever.[14]

However, any drugs, foods, or odors that by themselves can cause either nausea or disequilibrium, including alcohol, should be avoided. Also, it has been suggested that an empty stomach may slightly increase the risk of seasickness. Scientific evidence is not conclusive on this point, and it may not make any difference. It certainly doesn't matter what is put into the stomach, even though some people swear by certain foods, such as dry crackers or flat cola. Ginger has been recommended for prevention and treatment of seasickness, but studies examining its effectiveness have been contradictory. Ginger has been used for thousands of years as a treatment for a variety of gastrointestinal problems and most recently to counteract the nausea of chemotherapy. Since it probably functions primarily in the gastrointestinal tract, I would place it in the category of "possibly mildly effective," but it should not be depended on in a storm.[15]

Another therapy—which also has very little evidence to support its effectiveness—is the acupressure band. This is a device that is worn on each wrist, applied to the anatomical points on the wrist that purportedly diminish nausea. Like ginger, the acupressure band appeals to people who have a major aversion to taking medication. The acupressure band has never passed any kind of randomized controlled trial.[16] However, if the placebo effect helps you get through mild seasickness episodes, go for it.

One particularly contentious area, related to placebo, is the relationship between anxiety and seasickness. First, there are people who have *psychological* motion sickness. These individuals become nauseated and may vomit at the sight (or even the thought) of a boat. One writer has suggested the term emotion sickness. Second, fear or anxiety is a handy explanation, even though it is usually wrong. Most combat troops in World War II, for example, erroneously attributed their motion sickness to fear, even though they readily admitted that they did not remember feeling particularly fearful at the time.[17] The third origin is cultural. At least since the nineteenth century, seasickness has been regarded as evidence of a "lack of moral fiber" or, worse yet, a failure of "intestinal fortitude." This is evident from a few lines of the *HMS Pinafore* libretto:

> Though related to a peer
> I can hand, reef, and steer
> And ship a selvagee
> I am never known to quail
> At the fury of a gale
> And I'm never, never sick at sea![18]

The stigma of unmanliness continues to pervade our attitude toward the seasick individual. Although it is true that anxiety may worsen the situation, *the basic mechanism of seasickness is not psychological*. History certainly bears this out. Only four years before the Battle of Trafalgar, Lord Nelson (no shrinking violet) wrote, "Heavy sea, sick to death—this sea sickness I shall never get over." It is safe to say that he never did, since he was even seasick on the voyage to his final battle at Trafalgar![19]

Prevention

We cannot completely prevent seasickness. If the sea conditions are violent enough, almost everyone will succumb. However, before rushing headlong into drug treatment, there are some simple precautions that should be considered. If you are responsible for the safety of the boat and crew, it may be worthwhile to question the crew, prior to departure, about previous episodes of seasickness. If they have had no previous sea exposure, the presence or absence of car sickness or of other forms of motion sickness can serve as a rough guide. As a rule, if the crew member can read in a moving car, they are probably not overly susceptible. Conversely, susceptibility to car sickness indicates a propensity toward seasickness.

(In a similar vein, it is prudent to anticipate the sea conditions that will be encountered en route. For example, if the temperature is expected to fall or heavy weather is anticipated, crew members should be advised to err on the side of overdressing. It is far easier to shed excessive clothing and hand it below during rough conditions than it is to go below and change, especially to the forward cabin.)

As we have seen, anxiety does not cause seasickness—but it can exacerbate it. One experiment demonstrated that the incidence of seasickness is lower in subjects who were given a task to perform than in subjects who were not. In another experiment, subjects who were encouraged to pay attention to the abnormal motions were invariably sick. Thus, when feasible, crew members should be kept busy. It is no time for rumination.

Any maneuver that diminishes sensory conflict may ameliorate the seasickness. For this reason, staying on deck should be encouraged, and not simply to get fresh air as most people suppose. If during a rolling motion to starboard, for example, a person's vision is directed at a stationary point on land or at the horizon, sensory conflict does not occur (Figure 1.7).

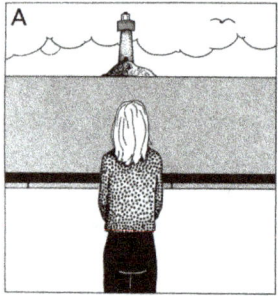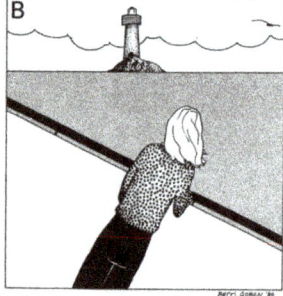

Figure 1.7 Rolling motion to starboard without visual-vestibular conflict

Both the vestibular system and the visual system register the same rolling motion. It is of no value to look at the mast or any other part of the boat. The object must be stationary with respect to the earth. Thus, seasickness is frequently lessened by taking the helm. The helmsperson has a task that distracts him or her from sickness and at the same time requires him or her to keep an eye on the horizon. This active role lessens the chance for seasickness and may even ameliorate the condition once it is present. Experimental evidence corroborates the fact that sensory rearrangement is facilitated by active participation. It is true of all forms of motion sickness that the operator of the vehicle (in this case, the boat) is less apt to become sick than are the passengers.

Parenthetically, car sickness in children is probably also due to sensory conflict. Since a child is often unable to see out of the front window, particularly from the back seat, he or she experiences an analogous vestibular-visual conflict. A car seat, that elevates the child high enough, may alleviate the problem.

If being below deck during turbulence cannot be avoided, it is advisable to keep the eyes closed to eliminate some of the conflict. If head movements are restrained, the conflict is lessened further. Several studies have now shown that restricting head movements eliminates signals from the third source of information—the neck position sensors. More importantly, it reduces the semicircular canal-U&S conflict to a great degree. Simply holding the head against the back of a seat, if high enough, is often sufficient neck restriction. If things continue to go from bad to worse, the best advice is to lie down, face up, eyes closed, as close to the middle of the boat as possible. This position will diminish most of the conflict, including some—but by no means all—of the semicircular canal-U&S conflict as well. Lying down, however, slows down the natural adaptation response. As we have seen, the adaptation response functions more rapidly as an active as opposed to a passive process. Therefore, if the crew member can "tough it out," preferably by keeping busy, he or she will be better off in the long run.

Other behavioral countermeasures include controlled and diaphragmatic breathing, listening to music, and choosing the right position in the vessel.[20] Adaptation schedules are useful in certain circumstances but less so for boating.[21] In one study, music which was perceived as "pleasant" no matter the genre showed a "trend" in reducing the severity of visually induced motion sickness.[22] See also Appendix A.

Seasickness "To Do" List

- **Skipper's Plan:** When preparing for the trip you should have some knowledge of each of your crew's experience with motion sickness (informal or questionnaire@);
    - Whether they have any medical conditions that could be worsened by severe seasickness – such as diabetes -or that would preclude the use of seasickness medication – urinary problems for example
    - What medication -if any- they have used in the past and plan to use if necessary
    - Since *all* the medications have some side effects it is always preferable to try one or two before embarking
    - **Avoid:** Large meals and excessive alcohol -eat moderately. Avoid noxious odors and other nauseogenic stimuli.
    - **Recognize:** It is important to recognize the early signs (see table 1.1) and treat as early as possible.
    - **Act:**
        — If you plan on taking medication – early is better. This is the time to let the skipper know that you have beginning seasickness symptoms and you should take the following steps if feasible.
        — Go on deck if feasible and try to fixate on the horizon.
        — Make sure you have sufficient clothing so that you do not have to go below later.
        — Try some of the behavioral modifications such as controlled breathing and listening to music
        — If you must stay below, try to get as close as possible to midships, close your eyes, stabilize your head, and if possible lie down.

Drug Treatment

Modern drug treatment for seasickness had an unexpected inception. In 1947, a woman was being treated for hives with the antihistamine dimenhydrate (Dramamine). She noticed that she was serendipitously cured of her car sickness every time she took the drug! Her physicians reported this phenomenon, and the next year "Operation Nausea," a full-scale trial of Dramamine was conducted on a troopship crossing the Atlantic during a storm. So began modern drug therapy for seasickness.

Although there is no single, ideal anti-motion-sickness drug, a number of drugs are very effective (Table 1.2). Of course, individuals vary in their response to each of these drugs; thus, the only way to determine the right drug or drugs, and the dosage that is best for any individual is by trial and error. To make an intelligent choice, these concepts should be kept in mind:

1. The goal is to maximize the anti-motion-sickness properties of a drug and to minimize its side effects. Because of a high recommended dosage, scopolamine (also known as hyoscine), the oldest and still the most effective anti-motion-sickness medication, has received unwarranted bad press for many years. Previously, the recommended dosage was about twice as high as is necessary, and nearly everyone experienced significant side effects as a result.

2. None of these drugs acts immediately. It takes time for the drug to begin to act, and even longer for it to provide maximal protection. For example, Dramamine requires at least one to two hours before there is any antimotion sickness effect. In a short-term situation, it would be illogical to expect Dramamine to be of any use. However, oral scopolamine, which is effective rapidly, would be an intelligent choice.

3. A corollary to number two is that different drugs have different durations of action. Oral Dramamine offers longer protection than oral scopolamine. For most of these drugs, the duration of action is inversely related to the time it takes for the drug to act. Obviously, a drug with a short duration of action must be taken at more frequent intervals than a drug with a long duration of action.[23]

All medications should be discussed with your primary care provider well in advance of embarkation. If you have not used a medication previously it would be wise to try it at your leisure on dry land to experience the side effects and customize the dose as best you can. For example, the oral form of scopolamine (Scopace) has several advantages over the better known Transderm Scop. However, it is infrequently used in medical practice and you may need to experiment with the dosage. Amphetamine (for a different set of reasons) may also prove a challenge (i.e., getting your doctor to agree). In that case, consider caffeine, which is discussed at length in Chapter 10.

The most effective preparation tested so far is the combination of 0.3 to 0.6 milligrams scopolamine (hyoscine) plus 5-10 milligrams dextroamphetamine. This combination has in fact been prescribed for astronauts suffering from space sickness. It has been thoroughly tested in seasickness, and, for susceptible people under rough conditions, this is the treatment of choice.

Drug	Brand Name	Rx / OTC	Form	Dosage (in mgs)	Duration / Frequency	Comments
Scopolamine	Transderm Scop	Rx	Transderm	1.5	72 hours	For prophylaxis. Needs to be applied prior to departure – up to 6hrs
Scopolamine (Hyoscine)	Scopace	Rx	Oral	0.4	1 - 2 tablets every 8 hours max 2.4 mgs/d	Discuss with your physician as this is infrequently used in practice. Begin 60 minutes before embarkation
Promethazine	Phenergan	Rx	Oral	12.5 - 25	Every 6 - 12 hours	Excellent anti-seasickness medication but may cause drowsiness.
Promethazine	Phenergan	Rx	Suppos	12.5 - 25	Every 6 - 12 hours	Probably treatment of choice when nausea and vomiting already present
Meclizine	Bonine, Antivert, Dramamine Less Drowsy.	OTC	Oral	12.5 - 50	Every 12 - 24	Probably the best of the OTC medications. Begin 2 hours before embarkation or night before
Dimenhydrinate	Dramamine, Gravol	OTC	Oral	50	Every 6 - 12; max 300mgs/d	Begin 60 minutes before embarkation
Cyclizine	Marezine, Bonine for Kids	OTC	Oral	50	Every 6 - 12	Begin 60-120 minutes before embarkation
Cinnarizine	Stugeron	OTC	Oral	25	Every 6 – 12 max 100mgs/d	Begin 1-2 hours before embarkation or night before. Not avail. In US/Can.
Amphetamine	Adderall	Rx	Oral	5-10	Discuss	Not usually given because it is a controlled substance.
Caffeine	Coffee or caffeine tablets	OTC	Oral	100- 200	Every 4 hours	The stimulant now commonly used in place of amphetamine

Table 1.2 Medication options for seasickness

All medications should be discussed with your primary care provider well in advance of embarkation. If you have not used a medication previously it would be wise to try it at your leisure on dry land to experience the side effects and customize the dose as best you can. For example, the oral form of scopolamine (Scopace) has several advantages over the better known Transderm Scop. However, it is infrequently used in medical practice and you may need to experiment with the dosage.

There are, however, some problems with the combination. The duration of action is only about four hours (which means that repeated doses are necessary), and it is becoming difficult to obtain dextroamphetamine because of its potential for misuse and abuse. The side effects of scopolamine (hyoscine) include drowsiness, blurred vision, and dry mouth (and sometimes dizziness, rapid heart rate, urinary obstruction, and worsening of glaucoma). But the side effects are usually a problem only with high doses or in very young or old people. Initially dextroamphetamine was added simply to counteract the drowsiness produced by the scopolamine, but recent experiments have demonstrated that dextroamphetamine has significant anti-motion-sickness properties of its own. In fact, it is second in effectiveness only to scopolamine. The important side effects of dextroamphetamine are insomnia and hyperactivity (sometimes with insufferable loquaciousness!). The scopolamine tends to counteract and modify both symptoms. Only slightly less effective is the combination of 25 milligrams promethazine (Phenergan) plus 25 milligrams of ephedrine (not available in the United States, and you would need to substitute amphetamine). The duration of action is approximately twice as long, which is a definite advantage. The side effects are similar, but not as marked. Promethazine alone may produce drowsiness, hence the dextroamphetamine. As in the first combination, these drugs were chosen to counteract each other's side effects. This combination is becoming very popular throughout the nautical community.

Three of the above drugs—scopolamine (hyoscine), dextroamphetamine, and promethazine—have proven effectiveness by themselves. Scopolamine and Phenergan (promethazine) can be given intramuscularly, and Phenergan is available as a suppository, a very effective route of administration.

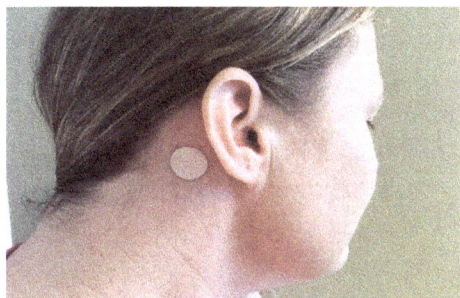

Figure 1.8 Transderm Scop placement behind the ear

There is a very popular option with scopolamine that straddles the line between prevention and treatment, and I am referring of course to Transderm Scop. Usage requires you to apply an adhesive, transdermal disk containing the drug to a hairless spot on the skin, usually behind the ear (Figure 1.8). The drug is slowly absorbed through the skin into the bloodstream. The idea behind the transdermal system is that a low-dose, continuous administration maintains an effective level in the bloodstream while reducing the side effects. The system delivers 1 milligram over a period of three days. Since it generally takes two to four hours after application to achieve an effective concentration, the disk must be applied at least that long before exposure. It has been recommended that the disk be applied up to twelve hours before, or the night prior to, departure. The disk is impervious to water and may be worn while swimming or showering. Once removed, however, it cannot be reused. The side effects do seem to be less, but they are still present. Dry mouth in two out of three cases and drowsiness in about one out of six cases are quite usual. Blurred vision is also common. Scopolamine tablets are also an alternative. Once the correct dose is determined, there tend to be fewer side effects than with the transdermal scopolamine.

There are three antihistamines (available without a prescription) that are about equally effective when used in mild-to-moderate situations: (1) dimenhydrinate (Dramamine), 50 milligrams; (2) cyclizine (Marezine), 50 milligrams; and (3) meclizine

(Bonine, Antivert), 12.5 to 50 milligrams. It is recommended that they be administered at least one to two hours before exposure, but there is evidence that pretreatment the day before may be even better.

We have not yet discussed cinnarizine (Stugeron). It is not available in the United States or Canada but is used widely throughout the world. It is the most commonly used drug in the Royal Navy. Beth Leonard, blue-water sailor / circumnavigator (who initiated her voyage with a severe case of seasickness!) has surveyed thirty-seven sailors and found cinnarizine to be the most recommended motion sickness medication based on effectiveness and side effects.[24] In fact, a German company has formulated a fixed combination of cinnarizine (20 milligrams) and dimenhydrinate (Arlevert; 40 milligrams), which has been effective in clinical studies and real-life experience for the treatment of all types of dizziness and vertigo.[25] The advantage of cinnarizine is that it has a lesser tendency to impair performance at sea than scopolamine.[26]

We are still learning about precisely how these drugs prevent or at least ameliorate seasickness. They appear to act at both the semicircular canals/U&S and in the brain itself. Functionally, the main activity is to "pacify" the motion analyzer, allowing the sailor to experience the abnormal motion for a longer period without becoming sick. This means that the brain has more time to adapt to the motion and *adaptation is the only cure*. If you are preparing a first-aid kit, it is important to include at least one drug that can be taken nonorally. Unless a physician or nurse is available, intramuscular injections (such as with promethazine) are not feasible, and it must never be given intravenously. However, promethazine suppositories are a rapid, effective, and practical alternative. So is the transdermal scopolamine system, although it takes at least two hours before a significant amount of the drug is absorbed. Except for the antihistamines, all the seasickness drugs discussed earlier require a prescription. At the recommended dosages, these drugs are safe for young, healthy adults. For very young children, older adults, or anyone with medical problems, *the choice of seasickness medication should be made in concert with a physician*.

One interesting, real-world evaluation of seasickness remedies was reported in 2000 by Dr. Paul Gahlinger.[27] There were 260 passengers on two expeditions traversing the Drake Passage from Argentina to Antarctica, encountering some of the roughest sea conditions in the world. The data was collected over the course of two voyages, each requiring two to three days of travel with gale force winds and sea swells up to 9 meters (30 feet). The subjects ranged in age from fifteen to eighty-seven years; 44 percent were male, and 56 percent were female. All passengers were informed about the sea conditions and the likelihood of seasickness and were offered a choice of meclizine, dimenhydrinate, or transdermal scopolamine. Many passengers brought their own medications including prescription medications and acupuncture wristbands. Several of the passengers had cinnarizine. All subjects were given a questionnaire covering the use of anti-motion-sickness remedies and subjective assessment of their benefits. Following the voyage, seasickness severity was evaluated with a standardized scale. The results revealed that sixty-nine passengers (26 percent) declined medication for a variety of reasons. Of the remaining one hundred ninety-one using medication, sixty-seven (35 percent) used meclizine, sixty (31%) used transdermal scopolamine, twenty-eight (15 percent) used dimenhydrinate (Dramamine), sixteen (8 percent) used cinnarizine, and twenty (10 percent) used acupuncture wristbands.

The most effective means of preventing or alleviating seasickness was clearly scopolamine, followed by meclizine, dimenhydrinate, cinnarizine, and acupressure. Side effects were common (Except in the acupressure subjects who reported no adverse effects!) and included drowsiness as the most common. Interestingly, the least effective medication was cinnarizine, which had a lower efficacy rating then either meclizine or dimenhydrinate (which are both nonprescription).

Performance and the "Sopite Syndrome"

Sopite syndrome (the unusual name is from the Latin *sopire*—"to lay to rest or put to sleep") is a neurologic disorder related to motion sickness and seasickness in which prolonged periods of motion produce drowsiness, fatigue, and change in mood.[28] The key symptoms are very similar to the head symptoms discussed above, but unlike seasickness, the head symptoms remain, and the gut symptoms never develop. The term was first developed at the Naval Aerospace Medical Research Laboratory in 1976 and has been studied and refined over the years.[29] The definition itself has been recently revised:

> Sopite syndrome is a symptom complex that develops as a result of exposure to real or apparent motion and is characterized by excessive *drowsiness, lassitude, lethargy, mild depression, and reduced ability to focus on an assigned task*. Sopite syndrome is most clearly distinguished in a healthy individual free from pathological conditions that engender similar symptoms and not suffering from sleep deprivation, mental or physical fatigue, or increased levels of physical activity.[31]

I believe it is reasonable to think of sopite syndrome as analogous to the head symptoms without the "autonomic" nervous system symptoms such as pallor, yawning, cold sweating, increased salivation, or dry mouth (see Table 1.1). The signs and symptoms seem purely psychological. And that is the problem. It is obvious to anyone that someone at sea who is in the throes of seasickness will have impaired performance in completing the task at hand. But sopite syndrome is more subtle. In fact, someone afflicted with it may appear depressed and just "want to be left alone." Unless this syndrome is kept in mind, it is likely that the cause of the performance decline will be totally misdiagnosed. In a recent study of mild motion sickness and sopite syndrome on multitasking cognitive performance, the authors found that multitasking declined even when the motion sickness and sopite syndrome were mild.[30] They postulated that both of these disorders (which appear to be closely related) reduce the ability of the sailor to focus on performing a task or tasks—and this became most apparent when shifting attention from one task to another as occurs in multitasking.

Correct recognition is important operationally because (1) the person may have impaired performance but not be identified as seasick; (2) drugs for seasickness may not improve performance due to the sopite effects; and (3) the side effects of many of the medications discussed above may actually exacerbate the effects of sopite syndrome—since many already produce drowsiness.

Coda

During a severe episode of seasickness, the feeling of hopelessness and despair can be overwhelming. If you should find yourself in such a state, you need only consider the fate of a young Englishman who became violently seasick during his first ocean voyage. In a letter to his father, who was a physician, the youth wrote:

> We sailed, as you know, on the 27th of December, and have been fortunate enough to have had from that time to the present a fair and moderate breeze. It afterwards proved that we had escaped a heavy gale in the Channel, another at Madeira, and another on the Coast of Africa. But in escaping the gale, we felt its consequence—a heavy sea. In the Bay of Biscay there was a long and continuous swell, and the misery I endured from sea-sickness is far beyond what I ever guessed at. I believe you are curious about it. I will give you all my dear-bought experience. Nobody who has only been to sea for twenty-four hours has a right to say that sea-sickness is even uncomfortable. The real misery only begins when you are so exhausted that a little exertion makes a feeling of faintness come on. I found nothing but lying in my hammock did me any good....
>
> In short, I find a ship a very comfortable house, with everything you want, and if it was not for sea-sickness the whole world would be sailors. I do not think there is much danger of Erasmus setting the example, but in case there should be, he may rely upon it he does not know one-tenth of the sufferings of sea-sickness.

Excerpted from a letter from Charles Darwin to his father on February 8, 1832, written aboard the *HMS Beagle*.[32]

Notes

1. J. E. Bos, S. N. MacKinnon, A. Patterson, "Motion Sickness Symptoms in a Ship Motion Simulator: Effects of Inside, Outside, and No View," *Aviation, Space, and Environmental Medicine* 76 (2005): 12

2. Antarctic explorer Ernest Shackleton took ponies with him. He recorded in his diaries that although they did not vomit (there is a valve that prevents this in ponies), they were in distress and displayed signs of seasickness and nausea.

3. Devices were invented that could be worn around the middle to restrict this motion. Someone even recommended that the passenger "should wear a pad in the epigastrium [abdomen] with an opposing one in the small of the back, and, at first qualms, should cause a mild galvanic current to pass between the two." Speculation that the inner ear and its connections with the brain were the source of motion sickness did not begin until the 1880s, and there were doubters well into the twentieth century.

4. Newton's first law of motion.

5. For you neuro-geeks, here is an overview of the inputs and outputs of the vestibular system. Much of the analysis (and our hypothetical "motion analyzer") is located within the vestibular nuclei, but as you can see, the connections to multiple different areas of the brain explain the difficulty the brain has in making sense of the sensory conflict. The multiple connections also explain the myriad symptoms—including all the emotional symptoms that are seen in seasickness. Most of the brain areas to the right of the vestibular nuclei are part of the so-called "limbic (emotional) system." I vividly recall the severe depression I experienced with my first seasickness episode.

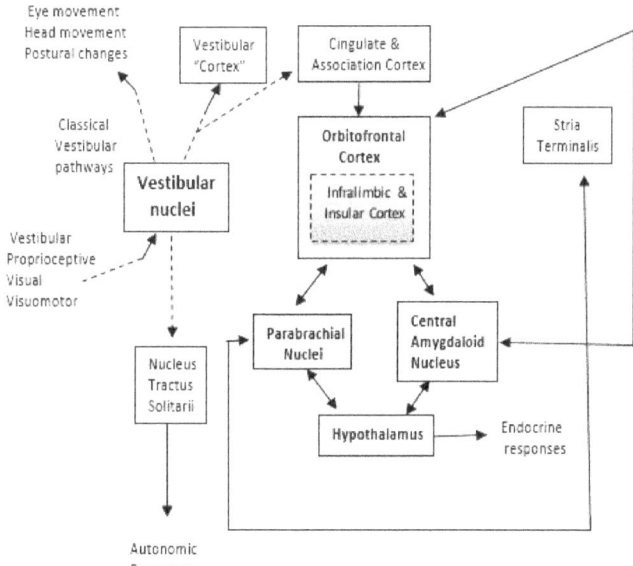

Redrawn from an illustration in C. D. Balaban, "Neural Substrates Linking Balance Control and Anxiety," Physiology and Behavior 7, no. 4-5 (December 2002): 469-475.

6. The astronauts aboard the International Space Station (and before that the Space Shuttle) have learned to keep their head still and mostly upright for the initial two to three days of their journey. See Michael Klesius, "Sick in Space," *Air and Space*, March 8, 2009, https://www.airspacemag.com/space/sick-in-space-56746153/.

7. The following note is for biology aficionados (others may safely skip). The most instructive and widely used paradigm for motion sickness is the Coriolis vestibular reaction. The Coriolis reaction is produced by simultaneous rotation about two perpendicular axes. If the term sounds vaguely familiar, it should, since the Coriolis force is in good part responsible for our weather

patterns. Because of the angular rotation of the earth, northerly or southerly air masses are deflected to the right in the Northern Hemisphere and to the left in the Southern Hemisphere. The Coriolis vestibular reaction is similar. As we have seen, horizontal rotation to the left, as in a rotating chair, initially stimulates the left horizontal canal and inhibits the right. However, if rotation is continued at constant velocity (zero acceleration), the endolymph will eventually overcome its inertia and acquire the same velocity as the canal itself. At this point the cupula will spring back to its neutral position. If, during this constant velocity rotation to the left, the person tilts his or her head to the right shoulder, a seemingly bizarre phenomenon occurs—motion sickness!

Most people need more than one tilt to become sick. The explanation lies in the incompatibility of the information the canals and U&S supply. When the head is tilted to the right shoulder, the U&S, unaffected by the rotation, signal right head tilt. All well and good. But with the head tilted, we now bring the two anterior canals into the plane of rotation and they are stimulated. But stimulation of the anterior canals usually occurs when the head is rotated forward. There's the rub. The U&S are signaling head tilt to the right while the canals are signaling forward head rotation. The only way this could occur is if the head were split down the middle and each half flew off in different directions! No wonder the brain becomes perplexed.

It might be asked how this is comparable to our experience on the water, since even in the roughest weather we are never subjected to this kind of stimulus. True, the assault on our vestibular system is not as regular or predictable; however, the same kind of semicircular canal and U&S "conflict" occurs on a smaller scale over a much longer period. The Coriolis vestibular reaction can produce nausea and vomiting in less than a minute, whereas seasickness usually takes about thirty minutes or more to occur.

G. Bertolini and D. Straumann, "Moving in a Moving World: A Review on Vestibular Motion Sickness," *Frontiers in Neurology* 7 (2016): 14, doi: 10.3389/fneur.2016.00014.

8. The most appealing explanation is the sensory conflict theory, as described above. According to this theory, which J. T. Reason, J. J. Brand, and others originally proposed, the motion analyzer eventually adjusts to the conflict by rearranging the sensory information. When the sailor is exposed to a situation that generates sensory conflict, whether among the vestibular, visual, and neck position systems or within the vestibular system or both, the motion analyzer searches its "memory" for previous similar episodes. If it finds a strong memory trace of sensory conflict comparable to the present situation, nothing happens. If it finds nothing appropriate, it does two things. First, it sets into motion the seasickness syndrome. Why this occurs, we do not know. Next, it begins to fill its memory bank with this new conflicting information (rolls plus heaves, yaws plus surges, and so forth).

With time, this conflicting information becomes the norm, and the motion analyzer eventually can search its memory and state categorically, "Yes, I am aware that this combination of sensory information may seem peculiar, but for this environment, which is my home at the present time, it is perfectly OK." This sensory rearrangement coincides with the second, or adaptation, phase; it is a form of unconscious learning.

The adaptation phase occurs only if the sailor continues to be exposed to the same abnormal motion. However, when the sailor, who has finally adapted, returns to a land, the motion analyzer is again confused. It searches its memory and on superficial perusal discovers that once again there is a conflict. The motion analyzer has come to expect the unusual combinations of movement, the "new normal." Again, it sets into motion the seasickness syndrome and searches through its memory more thoroughly. It soon discovers that this environment is not so foreign after all. Here we have the crucial difference between mal de mer and mal de debarquement. In the first instance, the process of sensory rearrangement or learning takes an appreciable amount of time to occur, during which the seasickness prevails, whereas in the second instance, the memory has been there all along, merely concealed beneath the more recent information. For this reason, mal de debarquement is never as prolonged as the original episode of seasickness.

    9. F. Schmal, "Neuronal Mechanisms and the Treatment of Motion Sickness," *Pharmacology* 91 (2013): 229-241, doi: 10.1159/000350185.

    10. J. R. Lackner, "Motion Sickness: More Than Nausea and Vomiting," *Experimental Brain Research* 232, no. 8 (2014): 2493-2510, doi: 1007/s00221-014-4008-8.

    11. Excepts from K. A. Coles, *Heavy Weather Sailing*, 3rd rev. ed. (Clinton Corners, NY: De Graff, 1981), 73-74, 82-83.

By dawn on Sunday (8 August) the wind had moderated, but in Cohoe's cabin conditions did not seem much quieter. For a while after a gale the sea is often more truculent than during its height. The yacht is no longer steadied by the wind and the motion is worse in consequence. At 0700 I got up. I felt amazingly well and refreshed, for I had had a good deal of sleep—more than we got at any other time in the race. I went forward through the cabin and tried the radio, as we wanted a weather report. It would not work. I tried various ways, but the only thing to do was to take it into the cabin for drying out and testing. I unscrewed it and carried it aft. At that moment I suddenly began to feel seasick. I handed the radio to Ross and lay down, feeling fit again at once. Ross played with its innards and inserted a new valve, but after sitting up he, too, suddenly felt ill. All of us were fit when lying down, but each felt seedy the moment he sat up and tried to do anything.

We started on a brilliant Sunday afternoon with a fine fresh breeze to shake us down. The wind headed in the early hours of Monday morning and by 0830 it had freshened so much that we had to take in a reef. We kept the genoa standing, but the bolt holding the runner plate sheared under the strain and repairs had to be effected. At 1000 the mainsail tore right across under the headboard. The sail came down with a run and the headboard and halyard went aloft to the masthead.

Cohoe's mast was solid, high and thin, and above the jumpers it was little more than the thickness of a big walking stick. A considerable swell was running and a fairly rough sea, so there was no prospect of swarming up the mast to retrieve the halyard. The burgee sheave was a strong one, so we tried to lead a wire rope through it by means of the burgee halyard, but the attempts were unsuccessful and finally the burgee halyard broke.

We then shackled the bosun's chair to the fore halyard and hoisted Dick Trafford, the lightest of the three of us, up to the forestay block. But the motion was so wild aloft and he was thrown about so much that he could not reach the peak and retrieve the main halyard. When he was lowered to the deck he was violently sick.

Deprived of her mainsail, the yacht was rolling tremendously in the seas. It was difficult to retain one's foothold even on deck, and aloft, even when secured to the mast, it was like being at the end of a pendulum, as it swung first one side and then the other over the sea. It was enough to make anybody seasick.

We abandoned the attempts to retrieve the main halyard and lashed the mainsail to the boom. Next we tried setting the trysail by means of the spinnaker halyard, but this failed because we could not get the lead right.

12. B. S. Hromatka et al., "Genetic Variants Associated with Motion Sickness Point to Roles for Inner Ear Development, Neurologic Processes and Glucose Homeostasis," *Human Molecular Genetics* 24, no. 9, (May 1, 2015): 2700-2708, https://doi.org/10.1093/hmg/ddv028.

13. G. Chan et al., "A Comparison of Motion Sickness Prevalence between Seafarers and Non-Seafarers Onboard Naval Platforms," *International Maritime Health* 57 (2006): 1-4.

14. In the past, a wide variety of absurd diets was prescribed for the embarking passenger. These varied between gastronomic austerity, dry toast or gruel, and gastronomic whimsy, "soup made of horse radish and rice, seasoned with red herrings and sardines." The latter was to be washed down with a "light, sparkling wine."

15. A. M. Bode and Z. Dong, "The Amazing and Mighty Ginger" in *Herbal Medicine: Biomolecular and Clinical Aspects*, 2nd ed., ed. Iris F. F. Benzie and Sissi Wachtel-Galor (Boca Raton, FL: CRC Press/Taylor & Francis, 2011), chap. 7; D. B. Mowrey and D. E. Clayson, "Motion Sickness, Ginger, and Psycho-Physics," *Lancet* 1 (1982): 655-657. The authors suggest that "ginger ameliorates the effects of motion sickness in the gastrointestinal tract itself. It may increase gastric motility and absorb neutralizing toxins and acids, so effectively blocking gastrointestinal reactions and subsequent nausea feedback."

16. K. E. Miller & E. R. Muth, "Efficacy of Acupressure and Acustimulation Bands for the Prevention of Motion Sickness," *Aviation, Space, and Environmental Medicine* 75, no. 3 (2004): 227-234.

17. The medications used in World War II are still somewhat of a mystery. It appears that many or most of the airmen (paratroopers) were given amobarbital (a barbiturate), presumably to calm their nerves, although it put many of them to sleep just before they were ready to jump (so-called "military intelligence"). Scopolamine was also starting to be used by both the Allies and the Axis, and there is some evidence that probably atropine and scopolamine were included with the amobarbital. The soldiers who made the sea crossing in terrible, rough seas were uniformly seasick. It is often reported that they were given Dramamine but that seems unlikely. Many were given "motion sickness" pills but the composition is still unclear. Eli Lilly and Company, the manufacturer, claimed in 2010 that it no longer has the information (I am too much of a cynic to believe that!), which suggests to me that the main ingredient may have been a barbiturate. The one thing we are certain of is that they were given a bag to throw up in! For further discussion, see "Battle Relic #7," Battledetective.com, http://www. Battledetective .com /battlerelic7.html.

18. *The Complete Plays of Gilbert and Sullivan* (New York: Garden City, 1938), 105.

19. Adm. Lord Nelson, who spent his life at sea and lost an eye and an arm in various nautical engagements, never entirely acclimatized to the sea. Just a year before his great victory and death at the Battle of Trafalgar, he wrote, "I am ill every time it blows hard and nothing but my enthusiastic love for the profession keeps me one hour at sea." "Lord Nelson Seasickness Letter Went on Display," *BBC News*, December 10, 2012, www.bbc.com/news/uk-england-20662931.

20. F. D. Yen Pik Sang et al., "Behavioral Methods of Alleviating Motion Sickness: Effectiveness of Controlled Breathing and Music Audiotape," *Journal of Travel Medicine* 10, no. 2 (2003): 108-111; S. E. Stromberg, M. E. Russell, C. R. Carlson, "Diaphragmatic Breathing and Its Effectiveness for the Management of Motion Sickness," *Aerospace Medicine and Human Performance* 85, no. 5 (2015): 452-457, doi: 10.3357/AMHP.4152.2015; A. Brainard, "Motion Sickness Treatment and Management" Medscape, updated November 10, 2017, www.emedicine.medscape.com/article/2060606-treatment.

21. In two other motion sickness situations (aircraft pilot sickness and spacecraft sickness), adaptation schedules have been developed. These individuals are gradually exposed in the laboratory to increasing stimuli of the sort that they are likely to encounter in the air or in space. In these two situations, the types of abnormal motion are limited and stereotyped, and adaptation exposures do confer some protection. Since the abnormal motion that occurs on the water is anything but stereotyped, adaptation schedules for sailors have not been very helpful. Perhaps sailors can hasten the adaptation response somewhat by sleeping aboard the night prior to departure. Yet it is doubtful whether this will offer much protection against really heavy weather.

22. B. Keshavarz and H. Hecht, "Pleasant Music as a Countermeasure against Visually Induced Motion Sickness," *Applied Ergonomics* 45 (2014): 521-527.

23. C. K. Sanchez and K. A. Lusk, "The Pharmacologic Management of Motion Sickness," *US Pharmacy* 40, no. 12 (2015): 34-44; A. C. Parrott, "The Effects of Transdermal Scopolamine and for Dose Levels of Oral Scopolamine (0.15, 0.3, 0.6, and 1.2 mg) Upon Psychological Performance," *Psychopharmacology* 89 (1986): 347-354.

24. B. Leonard, "Cures For Seasickness," in *Practical Sailor*, https://www.practical-sailor.com/issues/35_1/features/Seasickness-Medications_5724-1.html. I would point out that although promethazine (Phenergan) is in the phenothiazine class with the major tranquilizers, it effects primarily the histamine receptors of the brain and not the dopamine receptors. It has one tenth the potential—or less—of the major tranquilizers to cause the serious neurologic side effect known as tardive dyskinesia. I have used it personally and in neurology practice for more than forty years and have never had a case. *Nevertheless, as with all medical information, check with your personal physician or health care provider before taking any medication.* B. Leonard, Dealing with Seasickness, *Cruising World*, September 2010, 82-87.

25. A. W. Scholtz et al., "Cinnarizine and Dimenhydrinate in the Treatment of Vertigo in Medical Practice," *Wiener Klinische Wochenschrift* 128, no. 9-10 (2016): 341-347, doi: 10.1007/s00508-015-0905-5.

26. J. F. Golding, R. Strong, and R. J. Pethybridge, "Time-Course of Effects of Oral Cinnarizine and Hyoscine on Task Performance," *Journal of Psychopharmacology* 3, no. 4 (1989): 187-197.

27. P. M. Gahlinger, "A Comparison of Motion Sickness Remedies in Severe Sea Conditions," *Wilderness and Environmental Medicine* 11 (2000): 136-137, doi: https://doi.org/10.1580/1080-6032(2000)011[0136:LTTE]2.3.CO;2.

28. The phenomenon is probably analogous in adults to the physiologic effect rocking has on a newborn to help them to sleep (https://en.wikipedia.org/wiki/Sopite_syndrome).

29. A. Graybiel and J. Knepton, "Sopite Syndrome—Sometimes Sole Manifestation of Motion Sickness," *Aviation, Space, and Environmental Medicine* 47, no. 8 (1976): 873-882.

30. P. Matsangas and M. E. McCaukey, "Sopite Syndrome: A Revised Definition," *Aviation, Space, and Environmental Medicine* 85, no. 6 (2014): 672-673.

31. P. Matsangas, M. E. McCaukey, and W. Becker, "The Effect of Mild Motion Sickness and Sopite Syndrome on Multitasking Cognitive Performance," *Human Factors* 56, no. 6 (2014): 1124-1135.

32. F. Darwin (Ed.), *The Autobiography of Charles Darwin and Selected Letters* (New York: Dover, 1958), 135-137.

Chapter 2

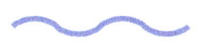

Sound, Smell, and Navigation

"You must learn to heed your senses. Humans use but a tiny percentage of theirs. They barely look, they rarely listen, they never smell, and they think that they can only experience feelings through their skin. But they talk, oh, do they talk."

—*Michael Scott,* The Alchemyst

"It's a poor sort of memory that only works backwards,"

— White Queen to Alice from *Lewis Carroll's,* Through the Looking-Glass

Sound at Sea

We would be remiss not to mention the importance of *hearing* at sea for two reasons: First, while we spent the last chapter discussing the *vestibular balance mechanism* (containing the utricle and saccule [U&S] and the semicircular canals)—the *cochlea*, or hearing apparatus, was biding its time right next door. The cochlea, which looks like a snail shell (cochlea is Greek for snail), is the sensory apparatus for hearing and sound discrimination. In fact, nerve impulses from both balance and hearing are sent over the eighth cranial nerve into the brainstem—for those of you keeping track of your cranial nerves. Second, appreciating and properly interpreting sound at sea could save your life. Consider this common nautical scenario—you are in unfamiliar waters in the midst of a dense fog. Visibility is zero and you have neither radar nor an Automatic Identification System (AIS). You hear a horn but have difficulty locating it. It seems off to the right, but is it in front or behind you? Is there anything you can do to pinpoint the sound? The problem of sound localization at sea is certainly not a new one.

In 1889, the president of the United States, in concert with a special provision of Congress, extended to the governments of all maritime nations an invitation to send delegates to the International Marine Conference. The conference was held in Washington, from October 16 through December 31, 1889, with the purpose of discussing and revising the rules and regulations and practice concerning vessels at sea and navigation generally (see Figure 2.1).

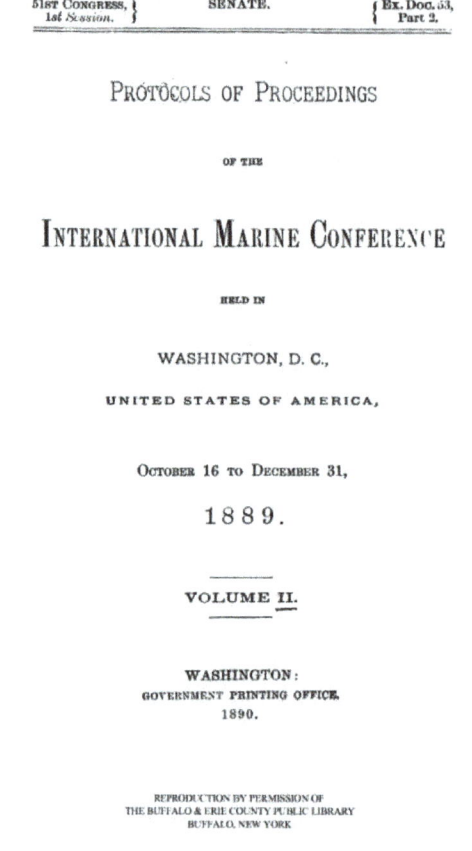

Figure 2.1 International Marine Conference of 1889

The following governments sent delegates to the conference: Austria-Hungary, Belgium, Brazil, Chile, Costa Rica, Denmark, France, Germany, Great Britain, Guatemala, Hawaii, Honduras, Italy, Japan, Mexico, the Netherlands, Nicaragua, Norway, Portugal, Russia, Siam, Spain, Sweden, Turkey, Venezuela, and the United States. The main concern was to codify *marine signals or other means of plainly indicating the direction in which vessels are moving in fog, mist, falling snow, and thick weather, and at night.* The conference made definite recommendations concerning rules for the prevention of collisions and rules of the road. There were three major areas of concern:

(1) Visibility, number, and position of lights carried by vessels
(2) Sound signals: their character, number, range, and position of instruments
(3). Steering and sailing rules

One resolution is pertinent to the discussion of sound at sea and the difficulty of localizing it—especially at times of impaired visibility when it would be most useful:

Resolved, That in the opinion of the Conference it is <u>inexpedient</u> to adopt course-indicating sound-signals in foggy or thick weather; inasmuch as among the other strong reasons presented by the Sound-Signal Committee, if such signals were used in crowded waters, danger would result from the uncertainty and confusion produced by a multiplicity of signals and from the false security that would be created in the minds of Mariners, and if vessels were navigated dependence on such signals, when neither could see the other, there would be danger that the officer in charge might read the signal incorrectly, or, if you read it correctly would interpret it wrongly.[1]

The take-home message is that whereas vision and by extension radar can signify *location* in space, sound waves are not nearly as precise in terms of localization. And therefore, in the nautical environment, sound waves are used mainly to signal *intent* rather than location. Even when coupled with aids to navigation, such as buoys, the sound of a bell or gong is primarily meant to signify danger, although the specific sound may help confirm the identity of a visible buoy.[2]

The following is from Boating Basics Online and contains the basic sound signals that should be second nature to any boater:

Are we able to localize sound at sea? Somewhat and within definite limits. Certainly not well enough to compete with vision during the day or radar at night. But in a pinch, our sense of hearing can come in handy. Localization depends mainly on two phenomena: the time difference between the sound reaching the two ears (Interaural Time Difference, or ITD) and the loudness difference experienced by the two ears (Interaural Level Difference, or ILD). You wouldn't think that there would be much difference in timing between sound waves reaching the two ears, and you would be correct. At sea level, sound waves travel at 340 meters per second and your head is only about 0.175 meters wide. The difference in the time it takes for sound waves to reach your left ear after they have reached your right ear is about *one half of a millisecond* (one thousandth of a second). The maximum difference would occur if the sound waves were coming directly from either side. Sound waves would obviously reach both ears at the same time if the sound were coming from directly in front or behind (Figure 2.3). How is the brain able to compute this infinitesimal difference almost instantaneously? Don't ask!

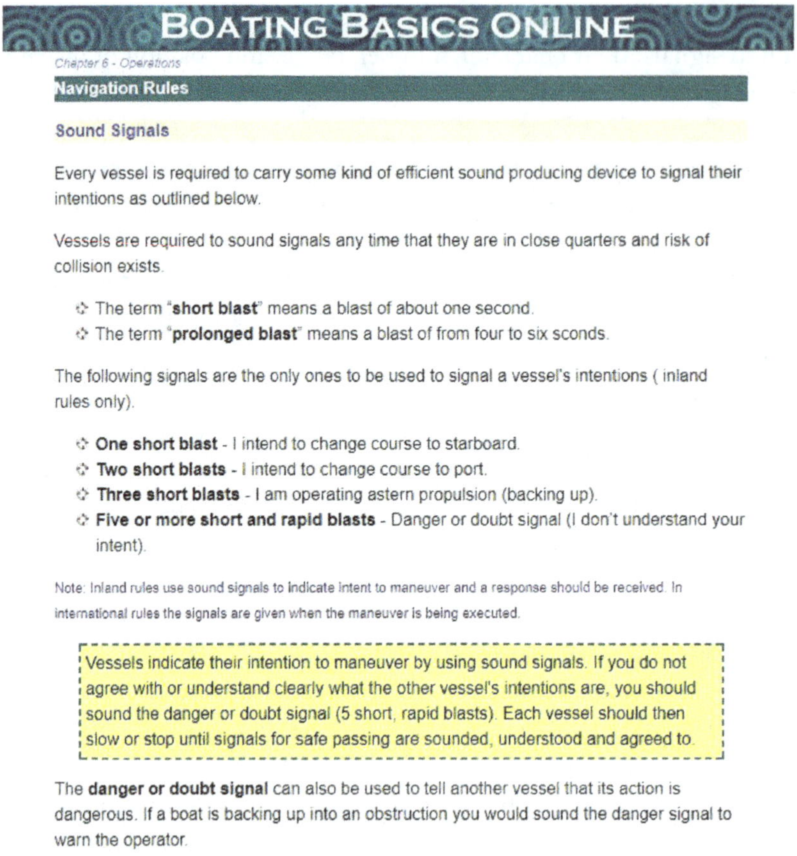

Healthy Boating & Sailing

BOATING BASICS ONLINE

Chapter 6 - Operations
Navigation Rules

Sound Signals

Every vessel is required to carry some kind of efficient sound producing device to signal their intentions as outlined below.

Vessels are required to sound signals any time that they are in close quarters and risk of collision exists.

- The term "**short blast**" means a blast of about one second.
- The term "**prolonged blast**" means a blast of from four to six sconds.

The following signals are the only ones to be used to signal a vessel's intentions (inland rules only).

- **One short blast** - I intend to change course to starboard.
- **Two short blasts** - I intend to change course to port.
- **Three short blasts** - I am operating astern propulsion (backing up).
- **Five or more short and rapid blasts** - Danger or doubt signal (I don't understand your intent).

Note: Inland rules use sound signals to indicate intent to maneuver and a response should be received. In international rules the signals are given when the maneuver is being executed.

> Vessels indicate their intention to maneuver by using sound signals. If you do not agree with or understand clearly what the other vessel's intentions are, you should sound the danger or doubt signal (5 short, rapid blasts). Each vessel should then slow or stop until signals for safe passing are sounded, understood and agreed to.

The **danger or doubt signal** can also be used to tell another vessel that its action is dangerous. If a boat is backing up into an obstruction you would sound the danger signal to warn the operator.

Figure 2.2 Boating Basics Online

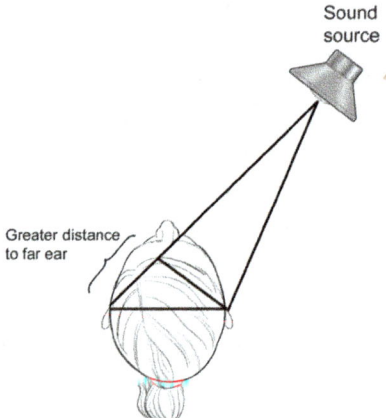

Figure 2.3 Interaural Time Difference (ITD). Copyright Jennifer M. Groh.[3]

The brain is also able to utilize the slight difference in loudness of sound coming from the side as the head produces an acoustic shadow, which decreases the loudness that reaches the far ear. This is most prominent for high-frequency sounds—not that commonplace in the nautical environment (Figure 2.4).

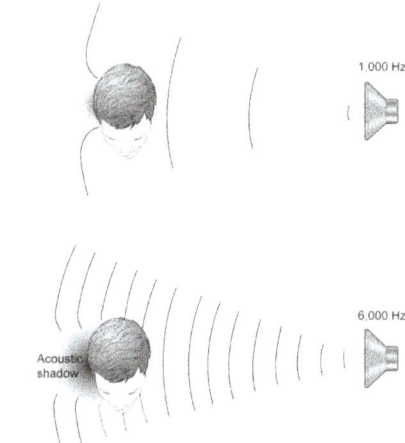

Figure 2.4 Interaural Level Difference (ILD; acoustic shadow). Copyright Jennifer M. Groh.

Getting back to our scenario: You are in thick fog, and there is the sound of a horn, but you cannot tell its precise location. If the sound is coming from the right, for example, but you are unable to tell if it is in front or behind, then head turning can help. If the sound is in front and you turn your head to the left, it will now localize to the right side. If it is behind and you turn to the left it will now be more midline (Figure 2.5).

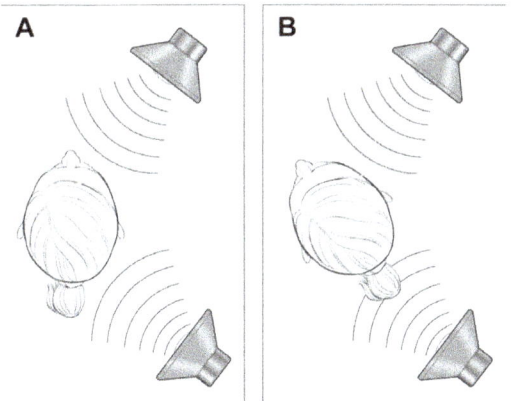

Figure 2.5 Head turning to disambiguate the location. Copyright Jennifer M. Groh.

Sound localization is a skill that can be practiced. If you are often boating in areas of reduced visibility or at night, then you *should* practice. How good can you become? Very good. Some of you may be familiar with the cases of blind children and adults who are able to use echolocation to navigate through space, just as bats do. These "echolocators" create clicking sounds with their mouth and then are able to interpret the sound waves that are reflected back from the environment (the echoes). With practice, and just by clicking rapidly, they are able to appreciate shape, contour, distance, and even texture from the environment. Some of the blind echolocators are skilled enough that they are able to ride a bicycle through town, avoiding obstacles. Blind echolocators are superior to their seeing counterparts in terms of utilizing this skill, but people with normal vision are *definitely* able to learn.[4]

If you are sailing close to a high, rock-bound coast in fog or at night, you can judge the distance offshore by the reflected echo you produce with a siren blast, gunshot, or even a loud shout. It helps to have a stopwatch. Since sound through the air will travel at a rate of roughly a mile (1.6 kilometers) every five seconds, each second between the sound and its echo means a distance of about 560 feet (170 meters) from the coastline bluff.

The above discussion takes care of azimuth location. In a nautical environment, we are less concerned with vertical location. There are similar techniques for helping to localize vertically, but if you are concerned with vertical location then you are probably too darned close! All that is required is that you tilt your head to maximize the Vertical Interaural Difference (Figure 2.6).

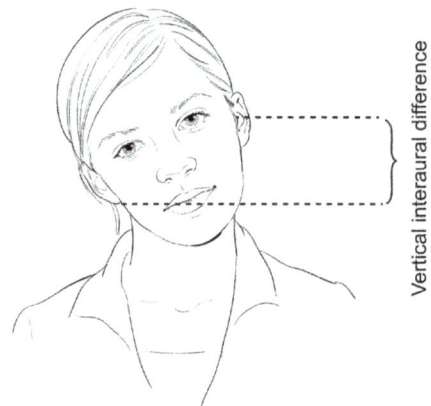

Figure 2.6 Head tilting to disambiguate the vertical. Copyright Jennifer M. Groh.

What about distance location? Yes, that would be *extremely* helpful information. The loudness of a sound is inversely related to the distance away from you. The farther away, the softer the sound. But unfortunately, the ear and brain are simply not able to distinguish a loud distant sound from a soft closer sound. Echoes are of some help, but

Sound, Smell, and Navigation

as with verticality, if you hear echoes at sea you are probably too darn close (or perhaps in a fjord).

To complicate matters further, sound waves sometimes travel differently over water than they do over land. Let's say you are sitting in your boat in the evening at the local marina and you unexpectedly hear someone speaking clearly from a distant shore. Your first thought may be *Oh, God, can they hear everything I have been saying?* Your second thought is probably *Why is their sound so clear? Is sound amplified when it travels over water?*

If the water is calm (as on a lake or a calm night on the ocean) you might guess that some of the sound waves skim over the surface of the water, adding to the amplification—*reflection*—off the surface of the still water. And you would be correct, but only partly so, as this is a relatively minor source of amplification. The main reason for the amplification is *refraction*. When a wave passes from one material to another it is frequently bent or refracted. We will revisit refraction in some detail in Chapter 8 since light rays are invariably refracted when light passes from air into water or water into air. The same kind of bending occurs when sound waves pass from cool air to warm air or vice versa. The temperature of the air just above the surface in a lake or ocean is often cooler than the normal air temperature further aloft (a type of temperature inversion that is very common on almost all calm clear nights and less frequently during certain daytime conditions). The cool air slows the sound waves near the surface. Next, as the sound travels from the cool air near the surface to the warmer air aloft, it speeds up and gets bent back down to the surface. This is the refraction (Figure 2.7). The result is that the amount of sound is much greater than it would be if the sound waves only took a direct path. The implication for the mariner is that sounds detected on the water *are often louder than would be expected.* This only confuses the issue when trying to estimate the distance to another ship blowing a horn or to a nautical buoy producing a sound.

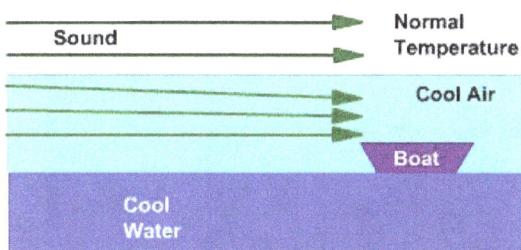

Figure 2.7 Refraction of sound rays over the water[5]

Therefore, the best way to judge the distance of a sound at sea is from *memory*. That is, by comparing the loudness of the sound to your memory of how far away you were when you last heard the sound at that level. It no doubt helps if you are a crusty old mariner who has traveled the same route many times.

There are a number of other techniques available to the "natural navigator." These have been enumerated by Harold Gatty in his classic text *Finding Your Way Without Map or Compass*.[6] This text highlights ways to listen for sounds of the land that can be heard at sea, including the sound of waves beating against the shore, trains, fog signals, and industrial activity. In the evening, birds are usually nesting or roosting on land. Therefore, it is safe to assume that in most parts of the world, seabirds will indicate the direction of land (since few seabirds feed at night).

The last health and safety issue regarding sound is noise and the decibel scale. It is important for boaters to realize that the decibel scale is logarithmic, rather than linear. Table 2.1 illustrates the scale.

Source	Intensity Level
Threshold of Hearing (TOH)	0dB
Rustling Leaves	10dB
Whisper	20dB
Quiet Room	40dB
Moderate Rainfall	50dB
Normal Conversation	60dB
Busy Street Traffic	70dB
Vacuum Cleaner or Alarm Clock	80dB
Garbage Disposal, Shop Tools	90dB
Large Orchestra	98dB
Headphones at Maximum Level	100dB
Rock Concert	110dB
Heavy Equipment, Chain Saw	120dB
Threshold of Pain	130dB
Jet Takeoff	140dB
Fireworks, Rifle, Handgun	160dB

Table 2.1 The decibel scale

The scale is logarithmic because the range of intensities is so large. Rustling leaves are measured at ten times the threshold of hearing (TOH). But the increase to whisper is ten times greater than that (20 dB), or one hundred times TOH. And a sound with a decibel level at thirty is ten times that, or one thousand times TOH. So, each increase of 10 dB multiplies sound intensity by another ten times. The National Institute for Occupational Safety and Health has recommended that the worker-exposure noise level should be at or less than 85 dB for an eight-hour day. Therefore, if you are working in the engine room or an equivalently noisy area for hours at a time, please obtain ear plugs and wear them! For a detailed discussion of ear protection: Wikipedia is a valuable source (https://en.wikipedia.org/wiki/ Earplug#Health _risks).

The Smell of the Sea

When you think of that "fresh sea air" or "smell of the shore," what word first comes to mind? Sulfur? Probably not. More likely you might think that it is the salinity (or "saltiness"), but you would be mistaken. The truth is that saltwater has essentially no smell. If you doubt this, just dissolve table salt in water and take a whiff—nothing. It turns out that the characteristic and distinctive smell of the sea is due primarily to small amounts of sulfur, and that sulfur in the atmosphere plays an important role in modulating our climate. Where does the sulfur come from? The two main sources are seaweed and phytoplankton.

Seaweed in the water is harmless, but once it is washed ashore onto the beach it starts to decompose, and during this process it will emit *hydrogen sulfide* (H_2S) gas. If the temperature is warm, the seaweed will decompose within forty-eight hours. Once seaweed is decomposed, it no longer emits the gas. Hydrogen sulfide is colorless, highly flammable, and produces an unpleasant odor much like the smell of rotten eggs. In small doses it is harmless, and in fact our bodies create and deal with very low levels of hydrogen sulfide all the time. Higher concentrations cause irritation of the eyes and respiratory system. At very high concentrations, it can cause loss of coordination, dizziness, vomiting, and even death (extremely rare). A much more common problem is that if large amounts of seaweed wash up on shore, especially in temperate and tropical climates, the beach must be closed and cleaned up. In lesser amounts, the hydrogen sulfide "littoral-ly" contributes to the "smell of the shore."

The more significant cause of that "fresh sea air"—present in all the oceans of the world—is a different sulfur compound known as *dimethyl sulfide* (DMS). It is a pungent sulfur gas that has been identified in the atmosphere only in the last thirty to forty years. How does it get there? Certain species of microscopic algae that engage in photosynthesis—phytoplankton—synthesize a molecule called *dimethylsulfoniopropionate* (DMSP) to protect themselves (it's tough being at the bottom of the ocean's food chain!). The DMSP molecule may act as a deterrent to being consumed, an antifreeze (phytoplankton are present in the Arctic as well as at the equator), and as an osmoregulatory molecule (too much water and they would expand; too little and they would shrivel like a raisin). When the phytoplankton cells are damaged by hungry zooplankton or viruses, they release their contents into the ocean. Bacteria (yes, there are loads of bacteria and viruses in the ocean[7]) convert DMSP into DMS, which leaks into the water and ultimately into the atmosphere. Seabirds and other ocean creatures can smell DMS and use it to locate areas that are rich in phytoplankton as well as home to other tasty marine animals further up the food chain. As mentioned previously, the importance of sulfur in the atmosphere has been appreciated only in the last few years. We now know that as DMS is further broken down, the sulfur molecules form an aerosol, attracting water molecules that then congregate in droplets to form clouds. In fact, there are now future proposals to "seed" the atmosphere with sulfur particles in order to increase cloud formation and reduce global warming.

Sulfur is not the only molecule to give the seaside its characteristic smell.[8] Returning to seaweed for a moment, most likely you were unaware that many species of seaweed have sexual relations and that seaweed sex involves pheromones. (No, I am not going to discuss the intimate nature of seaweed sexual relations.) Let's just say that the pheromones are released so that the seaweed eggs can attract the seaweed sperm and leave it at that. These chemicals when grouped together are called *dictyopterenes* and are found most abundantly in species of brown algae.

Bromophenols are another group of chemicals that give fish and seafood some of its "brininess" or fishlike smell. They are found most abundantly in the larger algae and may possess a variety of beneficial biologic traits, including antioxidant, antidiabetic, antimicrobial, and anticancer properties.

Navigation and Those Other Senses

What about using your sense of smell for navigating? We could do worse than the beginning of Harold Gatty's chapter "Using Your Sense of Smell" from *Finding Your Way Without Map or Compass*.

> Many early explorers were led to land beyond the horizon—by the nose. One wrote of the scent of rosemary off the coast of Spain more than ten leagues out at sea. Louis de Bougainville, when he was off the east coast of Australia in 1768, recounted that "a long time before sunrise a delicious odor announced the vicinity of the land which formed a great gulf open to the South-East."
>
> There were several explorers before de Bougainville who were led on their way by the perfumes of nature, by the breezes carrying the scent of sweet spring flowers, of new mown hay, of freshly turned earth. A journal of Sir Francis Drake's expedition in the Pacific in 1577 records that: "From hence wee directed our course toward the South-Southwest. . . . At which time wee had a very sweet smell from the land. . . . And wee had site of the land about 3 of the clocke in the afternoon of the same day."

It is reasonable to conclude that although we cannot navigate by smell alone, nor by sound alone, these senses provide useful information *if and only if we pay attention*. Which raises three questions:

(1) How did those Polynesian sailors navigate thousands of miles without a compass?
(2) Did they have a "sixth sense"?
(3) What's wrong with us, that we can't drive across town without using Waze?

Let's start by looking at the senses. How many do we humans have? Aristotle was close with four (he considered taste a form of touch). Following Aristotle and up to the present, however, the answer has been five. That's what you learned in school: the five senses—vision, hearing, smell, taste, and touch. There's one glaring problem with that (actually two), and they were discussed in the last chapter. You will recall that we have a sense of balance, the *vestibular system*, and a sense of where our body parts are, *proprioception*. Those additional two senses bring our total to seven. After that, opinions on what should be considered a human sense vary. There are two senses that other animals have but we do not—the ability to sense electrical fields and the ability to sense magnetic fields. But what about our ability to sense both pain and temperature? Absolutely. They are real senses that have specific receptors that convey sensory impulses to the brain. And there are more, but let's stop at seven since neither pain nor temperature nor any of the others will help us with the problem of navigation. The importance of the sense of vision is obvious. And it will be discussed in much greater detail in Chapter 8.

Can we really navigate long distances by just keeping our wits about us? ("Wits" is an older English word for our senses.) Marvin Creamer proved that it was possible. He set out in 1982 at the age of sixty-seven in his steel-hulled 36-foot boat to sail around the world *without any navigational aids*. Not even a compass or a wristwatch. Despite his share of mishaps—especially in the Southern Ocean where he suffered numerous knockdowns and a dislocated shoulder—this former professor at Glassboro State College (now Rowan University) completed the circumnavigation in just over five hundred days. How did he do it? It probably helped that he founded and was the chairman of the Department of Geography, so he was not a neophyte in terms of studying the earth.

Prior to departure, he spent years fine-tuning his celestial navigation skills and familiarizing himself with all of the other knowledge he would need: the currents, the prevailing wind patterns, the different colors of the ocean, and even the marine animals and birds in those regions to which he was sailing. In Tasmania, he even learned a celestial navigation pointer from a troop of Australian Boy Scouts. They taught him a mathematical equation based on the Southern Cross constellation—the southern hemisphere's equivalent of the North Star (Polaris)—which saved him days of sailing time. Creamer realized that there were two main approaches to navigation without instruments: the surface and the sky. As mentioned, he became very knowledgeable about celestial navigation but learned as much as he could about the wind patterns and the sea itself. There were many times, especially in the Pacific, when the weather turned overcast and the sun and stars were not available for days at a time. He then needed to depend upon his appreciation of the subtleties of wind and water.

Tristan Gooley refers to this type of navigation as "natural navigation."[9] It involves paying attention to the natural state of affairs so that your surroundings—wherever in the world—become your guide. This is not "pie in the sky" and is certainly not "primitive." Not only could it save your life, but it could give you a richer experience of the world.

Before we discuss the Polynesian navigators, let us turn to those other natural ocean navigators—the Vikings (Figures 2.8 and 2.9). By the standard of the Polynesians, the Vikings were only B+ navigators, although they did manage to navigate around much of the known world without any navigational equipment. (Most likely they would have been better navigators if they had spent more time studying the stars and less time raping and plundering.) To their credit they lived in relatively unforgiving circumstances.

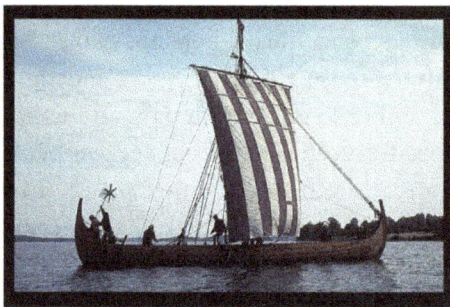

Figure 2.8 Viking ship[10]

The sun, moon, and stars provided a great deal of help to the Vikings, and they were aware of the concepts of north, south, east, and west. Navigation was based on the horizon, how high the sun rose, and where it was in relation to the horizon. But in overcast weather, celestial aids were of no use. Since the Vikings stayed fairly close to shore, they navigated by looking for familiar landmarks and taking note of objects along the coast that were particular or unique and would give them a clue as to where they were.

Birds were also particularly helpful, and there was one prominent early Viking sailor who allegedly traveled with the bird cage of ravens letting them go free one at a time. If they circled and returned to the boat, he knew the boat was still far from landfall. If the raven never returned, he followed them to the nearest shore (sounds suspiciously similar to Noah's shtick). The Vikings made use of all of their senses. They listened not only for the sound of birds but also the sound of waves breaking on shore. They used their sense of smell to detect plants, trees, and fire on land. Our sense of touch is helpful in registering changes in the speed and direction of the wind on the face; no doubt they made use of this information as well. It has been proposed that the Vikings also utilized taste. They routinely used a plumb bob to assess the depth of the water and may have collected a sample of the seabed or determined if fresh water flowed from the land into the seawater.

Sound, Smell, and Navigation

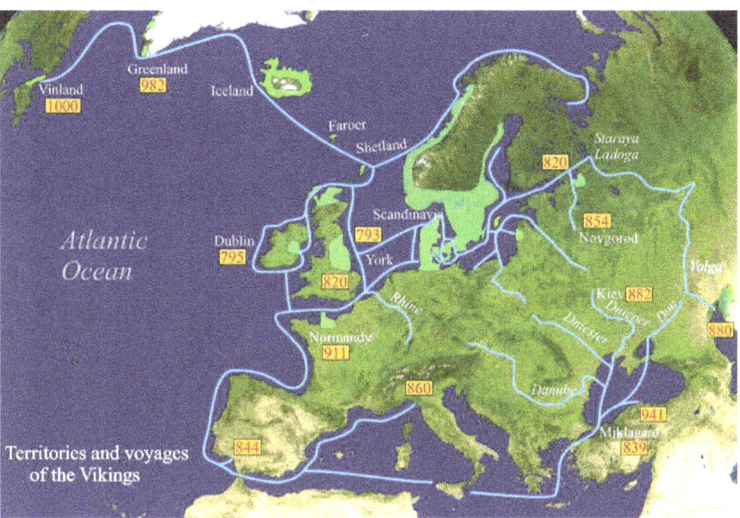

Figure 2.9 Viking navigation[11]

Since they had neither written descriptions of the journey nor nautical charts, the "travelogues" included narratives often with rhymes:

From Hernam [present-day Henno near Bergen] in Norway, head due west toward Hvarf in Greenland, and you will have sailed north of Hjaltland [the Shetland Islands], so that you just glimpse it in clear weather, but south of the Faroe Islands, so that the sea [the horizon] is right in between the distant mountains, and thus also south of Iceland."[12]

The Polynesians took natural navigation to another level. They combined an encyclopedic knowledge of every aspect of their surroundings with constant attention and observation. The sun was their main guide during the day. They knew its exact point of rising on the horizon and precisely where it would set, depending on the season. At night they would switch to the rising and setting points of the stars. A Polynesian navigator could identify many hundreds of stars, and they associated specific places with stars above the horizon.

Let's assume you're a Polynesian sailor. It is dusk and you are sailing to your cousin's island. You would sail in the direction of that star which was "right above" your cousin's island—that is, until that star moved. Then you would have to shift your direction of sail to another star or compensate for the movement of the original star. Figure 2.10 is an example of a star compass depicted with shells on the sand. The Polynesians had to commit the star compass to memory. There was no permanent star compass except in the brain of the navigator. (The map was only for teaching purposes; it was not taken on the voyage. The star compass was in the navigator's brain. Furthermore, in the navigator "guild," the information was proprietary and secret.)

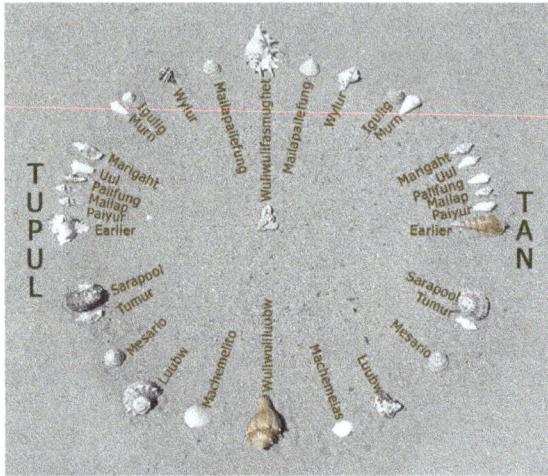

Figure 2.10 Recreation of a traditional star compass[13]

It may not seem that impressive until you realize that the sailing triangle of the Polynesian navigators represented a good portion of the Pacific Ocean—as much as 2 million square miles (Figure 2.11).

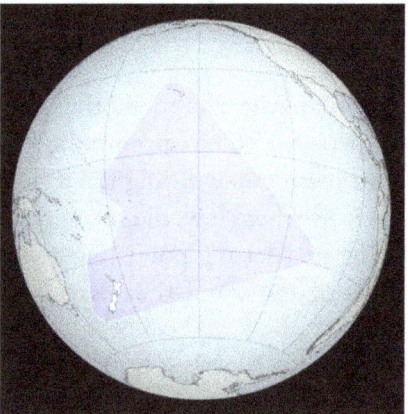

Figure 2.11 Polynesian Triangle[14]

The Polynesians also used wave and swell formations to navigate. This was information that was incorporated into their overall navigation system (in their brain), not a separate navigational tool to be used when the sun or stars were unavailable. Islands and island chains have predictable effects on waves, swells, and currents. The navigators would learn the effects the islands had on the shape and direction of the swells and would correct their course accordingly. Ripples and waves are the transient effect of the wind whereas swells represent the effect of the wind on the water over long stretches of the ocean. These long-range ocean swells will remain constant for days or weeks. The longer the wind blows in a constant direction, the longer the swell will last. Swell patterns are much more reliable than ripples or waves, and the knowledgeable navigator can distinguish the two even when the wave is traveling in a different direction than the more dependable swell. Winds may suddenly change, but the swell tends to be more stable. The Marshall Islanders developed stick charts to document the prevailing, predominant swells and the manner in which they were deflected by the islands (often represented by small shells). They would appreciate the swell as it traversed under their feet from right to left or vice versa. Sometimes they would lie down in the vessel and feel the swell in their "stomach." Like the star compass, these stick charts (made out of the ribs of coconut palms and tied together with coconut fiber) were developed for teaching purposes only. Like the star compass, the information on the stick figure was to reside in the brain of the navigator (Figure 2.12).

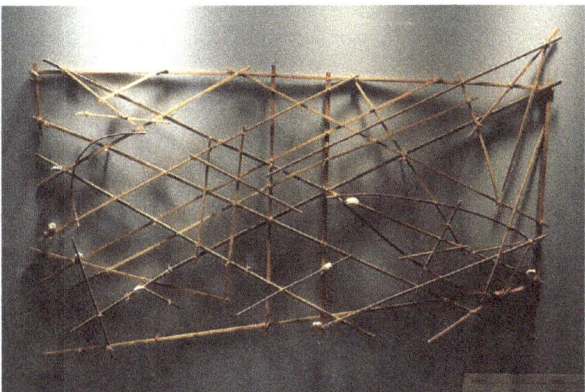

Figure 2.12 Stick chart[15]

What else did the Polynesians incorporate into their navigational toolbox?

- Speed: with constant observation comes the knowledge of the speed of the vessel
- Wind: knowledge of the prevailing wind, which, for example, might be southeast in the summer and northeast in the winter
- Color: sea color varies between green and blue and depends on its temperature, the organisms therein, the salt content, the bottom, and the depth
- Temperature: the practice of "thermometrical navigation," in a time before the chronometer; that is, dipping a hand in the water to appreciate a change in temperature (e.g., in the Gulf Stream in the Atlantic)
- Sea birds: the observation of sea bird habits (see the discussion of the Vikings earlier. Harold Gatty speculates that actual voyages of Polynesians followed the

flyway of birds. A voyage from Tahiti to New Zealand may have followed the migration of the "long-tailed cuckoo," and the voyages to Hawaii coincide with the migration of the Pacific Golden Plover.)

How unique were the Polynesians? M. R. O'Connor's recent book *Wayfinding: The Science and Mystery of How Humans Navigate the World*[16] answers that question. She studied not only the Polynesians, but also the Inuit and the Aborigines. These cultures are about as different as they can be—Oceanic, Arctic, and Australian desert. To the untrained observer, each of these landscapes appears to be bereft of unique features that would facilitate navigation. None were particularly colorful; all were more or less monochromatic: the ocean blue-green, the Arctic white, and the desert grayish brown. But in each culture, navigation was life or death. Because of the length of travel and the potential nautical mortality, the Polynesians depended upon a (revered) guild of navigators who were trained since childhood, whereas basically everyone who lived in the Arctic or in the Australian outback learned to be responsible for their own survival. How did they do it? Each group developed a number of skills including *remarkable attention to environmental detail that included appreciation of natural and manmade landmarks invariably beyond the perception of untrained eyes.* They used all of their senses to pick up clues. It might be that ocean swell reflecting off an unseen island. Or the subtle pattern of frozen snow in the Arctic. Or the grouping of rocks left in a particular place in the outback by nature or purposefully by their ancestors. With these landmarks, they could call up a mental map of the territory. And invariably, they would add mnemonics to help them remember all this information—often in the form of a story or stories, and sometimes in the form of a song. Space and stories —navigational maps and memory. As we will see shortly, this combination of maps and memory could only occur at one place in the brain.

The Aborigines took a somewhat different approach to navigation, merging map and memory. Their narratives were melded into their navigation so that the stories of and by their ancestors are in a very real sense woven into the landscape. They developed an excellent sense of direction, understanding north, south, east, and west. Knowing exactly where they started from, they would travel in a specific direction and follow the narrative that had been handed down for thousands of years. Their narratives incorporated both successes and importantly failures—ancestors warning against a certain route and describing the potential dire consequences of taking it. This system represents the interpolation of maps and memory.

Inuit navigation was in some ways even more challenging since the Arctic landscape was more formidable, and constantly changing with the seasons. Despite this, the Intuits paid astonishing attention to details in the often snow- and ice-covered Arctic landscape and never seemed to get lost. In fact, both the Aborigines and the Inuit understood the concept of getting lost very differently than we do, as it happened so infrequently. M. R. O'Connor relates:

William Parry, who also sought the Northwest Passage, praised the "astonishing precision" of the Inuit-created maps in the 1820s and their ability to masterfully depict every twist and turn of the arctic topography and coast. Without the help of a map made for him by a guide, Parry believed he never would have found a critical passage through the Fury and Hecla Straight.

Knud Rasmussen was equally surprised by the inland Inuit, who had never used paper or pencils before but were able to pick them up and draw accurate representations of the land and the best routes to get wherever he asked. . . . The historical record and modern cartographic research both agree that most Inuit maps, extensively tested through a century of use by non-Inuit explorers and field scientists, were extraordinarily accurate renderings of the landscape as sensually perceived, writes the geographer Robert Rundstrom.

The Inuit did not travel across the land randomly—they followed known routes. In most places around the world, routes have been indicated with roads and human-made landmarks, and these paths and locations are then laid out symbolically on maps. . . . Some environments are more legible than others because they have spatial coherence or an availability of landmarks that make navigation easier. The Arctic environment has ephemeral qualities that prohibit permanence—ice melts, snow is blown by changing winds, rivers flow and then turn to frozen ground come winter. Landmarks are either few and far between or difficult to distinguish and impermeable, so legibility depends on socio-cultural dimensions, the symbolic significance and meaning imparted to the landscape by the people who traverse it. . . . Certain routes for traveling across the land became favored over generations and knowledge of these unmarked trails is passed down from person to person, family to family, community to community, not in the form of maps but as oral descriptions that are memorized.[17]

I would again point out in both of these cultures the melding of memory and maps, maps and memory.

What about that "sixth sense"? As far as the "sixth sense" is concerned, the British zoologist Robin Baker[18] points out that the reason the concept of sixth sense lasted so long was that people in the West had *so many aids to navigation* that they forgot that there were natural strategies. It only took a couple of centuries to forget that environmental clues can be just as accurate as maps and instruments. Harold Gaddy wrote, "in our Western civilization, pathfinding and natural tracking are so little developed. . . . That notwithstanding all differences of innate ability, the man who has learned the simplest secrets of reading nature's signs is bound to outstrip the inexperienced observer, however intelligent he may be, and cannot only outstrip him, but frequently amaze him. Nature's signs can be read with a little practice by the average intelligent Western man just as clearly as if they were street signs."[19] Even Darwin was fooled into thinking that these "primitive" people retained some of the instincts that more civilized humans had gone beyond.

Some neuroscientists are concerned that with the advent of GPS and programs like Waze we will become less and less involved with our environment, offloading whatever navigational skills we still have to our computers and phones—or never develop them. As a result, the navigational part of our brain will shrivel up and atrophy. This is not a joke. In the last fifteen years, neuroscientists have identified the location of the major navigational portions of our brain. In fact, there are really two parallel systems for navigation, and we use both constantly. The first system we will discuss is the *spatial strategy*. It is the strategy we have been discussing—the making and using of mental maps. The second strategy is a stimulus-response strategy and will simply be referred to as a *response strategy*.[20]

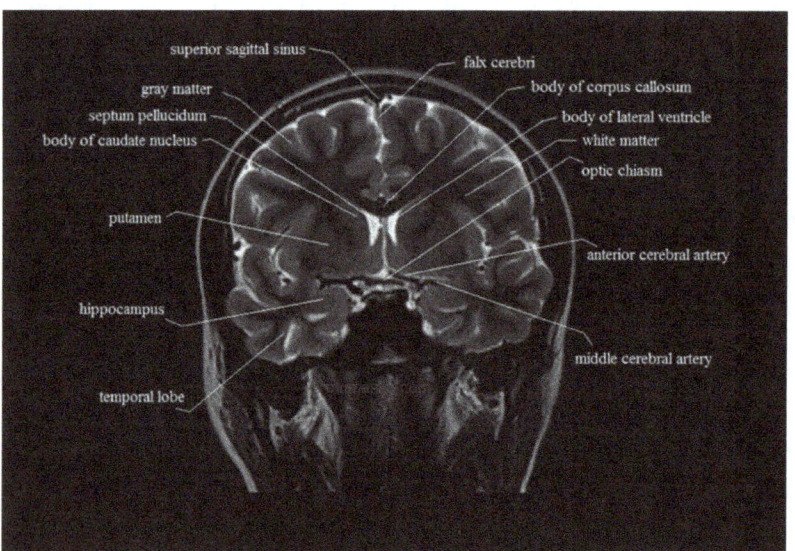

Figure 2.13 MRI scan (coronal plane) demonstrating the hippocampus and caudate nucleus[21]

The heart of the spatial strategy is the *hippocampus* (from the Greek word for seahorse, which this area of the brain resembles)—or rather the pair of hippocampi, as there is one on each side (Figure 2.13). The hippocampus and its immediate neighbors perform two basic functions:

1. They are critical for *memory* function (without a hippocampus, you cannot create ANY new memory).[22]

2. They comprise the *spatial* or *mapping* region of our brain. The hippocampus is responsible for creating a mental map of the environment. Within the hippocampus are a number of specialized cells that monitor different spatial functions. These specialized groups of cells are like apps that do one thing:

- *Place cells.* The place cells were discovered first in studies with rats, and these cells will fire if the rat (or presumably human) goes into a specific place in his or her environment. (Humans have similar place cells but some of the details are still being worked out since humans are more reluctant than rats to have electrodes placed into individual hippocampal cells.) If the rat is in a box or maze, individual place cells will only fire if the rat is in a specific location in the box—for example the top left corner. Other cells will only fire if the rat is in the bottom right corner, or the center, and so forth. Exactly how this works in sailors who walk from their relative "box" below deck onto the deck, surrounded by the vastness of the ocean, is unclear.
- *Grid cells.* These are a different group of cells that are arranged in patterns and that keep track of our movement—from place A to place B. They feed the movement information into the place cells to update the current place or location.
- *Forward-looking, boundary, and speed cells.* These other types of cells only respond when we face a certain direction, when we get near a boundary—for example a wall or cliff—or when we change speed. This information is sent into the grid cells, which are then updated and can update the place cells. The forward-looking (head direction) cells function as an "internal compass." Humans also appear to have grid cells, forward-looking, boundary, and speed cells.[23]

If we could do an MRI scan on a Polynesian sailor—preferably one from years ago—what would it look like? Would the brain, and specifically the hippocampus, look any different than ours? We can speculate with a high degree of certainty that the sailor's hippocampus—especially the back (posterior portion)—would be exceedingly large! How can we presume that? Well, the experiment has already been done. Professor Eleanor Maguire and her colleagues[24] performed MRI scans on the brains of London taxi drivers who were required to pass a rigorous test to become licensed. The test consists of many thousands of streets and landmarks throughout London referred to as "The Knowledge." It requires years of study. This kind of accumulated spatial navigation information is very similar to the years of study that the young Polynesian navigator had to undergo. When the MRI scan of the drivers who passed the test was compared with those who had not passed, the hippocampus in each of the successful group was found to be much larger. That is, the learning of spatial information had caused a demonstrable change in the cabbies' brains as they slowly and painstakingly created their own brain map. There is no evidence yet that the hippocampus will shrivel up if we don't use it, but the evidence for "use it or lose it" plasticity is at least highly suggestive.

So, is that all there is to human (and rat) navigation? No. There is another system—the *response* system. Think about your routine ride to work. You don't think in terms of a map, the way a Polynesian navigator might. In fact, if you are like many people, while driving the same route every day, you don't think about the route at all. No, you were *not* using a spatial strategy; rather, you were using a response strategy. What you were responding to were multiple (often unconscious) stimuli. It was, in psychologic parlance, a stimulus-response encounter. In reality, *multiple* stimulus-response encounters. At each point along your route to work, there was a stimulus and you responded. Behind the scenes, so to speak, this type of stimulus response was occurring: "At this traffic light where the gas station is, I need to turn left, and then I continue until I see the McDonalds, at which time I make a right turn." Or, since we are focused on the water, "When I motor into the harbor, I need to keep the red buoys on my right and the green on my left ("red right returning"). This system depends on a different part of the brain known as the *caudate nucleus* (Figure 2.12). This brain structure is very much involved in motor and emotional responses to a stimulus—and often, as in this case, the response or reward may be unconscious.

So, which is it? Spatial strategy, with its home in the hippocampus, or response strategy, which resides in the caudate nucleus? It turns out that *we humans can and do routinely switch between these systems.* The response strategy is quicker and easier—and if possible, we use that system. As everyone is aware, if you drive from your house to work or sail back into your home marina, you basically perform the maneuver on "autopilot"—your brain is responding unconsciously to various landmarks without even thinking about it. We have all had that experience. And it is (generally) very efficient. On the other hand, if we enter a harbor that is new to us, we need to consult our charts (or our mental maps) to figure out where we are and how to get to the anchorage.

The response system is trained by performing the same sequence over and over. The sensory input is training our motor system.

But what about training our spatial (hippocampal) system? That is more difficult, often more complicated, and requires a great deal of attention to the environment to "enlarge the hippocampus" with as much sensory information as it can get, in order to create those mental maps. Following the instructions from your GPS program to "prepare to turn left in 600 feet ... turn left now" isn't going to do it. As opposed to Gatty's "natural navigation," we might term this "unnatural navigation."

The point, of course, isn't that we need to get rid of GPS and "go back to nature." Rather, the key is to understand that these two systems are built into our brains, and we need to recognize which one we are using. That should motivate you to pay more attention to your environment, especially in less familiar waters, and to pick up whatever clues there are. And don't forget to look behind you as you are leaving if you plan to return to that location. You need to build that *return* mental map as well.

All of this is especially important for the younger sailor who can still build up quite a storehouse of information. Use GPS, set waypoints, but then open your senses to everything that is out there!

Notes

1. There have been additional conventions, including the Convention on the International Regulations for Preventing Collisions at Sea, 1972 (the rules are commonly referred to as 72 COLREGS). This has been amended most recently in 1989.

2. This reliance on vision for location, rather than hearing, is not universal in the animal kingdom. Dolphins, for example, use echolocation in addition to vision to locate prey, and barn owls have a remarkable auditory ability to locate prey by sound. But not humans. We use sound at sea mainly to signify intent rather than location. But I discuss human ability in greater detail throughout this chapter.

3. All four figures are with permission of Dr. Jennifer Groh. They are from her wonderful book *Making Space: How the Brain Knows Where Things Are* (Cambridge, MA: Belknap Press, 2014).

4. L. Thaler et al. "Neural Correlates of Motion Processing through Echolocation, Source Hearing, and Vision in Blind Echolocation Experts and Sighted Echolocation Novices," *Journal of Neurophysiology* 111 (2014): 112-127. One reason the blind echolocators have an "advantage" over the sighted echolocators is that they have all of that unused cortical real estate in the occipital lobe (our vision lobe of the brain). The occipital lobe is the primary visual cortex, but through the miracle of neuroplasticity, this unused cortical real estate is repurposed for sound. Imagine a large vacant space in any major city in the world—the auditory system swoops in and takes over that vacant occipital cortex faster than you can say "aggressive NY real estate developer"!

5. Ron Kurtus' School for Champions, accessed May 25, 2019, https://www.school-for-champions.com/science/sound_amplified_over_water.htm.

6. Harold Gatty, *Finding Your Way Without Map or Compass* (Mineola, NY: Dover, 2013). Originally published by Dutton under the title *Nature Is Your Guide: How to Find Your Way on Land and Sea by Observing Nature*.

7. There are not just a few marine viruses; there are, by the latest count, 195,728 viral populations! A. C. Gregory et al., "Marine DNA Viral Macro- and Microdiversity from Pole to Pole," *Cell* 177, no. 5: 1109-1123, doi: https://doi.org/10.1016/j.cell.2019.03.040. Every time you swallow a mouthful of seawater at the beach you will devour perhaps as many particles as there are people in North America, according to Jonathan Lambert at *Quanta*, https://www.quantamagazine.org/scientists-discover-nearly-200000-kinds-of-ocean-viruses-20190425/. And what about bacteria? There are loads of them as well. As far as human pathogens are concerned, there has been an increase in *Vibrio vulnificus* (popularly known as "flesh-eating bacteria") worldwide, and it appears that many species of bacteria are proliferating with the increasing temperature of the seas due to climate change. Also increasing with warmer water is methicillin-resistant Staphylococcus aureus (MRSA). MRSA has also been found in fresh water. So, with all these viruses and bacteria, what's going on? It turns out that most of the viruses are bacteriophages (viruses that infect and devour bacteria). That is, there is a long-standing war (good for the oceanic ecosystem) whereby the viruses chow down on the bacteria and in doing so add to the pool of dissolved organic matter in the ocean that in turn contributes to the ocean's ecologic food chain and health.

8. B. Wolfe, "Why Does the Sea Smell Like the Sea?" *Popular Science*, August 19, 2004, https://www.popsci.com/seasmells.

9. Two of Tristan Gooley's books should be on your bookshelf (if there are still bookshelves when you read this). The first is *How to Read Water* (New York: The Experiment, 2016) and *The*

Natural Navigator (New York: The Experiment, 2011). Both discuss natural navigation at length, including the nature of water in puddles, rivers, lakes, and oceans.

10. Björn Ambrosiani/ https://commons.wikimedia.org/w/index.php?curid=62935683

11. Bogdangiusca—Earth map by NASA; data based on w: File: Viking Age.png (now: File:Vikingen tijd.png), which is in turn based on http://home.online.no/~anlun/tipi/vrout.jpg and other maps, CC BY-SA 3.0, https://commons.wikimedia.org/w/index.php?curid=81232.

12. "How Vikings Navigated the World," *ScienceNordic*, October 9, 2012, sciencenordic.com/how_vikings_navigated_world

13. Newportm, https://commons.wikimedia.org/w/index.php?curid=11064414.

14. https://commons.wikimedia.org/w/index.php?curid=1886977.

15. https://commons.wikimedia.org/wiki/File:Stick_chart-BHM_1920.530.0032-P8260227.

16. M. R. O'Connor, *Wayfinding: The Science and Mystery of How Humans Navigate the World* (New York: St. Martin's, 2019).

17. O'Connor, *Wayfinding*.

18. R. R. Baker, *Human Navigation and the Sixth Sense* (New York: Simon & Schuster, 1982).

19. Gatty, *Finding Your Way*.

20. We are going to be discussing two navigational strategies, each depending on a different system. I will refer to the major group of cells that perform the task, but their precise location is not that important. It is important to realize that these structures do not work in isolation. Each structure (hippocampus and caudate nucleus) is interacting with numerous other brain areas—including virtually every lobe of the brain. And there is a noncompetitive interaction between the two systems so that they can work together and compensate for each other in health or if one system or the other is degraded by neurologic diseases such as Alzheimer's disease or Huntingdon's disease.

21. For you neuro-geeks, here is an MRI scan demonstrating among other structures both the hippocampus and the body of the caudate nucleus. Courtesy of MRIMasters.com.

22. A detailed discussion of memory is beyond the scope of this chapter, but some of you may be wondering: (a) why all this talk about memory in a chapter concerned with navigation and (b) what's with the Lewis Carroll epigraph? It may appear that memory and spatial navigation are totally different phenomena, but in reality, they are not. All of the navigational skills discussed above are totally dependent on memory. That shouldn't surprise us, as every day we struggle to recall where in "space" we left those car keys. And if we can't recall, we invariably travel back through all of the spaces (rooms) we have navigated through since returning home. But not only are navigational skills dependent on memory, but memory is often dependent upon spatial skills. Virtually every prize-winning memory champion uses a technique developed in Greece and Rome known as the "method of loci" in which memory items are stored visually in a well-known space with different rooms—such as the rooms of your house.

In fact, we can pose a more philosophical question: what is the purpose of memory? There is one school of thought that the real purpose of memory is to help predict the future. Indeed, patients who have lost their hippocampi to disease not only have a profound amnesia but have no future. They can't think about or imagine their future at all. They have lost both their past and their future. Think about that! And while you are doing that, recall that the navigators above, especially the Inuit and Aborigines, depended a great deal on their cultural narrative (memory) to help them navigate. Certainly, a prime example of memory of the past assisting with navigation into the future.

23. For additional discussion, see Groh, *Making Space*.

24. E.A. Maguire et.al., "Navigation-Related Structural Change in the Hippocampi of Taxi Drivers," *Proceedings of the National Academy of the Sciences USA* 97, no. 8 (2000): 4398-4403; E. A. Maguire, K. Woollett, and H.J. Spiers, "London Taxi Drivers and Bus Drivers: A Structural MRI and Neuropsychologic Analysis," *Hippocampus* 16, no. 12 (2006):1091-1101.

Chapter 3

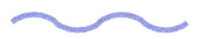

Cold Weather Sailing

"The sea lies all around us.... In its mysterious past it encompasses all
the dim origins of life and receives in the end ... the dead husks of that same.
For all at last returns to the sea, the beginning and the end."

—*Rachel Carson,* The Sea Around Us, *1951*

"Twenty years from now, you will be more disappointed by the things
you didn't do than those you did. So, throw off the bowlines. Sail away
from safe harbor. Catch the wind in your sails. Explore. Dream. Discover."

—Mark Twain

Consider the sinking of the *Titanic* in 1912. The water temperature was approximately 32 degrees Fahrenheit (0 degrees Celsius) when the ship foundered. When rescue vessels arrived two hours later, nearly all the people who had entered lifeboats were alive. In contrast, all 1,489 people immersed in the water appeared to be (and were presumed to be) dead. We now know that the victims suffered from hypothermia and that many could probably have been revived! Insufficient clothing, a lack of adequate flotation devices, and an absence of even a rudimentary knowledge of cold water survival procedures all contributed to the high death toll.

As sailors, we must learn to deal with the cold in two different circumstances. *On the water* while sailing, a foolhardy approach to the cold decreases comfort and impairs performance. Although our lives are not directly in peril, impaired performance certainly may have untoward consequences. *In the water*, we are engaged in a battle for survival. In either case, we have no excuse for not knowing how to keep ourselves warm.

Thermal Balance on the Water

We are *homoiothermic*, or warm-blooded, animals whose internal temperature is normally kept within narrow limits despite the vagaries of the climate. This is accomplished by balancing heat gain with heat loss. When successful, we are in thermal balance with our environment.[1]

In a cold environment, the human body is in danger of losing heat faster than it can be produced. Unless something is done, the body continues to cool off until a state of hypothermia supervenes. In order to decide upon appropriate measures to arrest this loss of body heat, let us consider the ways in which the body gains and loses heat (Table 3.1).

Heat Gain	Heat Loss
Metabolism	Radiation
Shivering or exercise	Convection
Radiation	Conduction
Ingestion of hot food	Evaporation

Table 3.1 Heat gain and heat loss

The most obvious source of heat is *metabolism*. An average active adult man produces about 2,500 calories of energy per day, whereas an active female performing various light activities such as sleeping, eating, dressing, and walking requires only about 2,000. About 95 percent of this energy is in the form of heat. Exposure to the cold does not affect the basic rate of metabolism very much but does have an effect referred to as *nonshivering thermogenesis*.[2] (For a full discussion of how this works, see endnote 2). After weeks or months in the cold, the rate of metabolism may increase a small amount, but this increase does not provide much protection against hypothermia. Interestingly, a few groups in the world had been able to adapt, with almost no protection, to extremely frigid conditions by increasing their metabolism, although the evidence for this is scanty. One such group, the natives of Tierra del Fuego (Cape Horn), lived in an intensely cold, windy, and wet climate. The temperature is near freezing the entire year. Darwin visited them during his voyage on the *HMS Beagle*, noting that the Fuegian men and women were almost completely naked. "A woman, who was suckling a recently-born child, came one day alongside the vessel, and remained there out of mere curiosity, whilst the sleet fell and thawed on her naked bosom and on the skin of her naked baby!"[3] Their higher rate of metabolism due to long-term adaptation presumably allowed the Fuegians to survive in this thoroughly unpleasant climate.

A second means of increasing heat production is muscular activity—either *shivering* or *exercise*. Shivering is involuntary and begins soon after exposure to the cold. It reaches a peak in about fifteen to thirty minutes and increases heat production. How does it do that? See endnote 2. Shivering and exercise are not additive, however, since exercise usually abolishes shivering.

There are two other means by which the body can gain heat—by the absorption of heat radiation and by the consumption of hot food and beverages. During the daytime, the body receives shortwave radiation from the sun, both direct and reflected. It also may absorb longwave radiation. Of course, the cold sailor could also sit in front of a heater. Finally, eating hot food or drinking a hot beverage supplies heat to the body. In *Two Years Before the Mast*, R. H. Dana describes that in a cold environment, sailors invariably prefer a hot beverage to an alcoholic one. "At the same time, as I have said, there was not a man on board who would not have pitched the rum to the dogs (I have heard them say so a dozen times) for a pot of coffee or chocolate; or even for our common beverage—'water bewitched and tea begrudged,' as it was."[4]

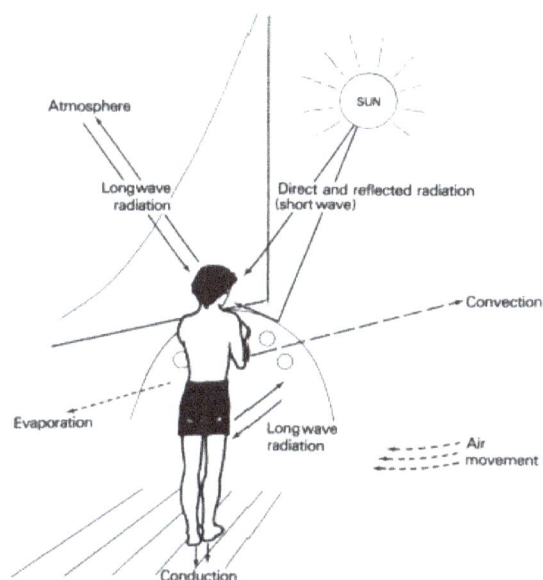

Figure 3.1: The four avenues of heat loss: radiation, convection, conduction, and evaporation

Conversely, there are four ways in which the body loses heat: radiation, convection, conduction, and evaporation—all of which are important on the water (Figure 3.1). Regardless of skin color, the human body not only absorbs but also emits longwave *radiation*. This exchange is not generally appreciated. When the surface of the body is not absorbing longwave radiation, it is actually radiating it back into the environment. The degree of radiation heat loss depends on the amount of exposed body surface, which is usually 80 percent or less, since certain areas such as the thighs and underarms tend to radiate heat back to the body. Curling up in a fetal position diminishes radiation heat loss. Lying spread-eagled enhances it.

Convection is the other important means by which the sailor loses heat. Air that is in direct contact with the skin is warmed. As it is warmed, air rises off the skin surface and is replaced by cooler air. These convection currents maintain themselves by transferring heat from the skin to the surrounding air (see Figures 3.1 and 3.8). The amount of heat loss depends on the temperature difference between the skin and the air; the larger the difference, the greater the heat loss. Wind velocity also plays a role. Although convection currents occur even when there is no wind whatsoever (e.g., below deck or even in a telephone booth—if you can find one), increasing the movement of air across the skin hastens the exchange of heat. Birds and some mammals can decrease convection heat loss to an enormous extent by fluffing up their feathers or bristling their hair. The goosebumps phenomenon we experience in the cold is a vestige of this response, although, unfortunately, it adds nothing to our insulation.

Conduction heat loss occurs when the body is in direct contact with a cooler object. Heat is transferred directly to the object. On the water, conduction is usually insignificant, since only the sailor's feet and/or buttocks are in contact with a cooler object, such as the boat. In the water, the situation is drastically different. Now, nearly the entire body is in contact with the colder water, and conduction becomes the most significant avenue for heat loss.

Evaporation plays a vital role in cooling the body in a warm climate, but it is of lesser consequence in the cold. In cold climates, sweating usually does not occur, although water vapor continually diffuses through the skin without wetting it. This evaporation, together with water vapor emitted from the respiratory tract, is known as *insensible water loss* because we are entirely unaware of it. Since the evaporation of water requires heat, this heat is lost from the body. In the cold, this evaporative heat loss generally is minimal. However, there are circumstances (discussed later in this chapter) when it may be a major source of heat loss.

Natural Defenses against the Cold

It is useful to think of the human body as a warm central "core" surrounded by a cooler "shell" (Figure 3.2). The core contains all the vital organs, whereas the shell consists of the skin, underlying subcutaneous tissues, and muscles. The shell provides the body with a layer of natural insulation, which *varies to suit the climate*. In warm climates, the shell is very thin so that heat from the core quickly dissipates. In cold weather, the core "retreats" to a more defensible position in the interior, leaving behind a thick shell to fight a rearguard action with the elements. The flow of blood controls the size of the shell, which can change very rapidly and constitutes our first response to cold and hot temperatures. Warm blood from the core may be directed toward or diverted away from the surface. When diverted away, the insulation of the outer inch of the body—the shell—approaches that of cork! Since the blood brings less heat to the surface, the temperature of the skin falls, and less heat is lost.

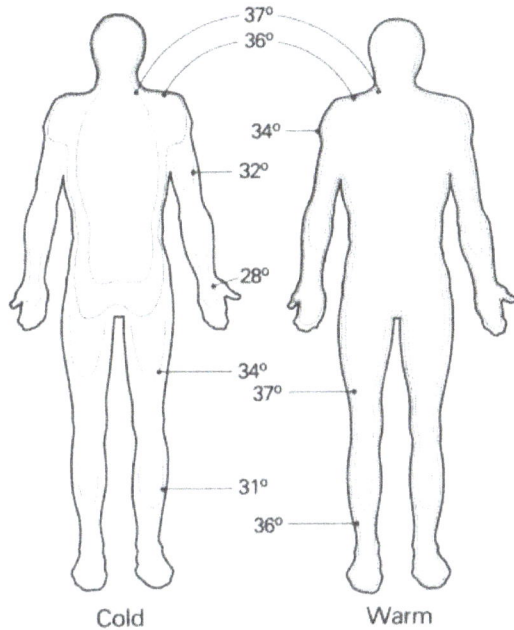

Figure 3.2 The distribution of the shell and core in cold and warm weather (in degrees Centigrade)

Sailors should be aware that *alcohol decreases the size of the shell and should be avoided in the cold*. It does this by dilating blood vessels, hence increasing blood flow to the skin—precisely what the body is trying to avoid! An account of a vessel's sinking in the North Atlantic during the month of October demonstrates the detrimental effect of alcohol. "There were forty of us on or clinging to a fifteen-man Carley float. Rescue came after seven hours. There was only one casualty, an able seaman who had drunk rum just before abandoning ship. He died after about three hours' immersion."[5]

If increasing the size of the shell fails to stem the tide, the body turns to its second line of defense, increased heat production either by shivering or exercise. Exercise is a potent resource, increasing heat production up to ten times; however, there are problems: First, exercise tolerance varies markedly among individuals depending on their physical fitness. Some people may be able to sustain vigorous activity for long periods of time (keeping themselves warm in the process), whereas others simply become exhausted. The second drawback is that some of the heat is wasted. During physical activity, blood must be supplied to the muscles, diminishing the insulation of the shell and nullifying some of the heat gain. As a rule, if the heat loss is modest, exercise may produce enough of a net gain in heat to keep the sailor warm. If the heat loss is proceeding at a rapid pace, chances are that exercise will be counterproductive. One situation in which exercise is nearly always counterproductive is during immersion in cool or cold water.

Healthy Boating & Sailing

Immersion Hypothermia

Most sailors never stop to consider hypothermia unless they are sailing in high-latitude waters in the wintertime. This is a mistake. Even when sailing in tropical waters, *hypothermia remains a potential hazard.* Figure 3.3 represents the change in body temperature of a thin man swimming in water of various temperatures. Note that his body temperature drops precipitously in cold water but that even in water temperatures as high as 83 degrees Fahrenheit (28 degrees Celsius), the swimmer continues to lose heat, albeit very slowly.

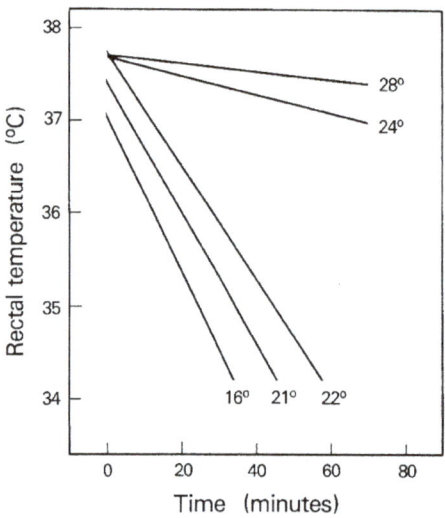

Figure 3.3 Body heat loss for a thin, unclothed man at various water temperatures. In colder water (16 degrees Celsius, 21 degrees Celsius, 22 degrees Celsius), heat loss proceeds at a rapid rate; in warmer water (24 degrees Celsius, 28 degrees Celsius), at a slow rate.

Figure 3.4 is a widely used diagram for estimating the survival time for a fully clothed, average-sized man in cold water. The two important variables are the temperature of the water and the duration of immersion. Thin men have shorter survival times, whereas fatter men and most women have slightly longer times due to the additional insulation of extra adipose tissue. Improving the type and amount of clothing and wearing a waterproof outer suit further increase survival time.

The following incident illustrates how a misunderstanding of some of the concepts of cold-water survival can be tragic. Adlard Coles documents it in *Heavy Weather Sailing*. A vessel, the *Dancing Ledge*, foundered during a midsummer gale in the English Channel. An experienced sailor, Lieutenant-Colonel H. Barry O'Sullivan, his wife, and two crew members were sailing her. The vessel broke up very rapidly, leaving little time for preparation. Coles shares the perspective of Mrs. O'Sullivan when recounting the tale:

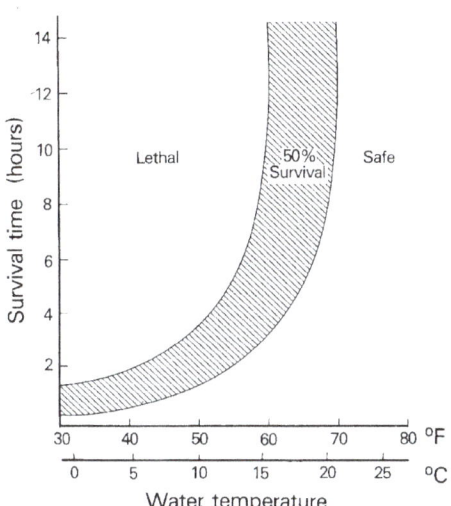

Figure 3.4 Predicted survival in cold water. The two most important considerations are: (1) time in the water and (2) water temperature. To use this graph, draw a line for a specific water temperature vertically until it intersects either curve. A horizontal line indicates the probable survival time. For example, if the water temperature is 55 degrees Fahrenheit (13 degrees Celsius), there is a 50 percent chance for survival at two hours. By six hours, the chance of survival approaches 0.

Once in the fresh air, we saw each other fairly soon, and also saw the dinghy, which must have broken from its chocks on the cabin top. It was upside down, but we hung on to it (aided by life-jackets) for nearly four hours and were carried inshore until we were close enough to see the window panes on the Ventnor houses. . . . Barry insisted that we should "bicycle" continuously with our legs to keep warm and avoid stomach cramp, which it proved successful in doing. The youngest member of the crew had only a kapok lifejacket. This proved to be totally inadequate and as he became cold and weak his head had no support. Colonel and Mrs. O'Sullivan held on to the dinghy with one hand and supported the crew's head with the other. The fourth member of the crew had already died.

A frigate, *H.M.S. Keppel*, approached at about this time. Colonel O'Sullivan took off his orange jacket to wave it above the spray to attract attention and this was seen as a tiny dot by the naval watch. He then attempted to put it onto the exhausted member of the crew to give him chin support, and he had therefore no jacket for himself.

When the frigate was maneuvered alongside (no mean feat), a rope was thrown to Mrs. O'Sullivan. She let go the dinghy with one hand to grip the rope. Her hand was so cold and rigid that she could not close it round the rope. She let go the dinghy with the other hand to attempt to get a stronger grip, but it was impossible to hold the rope and it ran through her hands as a wave, deflected by the bulk of the frigate, swept her along the length of the ship and she drifted away into the clear, supported by her life-jacket, and became unconscious. The frigate returned and Mrs. O'Sullivan was rescued by a man, secured by a lifeline, who went into the water and got her up the scrambling nets. The search was continued for the others, but there was no trace of the dinghy or the men.[6]

What should the sailor do when faced with the necessity of entering cold water? The foundering of the *Dancing Ledge* was exceptional in that the vessel broke up so rapidly. Usually there are at least a few minutes for preparation, during which time as much warm clothing as possible should be donned, including a cap and a waterproof outer suit if available.[7] A personal flotation device (PFD) is mandatory. It will help the sailor retain the energy—and thus the heat—to stay afloat. If the sailor should become unconscious, it will keep his or her head out of the water and prevent drowning. For want of a life jacket, the captain of the *Dancing Ledge* lost his life. Next, if the water temperature is below 50 degrees Fahrenheit (10 degrees Celsius), gloves and shoes should be worn. These are required because of a curious phenomenon known as *cold vasodilatation*. As we have seen, diverting blood from the shell to the core reduces heat loss. This diversion is caused by the constriction of the blood vessels of the skin (vasoconstriction). However, when the cold is severe enough to damage the hands and feet, vasoconstriction periodically gives way to vasodilatation (about every twenty minutes). Presumably this periodic "rewarming" of the fingers and toes developed to protect these exposed and vulnerable appendages. Unfortunately, in the process of saving the fingers and toes, a tremendous amount of heat is lost—thus requiring the need for gloves and shoes.

If there is time, it is worthwhile to take a rapidly acting seasickness preparation, since seasickness promotes heat loss.

Rather than jump in, the sailor should lower himself gradually if possible. Occasionally, strong, physically fit individuals have died almost immediately after entering very cold water. It is a physiologic response to the sudden exposure to cold often referred to as *cold shock* (gasp reflex, torso reflex, or inhalation reflex).[8] This cold-water reflex causes the person to inhale deeply and aspirate cold water into their airway and lungs. There is closure in the upper airway (laryngospasm), panic, disorientation, and uncontrollable gasping, which can bring more cold water into the airway and lungs. For those with cardiovascular disease, the additional stress may produce cardiac arrythmia or cardiac arrest. In addition to gradual entry into cold water, the sailor should cover the nose and mouth during entering, if possible.

As soon as the sailor enters the water, his or her body loses heat at a much more rapid rate. Since the sailor's head remains out of the water, it continues to lose heat at about the same rate as before immersion (primarily by radiation and convection). In the water, the body also loses some heat via radiation and convection, but now conduction plays the prominent role. *Water conducts heat twenty-five times faster than air.*

Clothing is crucial to preventing hypothermia. Most of the insulating effect of clothing is due to the layers of air trapped in and around the clothing rather than to the insulating property of the clothing itself. Once water permeates the clothing, much of the insulation is lost. Nevertheless, even wet clothing has a surprisingly large effect on the overall rate of heat loss. It can reduce the rate of fall in core temperature by 50 to 75 percent. Water trapped beneath and in the interstices of the clothing conducts heat from the body. As its temperature rises, the trapped water acts as a buffer between the body and the cooler water in circulation. Water immediately surrounding the sailor is also warmed and acts as a weak heat buffer.

It should be obvious why swimming is so detrimental to cold water survival. First, it defeats the body's attempt to increase the size of the shell by pumping warm blood into the muscles. Second, swimming pumps out the already warmed layer of water within and beneath the clothing. Third, the water in the immediate proximity, which has been heated at the sailor's expense, is replaced with cold water. Unless the sailor is certain he or she can make it to a nearby object or to land, the sailor is better off conserving body heat.

Remember the Rule of Fifties*:*

 50 yards in 50 degrees Fahrenheit water = 50:50 chance

There is another Rule of Fifty that has been attributed in the past to the U.S. Coast Guard:

 50 minutes (with PFD) in 50 degrees Fahrenheit water (10 degrees Celsius) = 50:50 chance

In fact, the sailor should avoid all exercise if immersed in the water. It is now well established that the heat loss is invariably greater than the heat that can be generated by exercise in cold water. The first mate of the *Dancing Ledge* survived despite bicycling, not because of it!

If alone, the sailor should adopt the *heat escape lessening posture* (HELP; Figure 3.5). This posture reduces heat loss from those areas that tend to lose heat the fastest: the head and neck, the sides of the chest, and the groin. The victim should lean back against the collar of the PFD, the arms drawing the PFD close to the body. The legs should be crossed below the knees. The older technique known as *drownproofing*, or the dead man's float, is no longer recommended. It consists of taking a deep breath and then allowing the head and arms to hang limply in the water, periodically raising the head above the water to take another breath. Although this maneuver conserves muscular energy, it allows a tremendous amount of heat to escape each time the head is submerged.

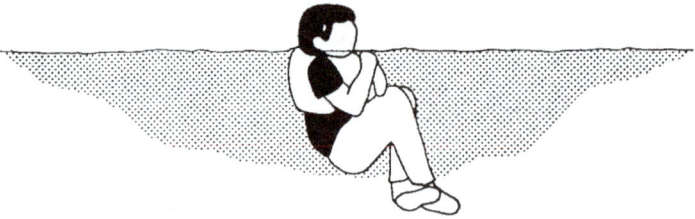

Figure 3.5 Heat escape lessening posture (HELP)[9]

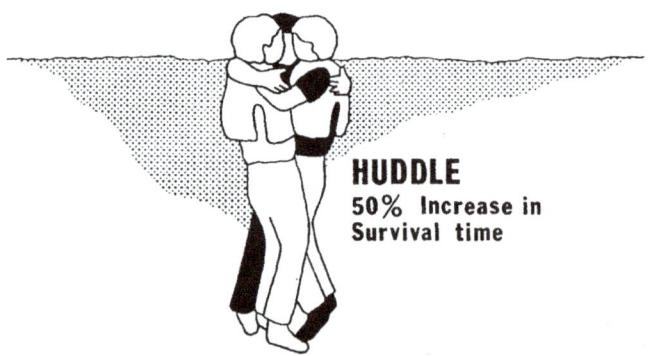

Figure 3.6 Huddle position for small groups[10]

When two or more people are in the water, they should huddle together with their chests in contact and their arms and legs wrapped around each other (Figure 3.6). This position is especially helpful for small children, who might perish quickly if left alone in the HELP position. Children already have a higher risk of developing hypothermia than adults since they have a greater surface area relative to their body weight from which to lose heat.

If the sailor is unsuccessful in his or her struggle to preserve body heat, the sailor becomes hypothermic. Figure 3.7 illustrates the signs of progressive hypothermia. Notice how the use of a PFD prolongs survival time. In addition to providing some insulation, the PFD keeps the head out of the water. Otherwise, once confusion, disorientation, and semiconsciousness are present, the sailor drowns.

Initially, the victim of hypothermia is often quiet and reluctant to communicate. Judgment may be impaired, an important fact since it potentially imperils the safety of others. The victim may become confused, resistant to aid, and even combative. Movement is slow and uncoordinated. The combination of clumsiness and slurred speech

Cold Weather Sailing

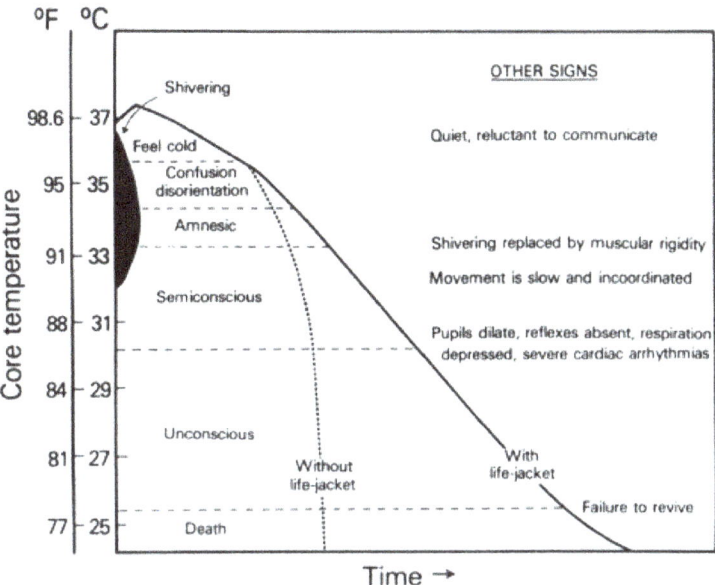

Figure 3.7 Signs of hypothermia. The signs correlate with body temperature, not with the time of immersion. The time at which the signs appear depends on many factors, such as the water temperature, duration of immersion, and the amount of clothing.

make the victim appear drunk. Shivering is an important sign, but it cannot be relied upon. It may not be present if the individual must engage in demanding activity (since exercise abolishes shivering), and as the core temperature declines, it is inevitably replaced by muscular rigidity.

When the core temperature drops to about 86 degrees Fahrenheit (30 degrees Celsius), the sailor may appear to be dead. There may be no sign of a pulse or of breathing. However, as Figure 3.7 illustrates, appearances can be deceiving. Often a long period of time elapses during which the person seems to be dead but can still be revived. A medical rule for this situation states, "No one is dead unless they are warm and dead." Until the victim is warmed and still has no pulse or breathing, the rescuer should not forgo treatment. Once the core temperature has reached 77 degrees Fahrenheit (25 degrees Celsius), the chances of successful revival become remote, although there are well documented cases of people who have survived core temperatures below 68 degrees Fahrenheit (20 degrees Celsius).

The Three Stages of Hypothermia

The *first stage is mild hypothermia* (32.2 degrees Celsius to 35 degrees Celsius or 90 degrees Fahrenheit to 95 degrees Fahrenheit). Common signs and symptoms include uncontrolled shivering mental changes, poor judgment, confusion, poor coordination, difficulty walking, clumsy use of hands, difficulty talking, and drowsiness.

The *second stage is moderate hypothermia* (27.8 degrees Celsius to 32.2 degrees Celsius or 82 degrees Fahrenheit to 90 degrees Fahrenheit). Common signs and symptoms include irregular heart rate, a slowed heart rate (about 50 percent of normal), and a slowed metabolism (about 50 percent of normal). Pupils frequently do not react to light, shivering stops, and loss of consciousness may follow.

The *third stage is severe hypothermia* (less than 27.8 degrees Celsius or 82 degrees Fahrenheit) with absent reflexes, lack of breathing, and no heartbeat.

(Note that the elderly and intoxicated may not demonstrate symptoms or signs reliably.)

If the victim is found with his or her head submerged in cold water, the victim may have activated the *mammalian diving reflex*, which will augment his or her chances for survival. This reflex occurs when the face (especially the area just above the bridge of the nose) is suddenly exposed to intense cold. The brain sets into motion a mechanism that rapidly reduces cardiac and respiratory activities to such a low level that they may not be discernible. This "instant hibernation," if you will, preserves the body for long periods of time and has been responsible for some of the dramatic recoveries reported from cold water drowning (so-called dry drownings). The mammalian diving reflex is independent of hypothermia, although they may coexist. The reflex is more likely to occur if the water is very cold and if the victim is young. Its incidence appears to decline as the age of the victim increases.

Treatment of Hypothermia

If hypothermia is mild and the survivor is alert enough to recount his or her experiences (despite dramatic shivering), it is necessary only to remove wet clothing and replace it with dry clothing or blankets. This treatment is known as *passive rewarming*. Sweetened, warm (but not hot) beverages such as cocoa should be given. Caffeine should be avoided initially and *in no case should the victim be given alcohol*. Alcohol has several deleterious effects: (1) it promotes heat loss, (2) it lowers blood sugar, and (3) it depresses the nervous system.

More severe cases require *active rewarming*. Hospital facilities have several means at their disposal for active rewarming, including those that selectively rewarm the core. Heat can be delivered by intravenous fluids, oxygen, dialysis, gastric lavage ("stomach pumping"), and even enemas; that is, *the victim can be warmed from the inside out*. If feasible, a victim who requires hospitalization should be prepared for evacuation at once. If the victim is semiconscious or unconscious, the first step is to transfer him or her gently to a warm environment. Unnecessary jostling must be avoided since it may precipitate fatal cardiac arrhythmias or cardiac arrest. Clothes should be removed with a minimum of movement—cut away if necessary—and they should be covered to prevent further heat loss. The legs should be elevated to counteract the effects of shock, and the head should be kept slightly lower than the body to facilitate blood flow to the brain.

If there has been no pulse or breathing for one to two minutes (both of which, remember, may be slow and difficult to detect), a person who is properly trained should begin cardiopulmonary resuscitation (CPR). The reason to delay CPR with the hypothermic victim until there is definitely no pulse or breathing is that the procedure is a double-edged sword. Although it may be lifesaving, CPR may precipitate cardiac arrhythmia or arrest and so should be avoided unless absolutely necessary.

Active rewarming of the hypothermic victim *on the water* remains controversial (unless on a large ship with medical facilities, such as a cruise ship or military ship). Otherwise on the water, the only practical methods are immersion in a hot tub or shower, selective surface heating with hot packs or towels, and person-to-person contact (buddy warming). The drawback to each of these procedures is that *the victim is not warmed from the inside out but from the outside in.* As a result, the victim may experience a phenomenon known as *afterdrop*.[11] In order to understand afterdrop, consider what would happen if one immersed the hypothermia victim in a tub of hot water. Since the arms and legs are part of the shell, they are maintained at a much lower temperature than the trunk by shunting blood away from them (see Figure 3.2). If the entire body is suddenly immersed in hot water, the blood vessels in the arms and legs will dilate and all the "coldness" will flow back to the body core, cooling it further. This sudden return of cold blood may produce cardiac arrhythmias or arrest and is probably responsible for some of the fatalities that have occurred after initial recovery from hypothermia.

If tub immersion is attempted, the suggested temperature is 105 degrees Fahrenheit to 110 degrees Fahrenheit (40 degrees Celsius to 43 degrees Celsius), or slightly warmer if the victim is clothed. *It is imperative to keep the arms and legs out of the bath.* The temperature of the bath water will drop almost as soon as the victim is immersed, so hot water must be added frequently.

Probably the safest procedure for active rewarming on the water is to apply warm to hot wet towels or packs to the head, neck, chest, abdomen, and groin. Depending on their temperature, they will at least retard further heat loss and may provide some heat to the body. In conjunction, exhaling warm breath into the victim's face (in unison with the victim's breathing) will supply some heat to the lungs, which are a part of the body core. Person-to-person is also an option. Both the victim and the volunteer must be naked, and contact should be restricted to the chest and back. A sleeping bag is ideal for buddy warming.

If transfer to a hospital is feasible, it certainly should be done for moderate and severe hypothermia.[12] Active rewarming on the water has risks, but the alternative treatment, passive rewarming, is slow, laborious, and potentially ineffectual. The victim may not generate enough heat to rewarm him- or herself, and the blankets may actually insulate the victim from the warmer environment.

Healthy Boating & Sailing

Keeping Warm on the Water

In order to develop a sensible approach to keeping warm—instead of merely wearing whatever clothing is at hand—the sailor need only consider a few principles. The processes of heat exchange (radiation, conduction, evaporation, and convection) still operate with the addition of clothing, only now they are somewhat modified. Whereas clothing prevents radiation from the sun from reaching the body, it also intercepts radiation that the body is emitting into the environment. The net effect in a cold environment is to conserve body heat. Since clothing is in direct contact with the skin, some heat is lost via conduction. In practice, this loss is insignificant. Evaporation heat loss in the cold is the least-understood process. Although usually it too is negligible, in certain circumstances (discussed later in this chapter) a tremendous amount of heat may be lost via this route. The most important avenue for heat loss is convection. Convection currents occur whenever there is a temperature gradient between the skin and the environment. Air that is heated through contact with the warmer skin rises to be replaced by cooler air (Figure 3.8). Thus, the body is constantly producing its own personal environment, or *microclimate*, of warm air. *The objective of all cold weather clothing is to preserve and augment this layer of warm air.*

Without clothing, convection currents inexorably play upon the skin, draining heat from the body (Figure 3.8A). If the clothing is to be effective, it must control these currents. It may surprise you to learn that only a small percentage of the insulation that clothing provides is due to the material itself. Most of the insulation is due to air trapped beneath and in the interstices of the garment and clinging in a layer to the garment's outer surface. Since air conducts heat very poorly, it is an exceptionally good insulating material. Keeping warm consists of utilizing the inherent insulating property of air!

Laboratory studies have shown that small laminations of "dead" air provide the best insulation for weight and flexibility (obviously important considerations for the sailor). This finding forms the basis of the "layer principle" with which we are all familiar. The small laminations are most efficient at a thickness of approximately 1/4 inch (6 millimeters). If the thickness of the dead air space is larger, the air rising on the warm side of the space (near the body) and settling along the cold side forms convection currents (Figure 3.8B). This circular motion rapidly increases heat loss. At 1/4-inch thickness, there is enough air to provide insulation but not enough to create convection currents (Figure 3.8C).

If the laminations of air become any smaller, the insulation is insufficient. The crucial concept, of which many sailors are not cognizant, is that for the layer principle to be effective, the layers of clothing must be worn *loosely*. Otherwise the air is squeezed out from between the layers, and much of the insulation is lost. Thus, each additional layer should be sufficiently larger than the one before to allow for the thickness of the garment as well as for the thickness of the dead air space.[13] Unfortunately, as layers are built up on the body, a point of diminishing returns is reached. We can think of the body as being composed of variously shaped cylinders. As clothing is added, the surface area (from which heat is lost) of each of the cylinders increases. Eventually the increased

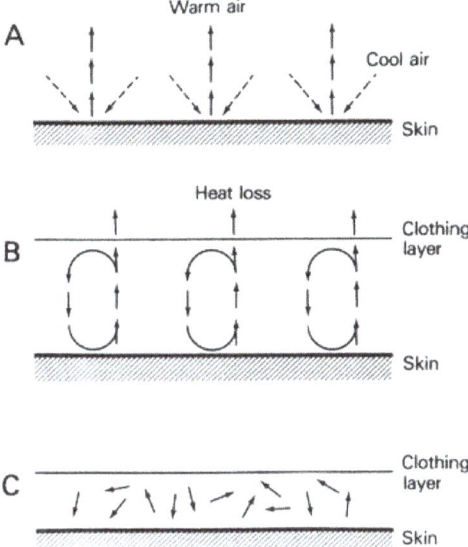

Figure 3.8 The influence of clothing on convection currents: (a) without clothing, there is continual heat loss; (b) very loosely worn clothing allows circular convection currents to form; (c) optimal-layered clothing at approximately 1/4-inch (6 millimeter) thickness prevents convection currents from forming.

surface area promotes more heat loss than the increased thickness can insulate. The fingers, as small cylinders, reach optimal insulation at about 1/4 inch, whereas the trunk, a much larger cylinder, is still deriving insulation up to 5 or 6 inches. The arms and legs, moderate-size cylinders, benefit up to about 2 inches. The feet, each a single cylinder of unusual shape since the toes tend to be cramped together, may be insulated to a thickness of 1/2 inch.

Boaters and other outdoorsmen tend to make the following mistakes:

(1) The legs tend to be neglected. In fact, they are larger cylinders than the arms and should have more insulation and not less, as is usually the case.

(2) The arms tend to be overly insulated in comparison with the trunk. Since the trunk can profitably accommodate much thicker insulation than the arms, vests should be exploited to provide the additional trunk insulation.

(3) The sailor whose feet are cold often incorrectly assumes that warmer footgear is the answer. Thicker footgear above the optimum will not improve matters. Rather, added insulation of the trunk may warm the feet. As the trunk is "over warmed," some of this blood is shunted to the feet, from which heat escapes from the body. The feet act as heat radiators and keep themselves warm in the process.

To preserve the laminations of dead air, they must be protected from the wind. Thus, a windbreaker is essential. By itself it provides an insignificant amount of insulation. However, by preserving the layers of dead air from the ravages of the wind, the windbreaker contributes enormously to the insulation process. It is foolish to go to the trouble of putting on layer upon layer of clothing to produce an "insulative edifice" without filling up the "chinks" to protect the layers from the wind. A windbreaker will also diminish the effect of the windchill factor, another misunderstood concept. Windchill is an estimate of the expected additional convection heat loss due to the wind. Since convection occurs most rapidly on exposed skin, the windchill factor (when stated in degrees of temperature) is strictly applicable to someone who is naked and exposed to the elements. It can accurately indicate, however, the subjective feeling of coldness over the exposed portions of the body such as the hands or face. Figure 3.9 is a simplified nomogram for calculating this subjective feeling. Notice that the left-hand scale for wind speed is "irregular"; that is, the rate of cooling is marked for the first few knots of wind, whereas the additional cooling produced by an increase from, say, 10 to 20 knots, is rather modest. This makes sense if we recall that in the absence of any wind, convection currents produce a layer of warm air that surrounds the body. Although most of this warm air is beneath clothing when worn, the still air on the exterior is also warmed. As soon as the wind begins to blow (from 0.1 to 1 knot), this layer instantly vanishes. As the wind speed picks up, additional heat is lost, but at lesser increments. Usually at least three layers are required in the cold:

- An inner or base layer, critical to keep the skin dry (should be moisture wicking, see endnote 12). This is the layer up against the skin. It is usually composed of wool or synthetic material, such as polyester, polyethylene, and microfiber. Synthetics often contain antibacterial, antiodor treatment.
- A mid layer—the main insulating layer. It should be more loose fitting to leave insulating air. A traditional mid layer material includes wool of course but also fleece, down, synthetic fill, and cotton.
- A shell or outer layer. This protects the other layers from wind and water. Ideally, the shell allows moisture through to the outside (it is "breathable") while not letting wind and water into the inside. There is always a trade-off between "breathability" and resistance to wind and water.

The face and head have yet to be considered. These areas can be a significant source of heat loss—to such a degree that they have been likened to "a hole in a bucket." The face and head, unlike the rest of the body, do not undergo blood vessel constriction (vasoconstriction). On the contrary, the skin vasodilates, producing the familiar rosy red color so typical of cold weather. Thus, a person usually suffers relatively little discomfort when exposing his or her face or entire head to very low temperatures. However, heat from the rest of the person's body is rapidly flowing out from these areas. If at the same time the person complains that his or her feet are cold, it may be more truth than jest that if the person put on a hat, he or she would keep his or her feet warm! In other words,

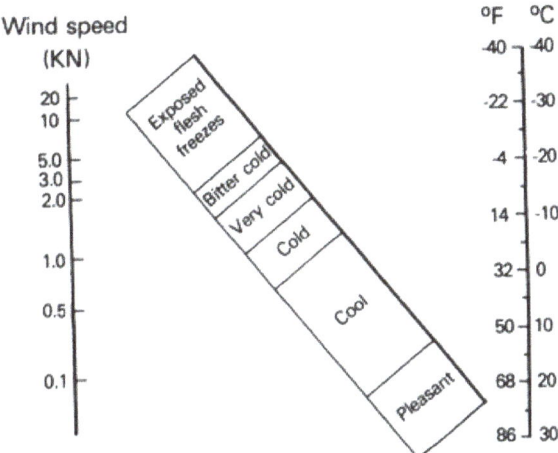

Figure 3.9 Windchill space factor. The subjective feeling of exposed flesh (such as face or hand) can be estimated with a straight edge. Line up the wind speed and the temperature. The intersection with the solid line in the center indicates the subjective feeling. For example, a temperature of 32 degrees Fahrenheit (0 degrees Celsius) with a wind speed of 20 knots will be experienced as "very cold."

when the face and head are provided with *protection*—even though they might not seem to need it—*more heat* is retained in the body, and warm blood is diverted to the feet, keeping them warm. A woolen cap can readily cover almost two-thirds of the head, and a thick "woolly" beard appreciably diminishes heat loss from the face.

Cold Weather Clothing

Keeping warm also depends on choosing the right clothing materials. Many different measurements can be made to compare various materials. It turns out that in still air, all fabrics provide about the same degree of insulation per inch of thickness. Is there any reason then for the universal preference for wool over other materials? The answer is yes and no. The explanation lies in the structure of the wool. Wool is distinctive because of its natural crimp. There are ten or more crimps, or undulations, per inch that impart a loftiness to the material, and this loftiness traps more air within the fibers. Natural wool also has microscopic surface scales that promote "aerodynamic drag," keeping the air in contact with the wool. Additional reasons for the superiority of wool are its elasticity and compressional resiliency, especially when moist. Dry cotton, for example, provides almost as much warmth as wool. But when moist, cotton loses its strength, is compressed, and consequently loses much of its insulative value. Wool tends to resist this compression better than the other natural or synthetic materials. However, synthetics that are spun to simulate wool perform almost as well as wool when wet, and they may dry faster and last longer!

Finally, in the effort to stay warm, there is one last requirement: clothing must have ventilation. The following case highlights this fact:

> A soldier (a newcomer) was brought to the Fort Wainwright Hospital in a state of collapse during the 1965 Operation Polar Siege; he had been pulling sleds and chopping timber under conditions where the temperature was -40°. The diagnosis at the hospital was heat stroke. He had been so alarmed at the thought of working in the cold that he had piled on every item of insulation he could borrow.[14]

Thus, it is necessary to provide not only warmth but also flexibility for a wide range of conditions. This is particularly true for sailors since periods of intense (sometimes frantic) activity alternate with periods of relative inactivity. For example, by increasing exertion from that expended sitting on deck to that expended in light duty, the sailor approximately doubles his or her heat output and halves the insulation requirement. (This is not precisely correct, since some of the heat that exercise generates is lost.) Unless about half of the insulation is eliminated, sweating begins, and *sweating must be avoided at all costs*. There are two alternatives: either some of the layers can be removed, or the whole "system" can be ventilated. The novice is generally reluctant to remove anything, whereas the old salt by habit avoids the danger of allowing sweat to accumulate in his or her clothing.

As soon as the sailor begins to feel hot, he or she should first remove his or her gloves and, if this is insufficient, cap. Then, prior to removing layers, the sailor should attempt to ventilate the system. The Inuit, who are constantly confronted with an identical problem, have arrived at this very solution by designing fur clothing with vents that can be opened to permit controlled ventilation. When an Inuit is stationary, he or she closes the apertures at the ankles, wrists, waist, and neck. As the level of activity increases, he or she opens these apertures, allowing upward ventilation through the neck region, so-called chimney ventilation. Most likely this was the original purpose of the necktie, with a knot that can be loosened without untying.

The reason that sweating must be avoided is that it can promote tremendous heat loss. It does this in two ways. First, the process of evaporation takes place. When the sailor begins to sweat, water vapor is produced at the skin's surface. Body heat is required to produce the water vapor, and this heat is lost. Second, there is a reduction in the amount of insulation. Once the sweat leaves the skin through evaporation, it meets the base or inner layer. As the inner layers become wet, air is displaced from the fabric. If the fabric is natural cotton, there is nowhere to go. It will become soaked.

Wool and the newer synthetic fabrics are designed to "wick" away water (sweat), and most of the clothing sold as active wear is advertised as "moisture wicking." To varying degrees, moisture wicking does work.[15] Wool was originally the best combination of wicking and water repelling and was often used (and still is) as a base layer—especially the softer Merino wool. Wool is naturally good at wicking. Moisture wicking relies on "capillary action" moving the moisture through tiny spaces within the fabric due to the molecular interaction between the liquid and the internal surface. As previously mentioned, wool is naturally wavy, and the natural fabric provides the "capillary" spaces. Most moisture wicking fabrics nowadays are synthetic and designed to be hydrophobic (resisting the penetration of water) so that the moisture travels through the interstices and out, as it does in wool. Cotton, on the other hand, is basically "non-wicking." It will soak up moisture and then take forever to dry. Some treated cotton fabrics are better than pure cotton, but they still lag way behind synthetics and wool in terms of moisture wicking capability.

But the process does not stop there. If the sailor is wearing waterproof foul-weather gear, the water vapor does not have ready access to the atmosphere. (Despite manufacturers' claims that the newer waterproof fabrics can "breathe," these fabrics are still relatively impermeable to water vapor.) This is where selective ventilation can be very helpful.

In a short period of time, unless there is some ventilation, the inner layers ultimately become soggy. When water vapor reaches the cooler semi-impermeable wall of the foul-weather gear, it reaches dew point, and condensation takes place. Condensation liberates heat to the inner surface of the rain gear, and much of this heat is eventually lost. Gradually, the entire space within the clothing layers reaches 100 percent humidity, and the liquid begins to soak backward. As it approaches the body surface, it is warmed and evaporates a second time, robbing the body of heat further. Once again, it condenses on the inner surface of the rain gear. This cyclic process of evaporation and condensation accounts for the extreme cooling that occurs when damp clothes are worn under foul-weather gear.[16]

Wet Suits and Dry Suits

Either of these may be useful to the sailor, depending on the type of sailing. Wet suits are composed of foamed neoprene rubber containing bubbles of air or nitrogen gas. Thus, the suit provides insulation due to the gas trapped within the neoprene material. However, as the name implies, the wet suit—which is relatively formfitting—does allow a thin layer of water to enter the suit. This water is trapped and warmed by the body, adding to the insulation. The water within the suit tends to prevent additional water from entering the suit, keeping the environment relatively stable.

Dry suits, on the other hand, are typically one-piece suits made of waterproof, "breathable" nylon with waterproof rubber seals at the neck, wrists, and feet. There is a waterproof zipper. These suits will keep the body completely dry—the warmth is due to insulation from the base layer as well as the air trapped between the base layer and the suit. The dry suit will keep a person much drier than the wet suit but at a cost—they are bulkier and more difficult to work in. However, if you enter the water, you can float around and will not feel the cold water much at all. For a full discussion of everything you might want to know about dry suits, consult the *Rescue and Survival Systems Manual* by the U.S. Coast Guard.[17]

Performance in the Cold

There is one final caveat for the sailor who must function in a cold environment: he or she must anticipate that his or her efficiency will suffer. This results from the effect of cold on the muscles, nerves, and even the central nervous system if hypothermia is present.

Experiments conducted aboard ships reveal a deterioration in the ability to perform various tasks simultaneous with a decrease in the skin temperature of the hand. The experiments tested handgrip strength and the ability to thread nuts onto screws and fasten screws into a metal plate—representative of the kinds of tasks that a sailor might be called upon to perform. When the temperature of the skin fell below 60 degrees Fahrenheit (15 degrees Celsius), there was a corresponding decline in both handgrip strength and manual dexterity. This decline cannot be attributed totally to the muscles. Many of the subjects also described difficulty in knowing what their fingers were doing! Subsequent experiments have confirmed that there is also a decrease in the sensation of the fingers at about 60 degrees Fahrenheit (15 degrees Celsius). These effects are clearly the result of local cooling of the muscles and nerves.

But what about the effects of cooling of the central nervous system (which is, after all, a part of the core)? Marked cooling produces the signs of hypothermia discussed earlier in this chapter (see Figure 3.7). Subtle cooling was evaluated in one experiment on watchkeeping proficiency in the winter. Carried out from the open bridge of a ship, the test consisted of monitoring two lights separated by 75 degrees, the task being to signal when a third, dimmer light appeared between the two. As a control, the test was repeated in a more temperate climate. In the cold, when the oral temperature (an approximation of the central core) fell as little as 1.2 degrees Fahrenheit (0.7 degrees Celsius), there was a reliable increase in the number of delays in reporting the third light. Brain wave (electroencephalograph, or EEG) studies have also demonstrated changes as soon as the core temperature cools as little as 2 degrees Fahrenheit (1 degree Celsius).

These findings have several implications for the sailor. When working in the cold, the sailor should make allowances for diminished efficiency. He or she will require more time for any given task, and, even if the task has been performed countless times before, visual cues may be needed to compensate for the diminished finger dexterity and sensitivity. Finally, if exposure to cold can be anticipated, it is advisable to complete the most complex tasks before the inevitable decline in performance occurs.

COLD WEATHER TIPS

(1) Stay active
(2) Stay dry—get reliable outer gear
(3) Think about your base and insulative layers and plan for ventilation
(4) Sleep in your gear—you have already warmed it

Cold Weather Sailing

(5) Avoid eating large meals
(6) Drink warm liquids to stay hydrated
(7) Empty your bladder frequently—why spend heat warming a "core" disposable product
(8) Make sure you have disposable hand and foot warmers
(9) Don't forget your neck and face
(10) Protect your eyes or they will dry out. Cold wind makes eye moisture evaporate, and your brain signals to create excessive tears to compensate. Use artificial tears.

Notes

1. There is no single "normal" temperature. Body temperature varies from one individual to another, as well as from one time of day to another for any given individual. It is usually highest at about 8 p.m. and lowest at about 5 a.m. The normal range for young healthy adults is 98 degrees Fahrenheit to 100 degrees Fahrenheit (36.7 degrees Celsius to 37.8 degrees Celsius) rectal or 97 degrees Fahrenheit to 99 degrees Fahrenheit (36.1 degrees Celsius to 37.2 degrees Celsius) oral.

2. It turns out things are even more interesting than we thought. All of us have stores of white fat (some of us more than others), but who knew we had brown fat and that it plays a major role in thermogenesis. Until recently, it was accepted that brown fat was present in newborns and other mammals but that adults had little or no brown fat. Not so. All of us have some brown fat (mixed in with our white fat)—the amount varies between individuals. Brown fat is good, lean fat.

When the boater is exposed to cold, an enzyme (FGF 21) is released, which reacts with brown fat to produce heat and convert white fat into brown fat. This is referred to as nonshivering thermogenesis.

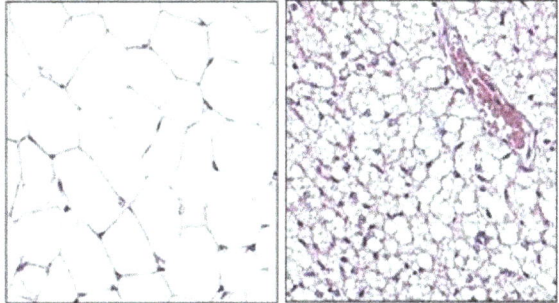

Figure 3.10 Typical white fat on the left and brown fat on the right

As the cold exposure increases, shivering begins, and the muscle contraction of shivering causes the release of a different enzyme (irisin). Shivering thermogenesis produces heat by two mechanisms: (1) by burning glycogen as the muscles contract (we knew that) and (2) by releasing irisin which helps to burn brown fat and, like FGF 21, convert white fat into brown fat. Shivering can burn one hundred calories in fifteen minutes, which is equivalent to the calorie burn of kayaking.

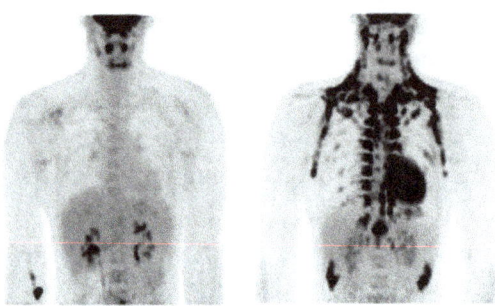

Figure 3.11 Demonstration of brown fat in a neutral environment (left) compared with brown fat in a cold environment. Notice that the distribution is not even close to your "trouble spots." (Mjw.hanssen, CC BY-SA 3.0, httpscreativecommons.orglicensesby-sa3.0)

To make matters even more confusing, the exercising muscle (no matter the temperature) not only burns glycogen for energy (while producing heat as we all know), but it also releases irisin just like shivering. It doesn't make a lot of sense as there is no need to produce more heat. It remains a bit of a puzzle, but it has been speculated that exercise is actually hijacking the shivering response, which is phylogenetically older (not aware of "Pilates for Primates," for example).

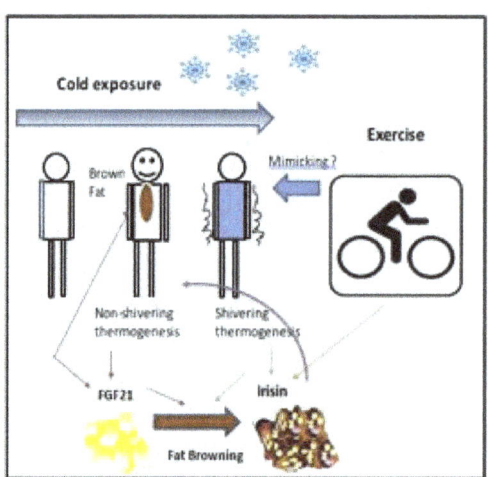

Figure 3.12 Shivering and nonshivering thermogenesis (and exercise) Illustration redrawn from P. Lee et al., "Irisin and FGF21 Are cold-induced endocrine activators of brown fat function in humans. *Cell Metabolism* 19, no. 2 (February 2014), 302-309.

3. D. Maclean and D. Emslie-Smith, *Accidental Hypothermia* (Oxford: Blackwell, 1977), 54.
4. R. H. Dana, *Two Years Before the Mast* (New York: Penguin, 1981), 393.
5. E. C. B. Lee and K. Lee, *Safety and Survival at Sea* (New York: Norton, 1980), 55.
6. K. A. Coles, Heavy Weather Sailing, Third revised edition, 1981 (Clinton Corners, NY: De Graff and London: Adlard Coles Ltd. Pp. 133-134
7. The head is responsible for one-third of the body's heat loss. Putting on a cap, even if the foul-weather gear includes a hood, helps prolong survival time considerably. Anyone who cruises

extensively should consider one of the many survival suits. They increase survival time five- to tenfold. Although they are somewhat expensive, a case could be made that not having them is an example of false economy.

8. "Cold Shock Response," *Wikipedia*, accessed January 15, 2019, https://en.wikipedia.org/wiki/Cold_shock_respose.

9. Reprinted by permission from Robert S. Pratt, "Hypothermia: The Chill That Need Not Kill," *American College of Surgeons Bulletin* 10 (1980): 26-35.

10. Reprinted by permission from Pratt, "Hypothermia."

11. "Afterdrop," *Wikipedia*, accessed January 15, 2019, https://en.wikipedia.org/wikipedia.org/wiki/Afterdrop.

12. K. Zafran et al., "Wilderness Medical Society Practice Guidelines for the Out-of-Hospital Evaluation and Treatment of Accidental Hypothermia," *Wilderness and Environmental Medicine* 25 (2014): 425-445.

13. Norwegian fishnet underwear is worth considering as the initial/base layer. It serves two functions: maintaining a layer of dead air adjacent to the skin and keeping the subsequent layer off of the skin. By preventing the clothing from coming into contact with the skin, the fishnet diminishes the amount of moisture that is absorbed into the base layer, allowing more of the body moisture to pass through to the mid layer. This keeps the skin dry and warm with the moisture ending up in the mid layer or beyond.

14. G. E. Folk, *Introduction to Environmental Physiology* (Philadelphia: Lea & Febiger, 1966), 103.

15. "Nike Shows Its Salty Side in Base-Layer Test," *Practical Sailor*, January 2006. In a more recent article, *Inside Practical Sailor* lists several practical recommendations; Darrell Nicholson, "Bracing for Cold and Wet Sailing," *Inside Practical Sailor*, September 26, 2018. The article discusses the following: base layers, including those from the 2006 issue that were not that effective; gloves; boots; and foul-weather gear.

16. The army has developed a mnemonic to assist their soldiers in the proper use of clothing: COLD. The "C" reminds the soldiers to keep clothing clean so it won't cling, become matted or greasy, and impair insulation; "0" suggests that the clothing be opened to avoid overheating; "L" recalls that clothing should be worn loosely and in layers; and "D" reminds them to keep the clothing dry.

17. https://media.defense.gov/2017/Mar/201723580/-1/-1/0/CIM_10470_10.G.pdf

Chapter 4

Heat and Dehydration

> "Water, water everywhere,
> And all the boards did shrink,
> Water, water everywhere,
> Nor any drop to drink."
>
> —*S. T. Coleridge,* The Rime of the Ancient Mariner, *1798*

Heat exposure presents the sailor with just as severe a challenge as exposure to the cold. The following account occurred during World War II on a prisoner-of-war ship in the Banda Sea, Indonesia. It clearly demonstrates one of the most feared dangers—heatstroke:

> All the men lay spread on the uneven bundles of firewood blistering horribly in the tropical sun. Tongues began to blacken . . . and all vestiges of sanity deserted many. . . . One youngster, delirious with sunstroke, shouted the thoughts of his disordered mind for thirty hours before he became too weak to utter another word. Just before he died, he grabbed a full tin, that was being used as a bed pan, and drank the contents greedily, before he could be prevented.[1]

In one respect, the challenge of heat exposure is even greater than that of the cold because there is less margin for error. As we saw in Chapter 3, the normal core temperature of the human body is approximately 98.6 degrees Fahrenheit (37 degrees Celsius). An average healthy adult may survive even when the core drops to 77 degrees Fahrenheit (25 degrees Celsius), a decline of 21.6 degrees Fahrenheit (12 degrees Celsius). Survival is rarely possible, however, if the core rises above 108 degrees Fahrenheit (42 degrees Celsius), an elevation of only 9.4 degrees Fahrenheit (5 degrees Celsius). Thus, over the range of core temperatures compatible with survival, the human "thermostat" is set high. The reason why this feature originally evolved will soon be evident.

Another crucial difference between heat and cold exposure is the body's requirement for water. The normal water intake and output for adults is shown in Table 4.1.

Intake (liters)		Output (liters)	
Water and beverages	1.2	Urine	1.3
Food water	0.9	Evaporation	1.0
Water of metabolism	0.4	Feces	0.2
	2.5L		2.5L

Table 4.1 Normal water intake and output for adults in liters

Food water refers to the water content of food. The water content of solid food is seldom less than 50 percent, and some fruits and vegetables may be as high as 95 percent.

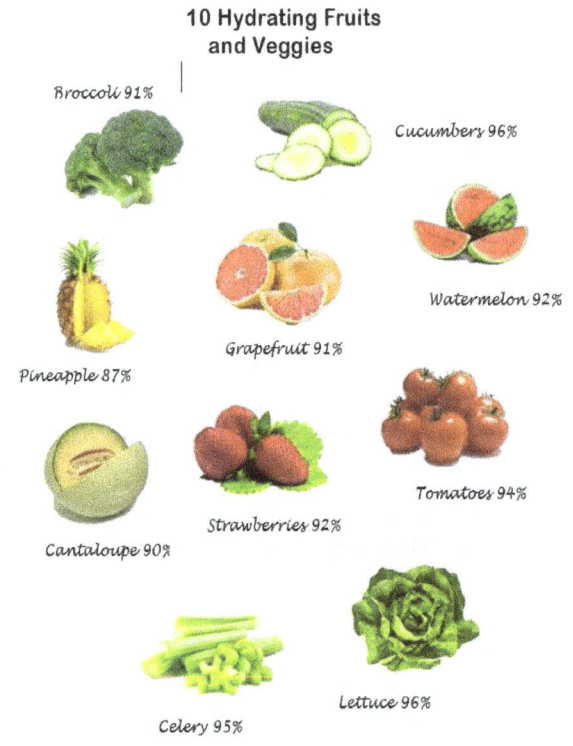

Figure 4.1 Hydrating fruits and vegetables and their water content

The amount of water produced during the metabolism of food (water of metabolism) depends on the type of food consumed (Figure 4.1). Fats yield the most water, carbohydrates somewhat less, and proteins the least. This is one reason why the dehydrated sailor should avoid protein when water is scarce. There is another more important reason, however. Fats and carbohydrates are metabolized into water and carbon dioxide (which the lungs excrete). The products of protein metabolism, primarily *urea*, must be excreted by the kidneys—and this process requires water. Thus, fats and carbohydrates are preferred when water intake is low. The *evaporation* listed in Table 4.1 refers to *insensible water loss*—you don't perceive it evaporating. This water loss is through the skin and from the lungs and is not the evaporation that heat stress produces, which is frequently much greater. The water loss from feces, although of small magnitude, is important for normal evacuation. Moisture reduction during periods of dehydration is partially responsible for the common sailing malady of constipation.

In the cold, requirements for water are minimal. In a hot environment, the only means of eliminating heat—via evaporation—is entirely dependent on water. Without water, evaporation fails, and without evaporation, the person rapidly perishes.

Evaporation

Humans are most comfortable when they neither shiver nor sweat. The range between the two extremes is known as the *thermoneutral zone* and is roughly when the environment's temperatures is from 77 degrees Fahrenheit (25 degrees Celsius) to 86 degrees Fahrenheit (30 degrees Celsius). Below 77 degrees Fahrenheit (25 degrees Celsius), either clothing or exercise is required to maintain body temperature. Without either, shivering will occur. Above 86 degrees Fahrenheit (30 degrees Celsius), sweating begins. Within the thermoneutral zone, temperature regulation is most efficient. This process is carried out exclusively by the varying amount of blood flow to the skin, which determines the skin's thermal conductivity (see Figure 3.2). At the cool end of the thermoneutral zone, the superficial blood vessels are constricted, increasing the natural insulation of the skin and subcutaneous tissues. When the air temperature reaches 86 degrees Fahrenheit (30 degrees Celsius), these vessels are fully dilated, promoting the transfer of heat from the core to the skin's surface, where it can be eliminated.

When the blood vessels are fully dilated, heat dissipation by radiation and convection is at a maximal level, and evaporation must make up the difference. Once the air temperature rises above 95 degrees Fahrenheit (35 degrees Celsius), the heat gradient reverses, and the body begins to gain heat by radiation and convection. Evaporation is now the only means of eliminating heat from the body. If any activity must be performed, evaporation must dispose of the heat generated from that as well. Fortunately, evaporation can eliminate tremendous amounts of heat.

Dr. Charles Blagden first demonstrated the remarkable capacity of evaporation two hundred years ago.[2] He, along with a few friends and a dog, entered a room heated to 260 degrees Fahrenheit (120 degrees Celsius). They remained in the room for forty-five minutes without ill effects, while the steak they brought in with them was thoroughly cooked in fifteen minutes. More recent experiments have confirmed his observations. For short periods of time, humans can produce sweat at a rate of 4 quarts (about 4 liters) per hour! The magnitude of this accomplishment can be appreciated when we recall that an adult has only 5 quarts (about 5 liters) of circulating blood at any one time. Obviously, there is a price to pay for this kind of energy efficiency, and it is paid in salt and water—especially water.

Sweat

The human body is endowed with two different kinds of sweat glands, the *apocrine* and the *eccrine*. The *apocrine glands* are located in the axillary, mammary, and pubic regions. They function primarily with regard to sex and reproduction, not in temperature regulation.

In the average adult, there are two million to four million *eccrine glands* concentrated in certain regions of the body. Sweat is most copious from these regions. The highest concentration (and hence the greatest sweating) occurs on the forehead, neck, trunk, and back of the hand. Lesser degrees of sweating occur on the cheeks and the remainder on the arms and legs. The underarms, palms, and soles sweat the least in the heat, in contrast to their production when the individual is under psychological stress. The eccrine glands lie deep in the skin and are connected to the surface by twisted coils (Figure 4.2). When blood passes through the glands, water and salt are extracted and secreted. At the skin's surface, the sweat evaporates, liberating heat from the body. *Sweating per se does nothing to cool the body. For heat to be liberated, the sweat must undergo evaporation at the skin surface. Sweat that drips from the skin without evaporating is entirely wasted.* The efficiency

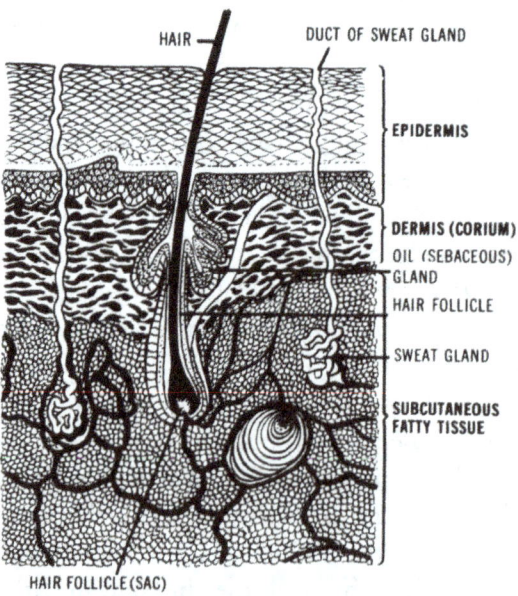

Figure 4.2 Skin with sweat glands surrounded by blood vessels (in black)

of evaporation is ultimately determined by the degree of atmospheric humidity. During periods of high humidity, the air is already holding a great deal of water, limiting evaporation from the skin, and making for an uncomfortable environment for humans.

Although the ability to sweat is taken for granted, there is a marked variation from one individual to another. Some people can produce sweat at a rate of 4 quarts (4 liters) per hour for brief periods of time, whereas others are capable of only a meager pint (0.5 liter) under the same conditions. Rare individuals are unable to sweat at all. This variation in sweating ability explains in part why certain individuals are more susceptible than others to some of the heat-induced disorders, such as heatstroke. Skin disorders such as prickly heat or rash interfere with sweating, as do several widely prescribed drugs, including many of those used to treat nervous and mental conditions.

Let us look at some of the categories of medication that could affect your body's ability to perform in the heat:

- Medications that are used to treat cold and allergy symptoms are known as either antihistamines or anticholinergic drugs. These medications directly decrease the body's ability to sweat and cool itself by acting on the nerve fibers that innervate the sweat glands. A common example is the medication dimenhydrinate (Benadryl).

- Major tranquilizers and antidepressants act directly on the portion of the brain that is the central thermostat—the hypothalamus. By impairing regulation, heat-related illness is more likely. Amitriptyline (Elavil) is a prime example.

- Ironically, many of the medications used to treat seasickness may also impair sweating. Scopolamine (hyoscine), our most potent seasickness medication, is one of the worst in this regard. To complicate matters, vomiting from seasickness will cause dehydration and worsen heat-related conditions.

- Medications like beta-blockers may slow heart rate and reduce blood pressure, both of which will reduce blood flow to the skin making it more difficult for evaporation to take place.

- Stimulants such as amphetamines (Adderall), methylphenidate (Ritalin), ephedrine, and cocaine will increase metabolism and increase the internal body temperature as well as constrict skin blood vessels. All of this will make it more difficult to release heat from the skin.

- Some antimigraine and antiseizure medications, such as topiramate and zonisamide, also impair sweating.

- Finally, diuretics (also known as water pills) will cause dehydration and make sweating more difficult.

For more information, see "The Hypertensive Sailor" section below in this chapter as well as Appendix B, which lists many of the medications that may impair sweating.

If there is a plentiful supply of water (and salt), a person can survive long periods of intense heat. In fact, with daily exposure, the sailor begins to acclimatize in four days and is fully adapted to the heat in about a week. Acclimatization improves the overall efficiency of the system. The threshold for sweating is lower, and the sweat is distributed more uniformly over the body, which promotes evaporation. In addition, body temperature and heart rate, which were initially elevated, return to normal.

It is worth noting that during an initial exposure to a hot environment, the body tends to become dehydrated even when salt and water are freely available. This common phenomenon is known as *voluntary dehydration*. For some reason, thirst is often satisfied before all the salt and water have been replaced. Therefore, if supplies are plentiful, the sailor should be encouraged to drink and replace his salt liberally.

When water is scarce, a problem most shipwreck survivors face, the sailor is in danger of becoming *progressively dehydrated*. You might assume that the rate of sweating would decline with progressive dehydration, but in fact the decrease is slight. By and large, *sweating continues at a rate determined by the temperature, rather than the degree of dehydration.* The sailor is clearly between the proverbial "rock and a hard place." If, on the one hand, sweating is reduced to preserve body water, body heat then rises to unacceptable levels. If, on the other hand, sweating continues, the sailor becomes increasingly dehydrated. Since the effect of uncontrolled heat gain has a more rapid fatal effect than dehydration, there is little choice but to accept a substantial amount of dehydration.

The sailor tolerates a certain amount of dehydration fairly well, giving time to search for sources of water. However, once the water deficit approaches 10 percent of body weight, the system begins to falter. Core temperature is now about 102 degrees Fahrenheit (39 degrees Celsius). The reduction in the blood volume due to the water loss compromises the heart and circulatory system. In addition, the viscosity of the blood increases, further taxing the system. If water is not available soon, the sailor will die of dehydration.

The degree of dehydration can be estimated as follows: at 2 percent weight loss, there is appreciable thirst; at 4 percent, the mouth and throat are exceedingly dry; at 8 percent, salivation stops, and speech becomes difficult; at 10 percent, the sailor is unable to care for him- or herself; at 12 percent, the sailor is unable to swallow and will recover only if water is given by stomach tube, rectal enema, or intravenously. Sweating fails at about 18 to 20 percent.

We can now make a guess at why our thermostat is set on the high side. If our body temperature were set at, say, 86 degrees Fahrenheit (30 degrees Celsius), it would not be physically possible to produce enough sweat fast enough to cool ourselves at an air temperature of only 100 degrees Fahrenheit (38 degrees Celsius)! With the thermostat set high, the onset of our efficient but costly evaporative cooling system is delayed as long as possible.

Not only is there a substantial loss of water in dehydration, but also a significant amount of salt loss. The body normally contains 160 grams of salt (give or take a pinch), the most important of which is sodium chloride, or table salt. The body is also rich in other salts, such as potassium and magnesium, but only sodium chloride is lost in large quantities in sweat. The concentration of salts in the body is just as important as—and sometimes more important than—the total quantity. The kidneys, the major arbiter of our internal environment, maintain this concentration within narrow limits at approximately a 0.9 percent solution.

Under normal circumstances if we ingest an excess amount of salt, three things usually occur. First, the increased salt concentration stimulates the thirst mechanism; second we increase water intake, and third, with this water, the kidneys excrete the excess salt in the urine, reestablishing a 0.9 percent solution. If there is a deficiency of salt, however, the kidneys selfishly conserve what is left by decreasing the amount of salt in the urine.

Not only is the rate of sweating variable, but so is the concentration of salt in sweat. The average concentration is 0.2 to 0.3 percent, with a range of 0.1 to 0.6 percent. In a very hot environment, the body, especially if under physical stress, usually begins to excrete sweat with a salt concentration of about 0.45 percent—about half the concentration found in blood. Sweating rates of 5 to 7 quarts (5 to 7 liters) per day (8 to 12 quarts [8 to 12 liters] per day are also possible) producing a salt deficit of about 20 to 25 grams—a loss of more than 15 percent! Clearly something must be done to reduce the amount of salt loss. The kidneys respond immediately by curtailing urinary salt altogether. In addition, over the next few days in a hot environment when exposed to physical stress, the concentration of salt in the sweat is reduced. By this time, however, the person already has a significant deficit in salt and water.

Ideally, salt and water should be replaced at the same rate and concentration at which they were lost in the sweat. Unfortunately, there is no easy way to determine such losses at sea. A practical approach to take is as follows: If water is readily available, the amount of salt in the diet should be increased from 10 grams to 20 to 25 grams per day. Slightly less is necessary if sweating is not profuse. This measure will satisfy the needs of all but the rare few who secrete a very concentrated sweat. Some of the salt can be replaced in the food (cooking and table salt), whereas the rest can be replenished with salt tablets, which are often 1 gram each.[3] Potassium supplements are usually not needed because the potassium loss in sweat is small. Anyway, a glass of orange or tomato juice replaces nearly all of the potassium, calcium, and magnesium excreted in about 3 quarts (3 liters) of sweat. There is no need to worry about overdose. In healthy adults, the kidneys easily excrete any excess salt. If water is not readily available, as in shipwreck situations, salt should be avoided. The reason is that even the most concentrated sweat is less concentrated than normal body tissues (0.9 percent), so the shipwrecked sailor with a limited water supply will always be more deficient in water than salt. *Only when they have replaced the water should they take salt.*

Heat-Induced Disorders

A common heat-induced disorder is *heat cramps*. Although quite painful, the condition is fortunately nearly always benign. Sir Francis Chichester describes it in *Gipsy Moth Circles the World*:

> I don't get hungry in these 85° F heats until the middle of the night, or early morning. . . . At night I was troubled by cramp in my legs which would hit me after I had been asleep about two hours and would let go only if I stood up. This meant that I never got more than about two hours sleep at a time. It was hot and I sweated profusely; I wondered whether my body might be losing too much salt. I decided to drink half a glassful of seawater a day to put back salt.[4]

The cramps begin suddenly and most frequently attack the legs and thighs, although they may also affect the abdomen, arms, hands, feet, or even the jaw. They last for hours at a time and continue until the salt deficiency is corrected. The cramps usually afflict the sailor who has been drinking large amounts of fluids without replenishing the salt. Gently stretching the affected muscle with steady pressure usually helps.

Heat syncope (fainting or loss of consciousness) occurs after long periods of time in the heat (such as at the helm). The boater may already be somewhat dehydrated, so there is less blood volume throughout the body, including blood going to the brain. With prolonged standing, blood pools in the legs (which may actually swell with leg edema), and this further reduces the blood volume traveling to the brain. What happens next is dizziness and sometimes passing out, referred to medically as syncope. Treatment is straightforward—lay the person down horizontally to make it easier for blood to go to the brain. Also, get the person to a cool place, administer fluids, and let him or her rest for a while.

Heat cramps and heat syncope may occur alone or as part of the disorder known as *heat exhaustion*. The boater who is working in the heat develops progressive salt and water deficiency, which temporarily diminishes the amount of blood circulating in the body. In addition, heat dilates the capillaries of the skin, allowing blood to pool there, further diminishing the amount of blood that the heart can pump to the rest of the body. As we have seen, sudden changes in posture, such as rising quickly, can result in dizziness and syncope. *Severe heat exhaustion* occurs with more extreme degrees of salt and water deficiency. In the absence of salt, water that is ingested does not replenish the blood supply but is instead excreted in the urine to maintain the proper salt concentration (0.9 percent). In other words, the blood volume can never be fully replenished until the salt is replaced. The symptoms of severe heat exhaustion resemble those of shock and in rare cases may be lethal. Sweating is profuse (Figure 4.3), the pulse is rapid and weak, blood pressure is low, there is malaise, along with weakness, dizziness, headache, nausea, and blurred vision. The body temperature may be normal, subnormal, or slightly elevated but

Heat and Dehydration

usually does not rise above 104 degrees Fahrenheit (40 degrees Celsius). The treatment requires rest, rehydration with salt and water, and cooling the body with cold packs along the neck, under the armpits, around the groin, and over the chest—anything to cool the affected individual off. Fanning him or her will help to evaporate any sweat, already present—and remember, *it is evaporation that cools the body, not sweating per se.*

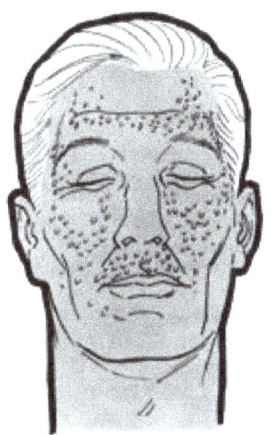

Figure 4.3 Heat exhaustion.   Figure 4.4 Heat stroke.

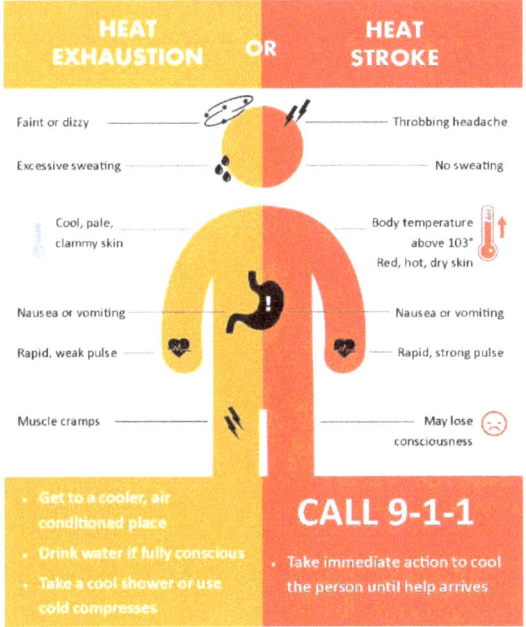

Figure 4.5 Heat exhaustion vs. heat stroke. Figure from the U.S. National Weather Service.

Whereas heat exhaustion is the end result of a normally functioning temperature-regulating system, *heatstroke* occurs when this system fails. Heatstroke is medically classified into two main types: *classic* and *exertional*. Classic heatstroke typically occurs among elderly persons who have difficulty dealing with heat stress. They are often chronically ill, often live alone, and may have limited means to cool off. Children are also at risk because they also have more difficulty dealing with heat stress—the well-known example is the infant confined in a closed car on a hot summer day. In classic heat stroke, the skin is typically dry and there may be a total absence of sweating (Figure 4.4). Exertional heatstroke is also a medical emergency that strikes sailors, athletes, and laborers in the heat. It can occur in the first hour and may occur out of the blue in sailors who have been in similar conditions uneventfully. The sailor's skin may be either sweaty (Figure 4.3) or red, hot, and bone dry (Figure 4.4). Either way, the temperature rises to above 104 degrees Fahrenheit (40 degrees Celsius) or higher. Periods of delirium (as described in the excerpt at the beginning of this chapter) are quite common, as are convulsive seizures and eventually coma.

Although heatstroke may occur with dramatic suddenness (hence the term *stroke*), it is often preceded by numerous warning signs, such as faintness, headache, staggering, and brief episodes of mental confusion. A few sailors have noticed that their sweating capacity has declined in the days prior to heatstroke. Unfortunately, this important warning is often overlooked. It is vital to recognize the early warning signs of heatstroke because the mortality rate is as high as 50 percent! Even if the individual survives, they may sustain permanent damage to the brain, heart, kidneys, or liver.

The cause of heatstroke is still unknown. Commonly, it has been attributed to "sweat-gland fatigue," but since sweating may continue until it fails—all at once over the entire body—this seems unlikely.

Although the cause is unknown, some factors seem to predispose its development, including poor overall health, increasing age, obesity, lack of acclimatization, peer and coach pressure with "killer workouts," extensive prickly heat or other skin diseases, alcohol, and finally, drugs that inhibit sweating (Appendix B). Previous, even mild, episodes of heatstroke may also be a predisposing factor (Figure 4.5).

> The treatment of heatstroke consists of reducing the body temperature as rapidly as possible. Heatstroke is a systemic disorder. As it progresses, it produces an inflammatory response as well as coagulation throughout the body and shock—ultimately leading to multi-organ failure.[5]

Upon exhibiting symptoms of heatstroke, the sailor should be undressed and placed in a tub of ice water. If that is not feasible, the sailor should be covered with ice packs or sponged with cold water until his or her temperature drops. The skin should be massaged vigorously at this time to prevent constriction of the blood vessels of the skin (due to the cold water) and to stimulate the return of cool blood to the body core. After the body temperature has dropped, the victim should be placed in a cold room or the coolest place on the boat. If the body temperature starts to rise again, it will be necessary to repeat the cooling procedure. The sailor should be kept in bed for several days after an episode of heatstroke and should avoid heat exposure for some time. If transfer to a hospital is possible, then evacuate, but still perform the above actions while waiting to transfer the victim.

Heat and the Hypertensive Sailor

Any sailor who has a diagnosis of hypertension (high blood pressure) must exercise particular caution in the heat. Most hypertensive individuals are kept on a low-sodium diet, which, of course, restricts salt intake. This produces a dilemma. If the sailor reduces salt intake, he or she will become more susceptible to the heat-induced disorders described above. Yet if the sailor increases salt intake to compensate for his or her losses, the sailor may aggravate the hypertension. There is no simple solution. The sailor may circumvent the problem, however, if he or she pays special attention to the rate of sweating and attempts to replace only his or her salt losses. The sailor cannot be quite as liberal in his or her salt replacement as can a nonhypertensive mate.

The hypertensive sailor may have to face an additional dilemma. If the sailor is being treated with a diuretic, or "fluid pill" (the medication of choice for certain types of hypertension), his or her tolerance to heat is even less, since the sailor is already slightly dehydrated even before beginning to sweat. Some physicians try to compensate by prescribing a slightly lower dose of diuretic for those patients who will be exposed to intense heat. However, this is hardly a satisfactory solution to the problem.

Thermoregulation and Athletic Performance

Let us turn our attention to the sailing athlete. When the first edition of this book was published in 1983, there was very little information about the physiology of the sailing athlete. Things have definitely improved, but there are tremendous inherent problems in understanding this subject, including the following:

- It is extremely difficult to perform science in a nautical environment.
- Scientists attempt to limit the number of variables—a difficult proposition on the water. The thermal load for sailing athletes depends upon wind currents, solar radiation, humidity, ambient temperature, and water temperatures—all of which vary during training and races. Even the course has an effect—the heat stress may be very different when sailing into the wind versus running before the wind.
- Unlike most other sports, there is a tremendous variability in the type of activities that must be performed.[6] A Laser sailor has a very different set of physiological

needs and heat responses when compared with a sailboarder, or an America's Cup crew.

One point upon which all of the recent studies agree is that increases in heat stress produce increases in core body temperature, and that an increase in core body temperature is associated with a decrease in the performance of sailing athletes. That is, *there is an inverse relationship between core body temperature and performance on the water.* A recent study also demonstrated large interindividual differences observed across athletes. That is, some elite sailors were better able to handle the thermoregulatory burden during exercise in the heat than were others.[7]

As we saw earlier in this chapter, there are four mechanisms by which the body can regulate temperature:

- Radiation
- Convection
- Conduction
- Evaporation

If the outside temperature and humidity are high, then radiation, convection, and conduction are ineffective; all that remains is sweating and evaporation. For athletes who are focused on performance, the signs of dehydration may not be recognized since many of the signs of dehydration mimic exercise fatigue.

So, how does hydration affect performance? There are two ways. First, as the sailor becomes increasingly dehydrated, there is a decrease in the volume of blood that can be sent to the brain and muscles (both of which require high levels of oxygen and glucose to function properly). Second, as one loses water (fluid), the blood becomes more viscous, making it more difficult for the heart to pump blood throughout the body. On any given day, a 70-kilogram (154-pound) person will lose about 2 liters of water each day, mainly through urine and also through the lungs. How long does it take to become mildly dehydrated in the summer heat? Hiking on land at moderate intensity for one hour can cause one to be 1.5-2 percent dehydrated. *The general rule is that losing approximately 2 percent of body weight fluids produces a 4 percent decrement in performance—in both muscular strength (anaerobic) and endurance (aerobic) events.* Racing in hot, humid, and windy conditions can result in an 80-kilogram (180-pound) sailor losing approximately 4 pounds of fluid body weight. This results in an approximate 4 percent performance decrease.[8]

Recall the concept of voluntary dehydration discussed earlier. That is, despite losing the significant amount of water while sweating, we tend to *underestimate* the degree of dehydration, so thirst does not kick in until the sailor is well on the way to becoming dehydrated.

How much water does a sailor need? In moderate conditions, at least 750 milliliters (25 fluid ounces) per hour is a good starting point. But remember, it is not just one's muscles that determine performance, but also a fully functioning brain. In a study from the Yale School of Medicine, dehydrating young healthy adults by about 1 percent of their body weight produced a measurable decline in their executive function—improving back to normal once they were rehydrated. This study found that dehydration resulted in a 10 to 12 percent increase on errors during complicated tests and tests of attention (reaction time did not decline). A 10 percent error rate could certainly be the difference between winning and losing a race.[9]

Preventing Dehydration

The best way to prevent dehydration is to consume plenty of fluids before, during, and after a workout or competition. *Weighing before and after practice is extremely helpful.* For every kilogram (2 pound) loss during exercise, the sailor needs to drink approximately 1.5 liters (32 ounces) of fluid. In addition to weighing, the sailor needs to *check the color of his or her urine*. A normally hydrated athlete produces a clear or mildly yellow-colored urine (Figure 4.6). As the sailor becomes increasingly dehydrated, the urine becomes a deeper yellow and eventually transitions to brown.

The American College of Sports Medicine has addressed the issue of hydration and physical activity.[10] The organization provides general guidance that every sailing athlete should be aware of. The goal is to avoid dehydration of more than 2 percent of body weight, the point at which performance decline is noticeable. Since every sailor's physiology is different, the best course is to develop an individualized program using pre- and postexercise weight and urine amount and color to *personalize* replacement requirements. See also Appendix C.

Prehydrate Before Exercise

(1) The goal of pre-hydrating is to start the activity euhydrated (i.e., normally hydrated) and with normal electrolytes.
(2) Prehydrating should be initiated several hours before the exercise/event. If recovery has been eight to twelve hours, then slowly drink beverages four hours before the event—at 5 to 7 milliliters per kilogram (1 kilogram = 2.2 pounds and 70 kilograms = 154 pounds). If the individual either doesn't produce any urine after two hours or if the urine color is dark or highly concentrated, then at two hours before the event, drink another three to five milliliters per kilogram. Consuming salty snacks will help to stimulate and retain the fluid.

The average, moderately active individual requires 2 to 2.5 liters of fluid per *day*. An active America's Cup sailor in a tacking duel may require up to 2 liters per *hour*, or 10 to 15 liters per day.[11]

The Human Performance Resource Center—an educational arm of the Consortium for Health and Military Performance at the Uniformed Services University of the Health Sciences—has a number of recommendations for hydration.[12]

Healthy Boating & Sailing

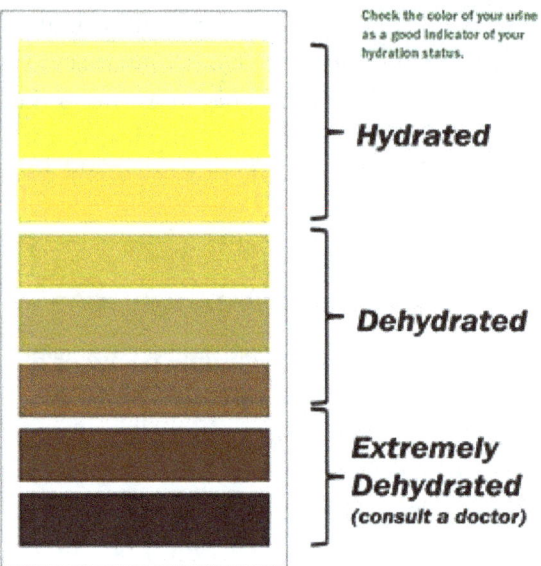

Figure 4.6 Urine color as a rough measure of dehydration. Figure from United States Marine Corp.

Rehydrate During Exercise

For exercise lasting up to one hour:
Drink water—about 3 to 8-ounces of water every fifteen to twenty minutes. (A gulp is about 1 to 2 ounces.)

For exercise lasting longer than one hour:
Drink 3 to 8-ounces of water + carbs + electrolytes—basically, a good sports drink—every fifteen to twenty minutes.

A sports drink should contain (per 8 ounces):

- Carbohydrates: 12 to 24 grams
- Sodium: 82–163 milligrams
- Potassium: 18–46 milligrams

In general, limit fluid intake during exercise to about one quart per hour, or as much as 1.5 quart per hour in hot weather. However, when you're active in extreme environments such as heat, humidity, cold, or altitude, your fluid needs might be much higher. But in any environment, do not exceed 1.5 quarts per hour, or 12 quarts per day, during work in the heat.

Rehydrate After Exercise

Rehydrate with fluids and foods. For every pound of body weight lost, consume 16 to 24 ounces by drinking fluids and eating high-water-content foods throughout the day. These include:

- Fluids—water, sports drinks, 100 percent fruit juice (diluted), milk, and milk alternatives (soy, almond)
- Foods—fruit (watermelon, grapes, peaches, etc.), high-water-content vegetables (zucchini, celery, cucumbers, tomatoes, etc.), soup, yogurt, and sherbet/sorbet

Replenish sodium by consuming beverages or foods that contain salt. Drinking too much plain water and/or not consuming enough sodium can result in *hyponatremia* (low sodium levels in your blood), which can be very serious if not treated. Be aware of the signs and symptoms: headache, vomiting, swollen hands and feet, confusion, and wheezy breathing.

For a quick method to calculate your "sweating rate," see Appendix C. Yes, fluid and electrolyte balance does require mathematics. (That may be the reason I went into neurology rather than nephrology.)

Is there anything that can be done to improve acclimatization? Yes.[13]

- Practice once a day for the first five days when in an unfamiliar climate
- Avoid working out more than three hours a day
- Dress with lightweight clothing for the first five to six days
- Follow days of multiple practices with a rest day or single practice day
- Increase the intensity of practice slowly over the first few days
- Increase sodium in the diet for the first few days
- Have cool-off periods and plenty of breaks throughout the first few days

Survival

An altogether different problem confronts the sailor who is forced to abandon ship—a restricted supply of water. In one sense, there is never a shortage of water in a marine environment—only a shortage of *potable* water. The high salt content, or salinity, of seawater generally prohibits its consumption.

The salinity of seawater varies little around the globe. It ranges from a 3.5 to 3.7 percent solution, except in the Mediterranean Sea and the Red Sea where it is slightly higher (3.7 to 4.1 percent). This 3.5 percent solution consists of primarily sodium chloride (2.8 to 3.0 percent), as well as smaller amounts of such salts as calcium chloride, magnesium chloride, magnesium sulfate, and potassium chloride.

Animals have established an accommodation with nature and are able to extract water from the "hostile" environment. Most species of saltwater fish simply excrete excess salt through their gills directly back into the ocean. Oceanic birds such as the cormorant, pelican, and albatross are able to tolerate drinking seawater by excreting most of the ingested salt through specially developed salt glands (nasal glands). Since this salt solution is more concentrated than seawater, the birds end up with a net gain in water.

Whales, dolphins, and seals have adopted a different strategy altogether. These animals obtain virtually all of their water from the metabolism of food, particularly fat. There is no evidence that they can tolerate seawater any better than we can. Other animals, especially some desert-dwelling mammals that are in constant need of water, possess kidneys of great concentrating power. The kangaroo rat, for example, excretes a urine that is four times as concentrated as ours. This animal can thrive on a diet of seawater.[14]

How much water is necessary for a human to survive? Obviously, the requirements vary with the climatic conditions and the amount of work that must be done. With no water whatsoever, the following survival times may be expected. They are rough approximations based on mean air temperature, which takes into account the lower nighttime temperature at sea:

- 98 degrees Fahrenheit (37 degrees Celsius)—two days
- 89.6 degrees Fahrenheit (32 degrees Celsius)—three days
- 78.8 degrees Fahrenheit (26 degrees Celsius)—four days
- 69.8 degrees Fahrenheit (21 degrees Celsius)—eight days
- 59.0 degrees Fahrenheit (15 degrees Celsius)—ten days

These figures are applicable to a sailor who does not have to perform an appreciable amount of work. Hard work requires more water. According to previous dogma, 1 pint (0.5 liter) per day was required to sustain a sailor for longer periods of time. However, recent survival accounts indicate that this figure can probably be revised downward to about 0.33 pint (0.16 liter) per day (see the discussion of the Robertsons and the Baileys later in this chapter).

Many sources of water are available to the shipwreck survivor. These can be divided into *freshwater* sources (which are preferred) and *other* sources. There are five sources of fresh water: (1) water rations stored in or brought aboard the survival craft, (2) rainwater, (3) water that has been chemically desalinated, (4) water produced in a solar distillation unit (or "solar still"), and (5) water produced by "reverse osmosis"—a so-called watermaker.

Solar stills have been a method of desalination used at sea since Elizabethan times. Sir Richard Hawkins in his *Observations on a Voyage to the South Seas* reported:

Although our fresh water had fayled us many days before we saw the shore, by reason of our long navigation and the excessive drinking of the sicke and the diseased, yet with an invention I had in my shippe, I easily drew out of the water of the sea sufficient quantity of fresh water to sustain my people, with little expense of fewell

[fuel]; for with foure billets [of wood] I stilled a hogshead [more than 63 gallons] of water and therewith dressed the meat for the sicke and whole. The water so distilled we found wholesome and nourishing.[15]

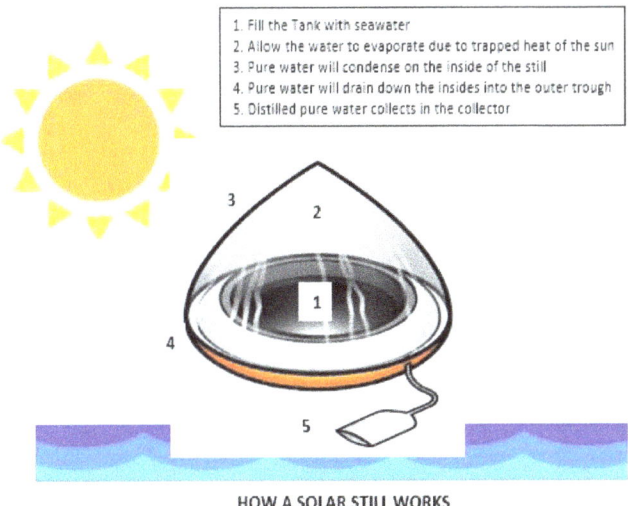

Figure 4.7 Solar still. Figure from How Stuff Works.

Unfortunately, solar stills (Figure 4.7) are a bit tricky to use and are limited in output to about 1 quart (1 liter) per day (depending on the latitude). Steven Callahan, in his wonderful book *Adrift: 76 Days Lost at Sea*,[16] documents in great detail just how finicky and undependable a small portable solar still can be, especially when used in the open ocean. He spent countless hours repairing and fidgeting with his solar stills (he had two) and still depended upon collecting rainwater and utilizing other sources. He was also assisted by the survival experiences of the Robertsons and Baileys, discussed below.

Chemical desalination is possible but is limited to the number of packets contained in the "desalting" kit. One of the most popular is the U.S. Military Emergency Desalting kit, which has been in use since World War II and is still standard equipment on many U.S. Navy and Air Force planes as well as private aircraft. One compact kit contains eight packets of desalting chemicals, which yields more than 7 pints of drinkable water. The kit will produce treated water with reduced sulfates and chlorides, and although it is not "fresh" water, it is acceptable emergency drinking water.

To be certain of a continuous supply of fresh water, every offshore sailor should purchase a manual (hand pump) desalinator—or "watermaker," such as the Katadyn Survivor 06 or Survivor 35 Desalinator (Figure 4.8). They are hand-pumped, reverse osmosis desalinator units. The "06" will produce 890 milliliters (30 ounces) of drinking water per hour and it only weighs 2.5 pounds. They work by forcing seawater through a semipermeable membrane that allows water molecules through the membrane but not salt, particulate matter, bacteria, or viruses. What emerges is fresh, clean, drinking water. Many boaters may be aware of larger units such as those sold under the brand name Rainman (Figure 4.8), which are powered by a small generator. And of course, larger vessels will have installed desalination units. The hand-pump unit is appropriate for a life raft.

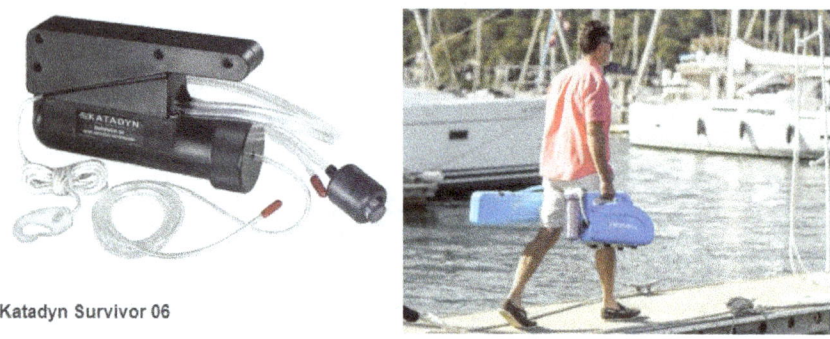

Katadyn Survivor 06

Figure 4.8 The Katadyn Survivor 06 is a basic hand-pumped desalinator. The Rainman unit to the right is a portable electric desalinator requiring a generator or inverter.

Water can be coaxed from other sources in the environment, including the tissues of marine creatures such as fish, sea turtles, and marine birds. Two splendid discussions of these sources are *Survive the Savage Sea* by Dougal Robertson and *Staying Alive* by Maurice and Maralyn Bailey.[17] Since the Robertsons were in worse shape with regard to water stores, let us examine their story.

Robertson, his wife (a nurse), and four children were shipwrecked when killer whales attacked their schooner west of the Galapagos Islands on June 15, 1972. The boat sank in 60 seconds, leaving little time for coordinated preparation. They survived and were subsequently rescued from their dinghy 38 days later, although it seems likely that they would soon have made a landing on the coast of Costa Rica. Their survival (and that of the Baileys, who survived 117 days in virtually the same region of the Pacific) is a testament to humans' ability to wrest sustenance, especially water, from the sea. The Robertsons were equipped with emergency rations of food and water for only three days and lived almost entirely on rainwater and marine life.

Rainwater was their most highly prized commodity, and with Robertson's ingenuity, they were able to use almost all of it. Because of the improvisational nature of their rain-catching system, the initial part of the collection, although technically potable, was not palatable. This portion was separated from the rest and given via a plastic tube as a water-retention enema. Up to 1 pint (0.5 liter) of water can be readily absorbed in this fashion. As Robertson's wife pointed out, this technique is only effective for unpalatable fresh water, not seawater. Seawater given via retention enema causes just as much havoc as it would if taken orally.[18]

Sea turtles and fish were the mainstays of the Robertson's existence. Each 75-pound (34-kilogram) turtle yields 3 to 4 pints (1.5 to 2 liters) of blood. The blood coagulates in about a minute, so it must be drunk immediately. The cerebrospinal fluid from the spinal cavity and the eyeball fluid, although limited in quantity, are even purer sources of water (lower salinity). These fluids can be obtained from turtles, fish, and even marine birds! Both the Robertsons and the Baileys utilized them. Curiously, neither of these books mention extracting "fish juice" (see the discussion later in this chapter).

The metabolism of food also produces water. As discussed earlier in this chapter, either fat or carbohydrate is superior to protein. According to classical teaching, it is best to avoid protein when less than 2 pints (1 liter) of water is available, although Robertson suggests that small amounts of protein can be eaten with somewhat less water than this. Nevertheless, if there is a choice, fat or carbohydrate is preferable. In maintaining fluid balance, it is equally important to reduce the losses. The output of urine is already reduced to a minimum, and nothing further can be done. Some water continues to be lost via evaporation from the lungs, but it is relatively insignificant. What is significant is sweating. The sailor should take every opportunity during the day to keep his body as cool as possible. Keeping out of the sun is most important. Robertson states, "The double canopy alone was worth a gallon [4 liters] of water a day to us in keeping out the heat of the sun."[19] Strenuous work should be done at night if possible. The Baileys, during the early days of their ordeal, decided to try to row to safety. They realized that this could only be done at night. Brief baths in the ocean are possible, but the sailor must be careful to avoid the twin dangers of sharks and separation from the craft. Cool water compresses and wrapping portions of the body with cool, wet cloths can be tried. The sailor should avoid overdoing it, however, since constant contact of the skin with seawater tends to produce boils, which are quite painful. Continuous immersion eventually causes the skin to break down. Once this happens, the sailor is in serious trouble, since water losses increase tremendously in the presence of denuded skin.

Finally, it should be noted that the Robertsons survived for seven days on as little as 0.33 pint (0.16 liter) of water per day and, except for brief respites, the remainder of their ordeal with 1 pint (0.5 liter) or less per day! This experience, and others like it, should be kept in mind when considering the seawater controversy.[20]

The "controversy" over whether or not the castaway should ever drink seawater seems finally to be over. What probably kept it alive is the supreme irony of suffering and dying from thirst while surrounded by water. There is now virtually unanimous international medical opinion regarding this topic. The British Department of Trade clearly summarizes this position:

> Seafarers are reminded that if cast away they should never under any circumstances drink sea water which has not been through a distillation plant or desalinated by chemical means. A belief has arisen that it is possible to replace or supplement fresh water rations by drinking sea water in small amounts. This belief is wrong and dangerous.

Drinking untreated sea water does a thirsty man no good at all. It will lead to increased dehydration and thirst and may kill him.

Even if there is no fresh water at all it should be remembered that men have lived for many days with nothing to drink, and therefore the temptation to drink untreated sea water must be strongly resisted.[21]

Dr. Alain Bombard, a feisty French physician, took the contrarian view. In 1952, Bombard, recently out of medical school, decided to prove that man could live entirely on the sustenance the sea provided and so became a "voluntary castaway." He spent sixty-five days at sea in an inflatable life raft traveling from Las Palmas in the Canary Islands to Barbados without relying very much on supplies of food or water (this has long been a matter of some dispute). He stated that his only water for the first twenty-four days at sea consisted of seawater and fish juice. After this period, squalls were frequent enough to provide a reserve of fresh water. He publicized his findings and became famous in France, but his position was later scorned by the French medical and maritime communities. His position about the use of small amounts of diluted seawater early in the survival is currently untenable.[22] So let's be clear—DO NOT DRINK SEAWATER.

In order to appreciate the risk of drinking seawater, let us first examine a situation in which the use of seawater is indisputably contraindicated—the case of the severely dehydrated survivor.

The normal salinity of most human and animal body fluids is about 0.9 percent. Any fluid that has this concentration of dissolved salts is referred to as *isotonic*. Seawater (3.5 percent) has almost four times as much dissolved salt and so is *hypertonic*. A liquid that is less concentrated than 0.9 percent is *hypotonic*. Pure fresh water is as hypotonic as you can get.

In every instance, the dehydrated sailor, although deficient in both salt and water, will be much more deficient in water. This causes the concentration of salt in the body to be higher than normal—a condition known as *hypernatremia*. What if the sailor now drinks seawater? Under the best of circumstances, the kidneys are able to excrete a urine almost as concentrated as seawater. However, salt accounts for only a little more than half of the dissolved substances in the urine, approximately a 1.5 percent solution. The other half is practically all urea, the main end product of protein metabolism. Thus, if the sailor drinks a 3.5 percent solution and is able to excrete only a 1.5 percent solution, he or she will end up with a net loss of water. In addition, if the urine is to remain maximally concentrated, the kidneys can only deal with small amounts of dissolved substances. If the kidneys have to get rid of large amounts of dissolved substances —either salt after the drinking of seawater or urea after a large protein meal—they are no longer capable of producing a maximally concentrated urine. In other words, the more salt the kidneys have to excrete, the lower the concentration and the greater the net loss of water.

The increasing salt concentration in the body (hypernatremia) has drastic consequences including delirium, hallucinations, epileptic convulsions, coma, and death.

Many of the crew drank sea water; although I threatened to stop their fresh water if they continued to do so, many of the men continued to drink it at night; I could always tell when a man had been drinking saltwater because the guilty ones suffered from hallucinations. During the tenth day the second cook became insane probably through drinking of sea water.[23]

What about drinking straight seawater soon after shipwreck, perhaps two to three mouthfuls every three hours? This is also a bad idea. Since the sailor is not yet deficient in either salt or water, all of the salt will have to be excreted, thereby increasing again the rate of dehydration. If the only other option is drinking straight seawater, the sailor is better off having nothing.

If the survivor has some fresh water, should he or she attempt to extend it by mixing it with seawater? No. We must keep in mind the distinction between what the body can tolerate and what is beneficial. There is no question that the body can tolerate dilute salt solutions—the more dilute or hypotonic the better. If we dilute seawater in a ratio of two to one, the concentration is reduced to about 1.2 percent, below the kidneys' maximum of about 1.5 percent. But we must remember the kidneys excrete 1.5 percent only if there is not too much salt to contend with. A three-to-one dilution produces an isotonic (0.9 percent) solution. However, since the average concentration of sweat is only 0.2 to 0.3 percent, in order to replace his or her losses with seawater, the sailor should ideally dilute it at about ten to one.

One problem is obvious. The more the sailor dilutes the seawater, the less he or she is going to extend freshwater supplies. It's just not worth it. But there is another, more dangerous problem which is establishing a precedent of drinking seawater in the first place. Robertson addresses just this point:

Since the castaway has to adopt some personal attitude to this argument perhaps our experience can be of some assistance to him in arriving at a decision. All evidence, from both sides of the argument, points to the fact that if the body of the survivor is at all dehydrated, sea water can not only cause damage to internal organs and sickness, but it will intensify the dehydrated condition. Most advocates of the sea-water theory qualify their advocacy by stating that it can only be usefully assimilated by a body that doesn't really need it. During periods of severe thirst when we were on raft and dinghy, Lyn [his wife] and Douglas [a son] both admitted to an almost overwhelming desire to drink sea water, both by day and night. Only their own moral fiber prevented them from doing so, but how much would that moral fiber have been weakened if they had drunk some sea water in the initial stages after the disaster?[24]

Instead of posing the question, "Should I, or should I not, drink seawater?" (in case I was unclear, the answer is still NO), it would probably be better to rank according to potability all of the possible sources of water available (Table 4.2).

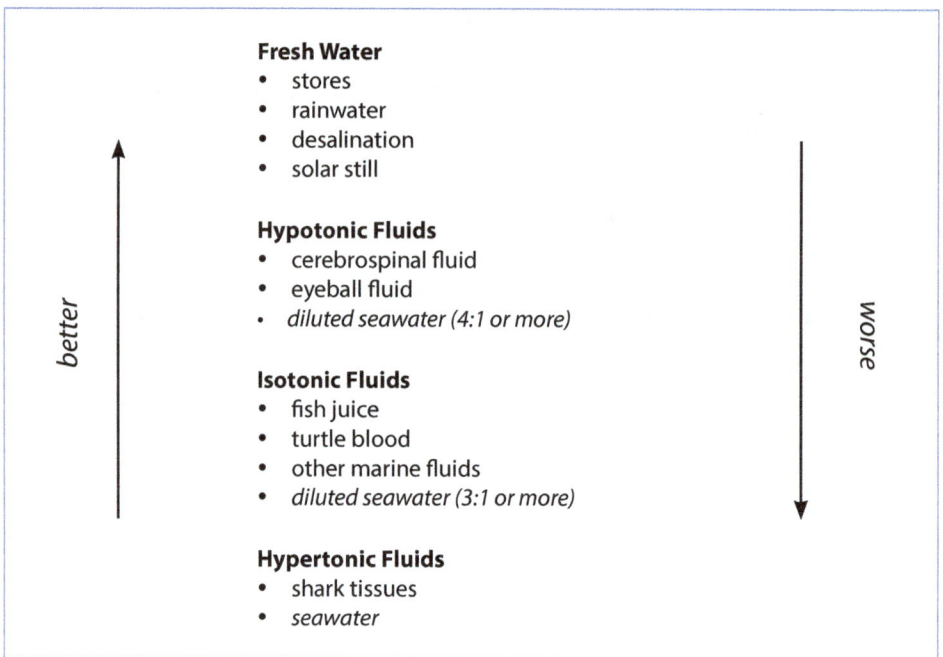

Table 4.2 Sources of water in a marine environment

The advantage of thinking about sources of water as in Table 4.2 is that it avoids classifying seawater as an absolute "poison" and prompts the castaway to think twice before discarding fresh water that has been adulterated with it. The Baileys apparently made this error when on their second day they discovered that 4 gallons (16 liters), or 40 percent, of their water supply had been contaminated with seawater. Since the water containers were presumably almost full at the time, it is likely that the adulterated water would still have been quite useful.

How can one estimate the salinity? The only rule of thumb is that if a fluid tastes salty, its concentration is probably 0.9 percent or greater. This is about the threshold for the appreciation of salt. But as the sailor becomes dehydrated and his or her salt concentration rises, the sailor's threshold also rises. This phenomenon explains why blood tastes a bit salty to people under normal conditions but not at all to the dehydrated sailor! Although there is some variation from species to species, the fluids and tissues of most marine animals are approximately isotonic. Fish juice (the fluid drained or squeezed from the body of a freshly caught fish) and sea turtle blood are good examples of isotonic marine fluids that can be utilized. Surgeon Captain J. D. Walters states that some species of turtles have hypotonic blood.[25] So much the better: hypotonic fluids are clearly superior. The cerebrospinal fluid of fish and turtles is hypotonic, as is a human's. The same applies to eyeball fluid. Although both of these sources are small, in survival situations, all sources become important.

One animal should be avoided unless there is plenty of water available—the shark. Both the Robertsons and the Baileys caught small sharks. The sharks (and related species) are unique in that they have a tissue concentration that is the same as seawater! They achieve their 3.5 percent concentration not with salt but with urea, which is present in enormous quantities. Because our kidneys must excrete urea directly, consuming fluid from shark tissue tends to produce dehydration just as much as seawater.

Notes

1. E. C. B. Lee and K. Lee, *Safety and Survival at Sea* (New York: W. W. Norton, 1980), 90

2. C. Blagden, "Further Experiments and Observations in a Heated Room," *Philosophical Transactions of the Royal Society A* 65 (1775): 484-494.

3. Some individuals find it difficult to tolerate salt tablets because of nausea. On the other hand, they are life changing for patients with chronically low sodium and patients with postural orthostatic tachycardia syndrome. It remains a simple, inexpensive way of increasing salt in people who cannot tolerate excessively salty foods.

4. Sir Francis Chichester, *Gipsy Moth Circles the World* (London: Hodder & Stoughton, 1967), 46.

5. Y. Epstein and R. Yanovich, "Heat Stroke," *New England Journal of Medicine* 380 (2019): 2449-2459.

6. V. Neville, N. Gant, and J. P. Folland, "Thermoregulatory Demands of Elite Professional America's Cup Yacht Racing," *Scandinavian Journal of Medicine and Science in Sports* (2009), doi: 10.1111/j.1600-0838.2009.00952x. In a study of America's Cup yacht racing, the authors evaluated athletes exposed to hot and humid conditions for prolonged periods of time. The aim was to assess the thermoregulatory responses of elite professional racers according to crew position and upwind and downwind sailing. Environmental conditions were as follows: 32 degrees Celsius, 52 percent relative humidity, and 5 meters per second wind speed. The race intensity was moderate. The crew was divided into five groups including bowmen, grinders, utilities (these three groups were considered highly physically demanding roles), and after guard, such as helmsman, navigator, tactician, and trimmers (these were considered moderately demanding roles). For a number of reasons, bowmen had the highest thermal stress. The mean sweat loss during racing was 1.34 +/- 0.58 liters per hour. The mean fluid intake was highly correlated to sweat loss, with a significant loss of sodium chloride.

7. M. van Delden et al., "Thermoregulatory Burden of Elite Sailing Athletes during Exercise in the Heat: A Pilot Study," *Temperature*, doi: 10.1080/23328940.2018.1540964.

8. J. Norton, "Understanding the Importance of Hydration," August 21, 2017, https:/internationalsailing-academy.com/author/justin/.

9. Allison Aubrey, "Off Your Mental Game? You Could Be Mildly Dehydrated," National Public Radio, July 30, 2018.

10. D. J. Casa, P. M. Clarkson, and W. O. Roberts, "American College of Sports Medicine Roundtable on Hydration and Physical Activity: Consensus Statements," *Current Sports Medicine Reports* 4 (2005): 115-127; M. N. Sawka, "Exercise and Fluid Replacement—Special

Communication Position Stand," *Official Journal of the American College of Sports Medicine*, http://www.acsm-msse.org.

11. Jennifer Langille, "Dehydration May Be the Cause of Poor Sailing Performance," FloTrack, December 10, 2008, https://www.flotrack.org/articles/5017002-dehydration-may-be-the-cause-of-poor-sailing-performance.

12. "Hydration Basics," *Human Performance Resources*, accessed January 21, 2019, https://www.hprc-online.org/articles/hydration-basics.

13. Administrator, "How Thermoregulation Can Give Athletes An Edge (Mission Athletecare)," *Korey Stringer Institute*, May 17, 2015.

14. The different lifestyles that have evolved in response to the ever-present need to preserve salt and water are beyond the scope of this chapter. Refer to the works of Homer W. Smith for more details on this topic, in particular the classic *From Fish to Philosopher* (Garden City, NY: Anchor, 1961).

15. L. H. Roddis, *A Short History of Nautical Medicine* (New York: Hoeber, 1941), 106.

16. Steven Callahan, *Adrift* (New York: Houghton Mifflin, 1986). This is my favorite of the recent nautical survival books. The Robertsons' *Survive the Savage Sea* (New York: Praeger, 1973) and the Baileys' *Staying Alive* (New York: McKay, 1974) are also wonderful. A more recent volume by William Butler entitled *66 Days Adrift* (Camden, ME: International Marine, 2005) is also well worth reading. In particular, the Butlers experience contrasts with all of the others since William Butler was able to salvage his "watermaker" at the very last minute as his ship was sinking, so they had a relatively continuous supply of fresh water throughout their ordeal. That alone should endorse the requirement that every life raft be equipped with a manual desalinator when open ocean sailing.

17. Robertson, *Survive the Savage Sea*, and Bailey and Bailey, *Staying Alive*.

18. Some authorities have misrepresented the Robertsons' position, suggesting that they advocated using seawater. This is puzzling, since in both *Survive the Savage Sea* and *Sea Survival* (New York: Praeger, 1975), a second book by Robertson, it is clearly stated that seawater should not be given in this manner!

19. Robertson, *Survive the Savage Sea*, 52-53. See also Callahan's *Adrift*.

20. Bernard Robin has collected thirty-one shipwreck stories in a fascinating book entitled *Survival at Sea* (Camden, ME: International Marine Publishing, 1981). The second part of the book is devoted to an analysis of a number of aspects of survival.

21. British Department of Trade, "Drinking of Seawater by Castaways," Merchant Shipping Notice no. M.729 (August 1975).

22. Frank Golden and Michael Tipton, *Essentials of Sea Survival* (Champaign, IL: Human Kinetics, 2002), 150-154.

23. Lee and Lee, *Safety and Survival*, 152.

24. Robertson, *Survive the Savage Sea*, 244.

25. Surgeon Captain Walters, as quoted in Bailey and Bailey, *Staying Alive*, 187-191.

Chapter 5

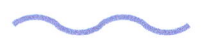

Sailor's Skin

> "Mad dogs and Englishmen go out in
> the midday sun:
> The Japanese don't care to, the
> Chinese wouldn't dare to;
> Hindus and Argentines sleep firmly
> From twelve to one."
>
> —*Noel Coward*, Mad Dogs and Englishmen

In my lifetime a quiet revolution has occurred that has radically altered our attitude toward the sun and its effect on our skin. Unabashed sun worship, only to achieve the darkest suntan in the shortest time, has given way to an increasing awareness of the long-term consequences of sun exposure with the major risks being—premature skin aging and an increased risk of skin cancer. Nowhere is this revolution more visible than in the cosmetics industry's marketing of sun lotions. Whereas the emphasis in the past (during my youth, for example) was on quick tanning (which we will see is not possible anyway), manufacturers now advertise their products' protective value as sunscreens.

This raised level of consciousness comes none too soon for boaters, who have always been at risk of sustaining solar (actinic) skin damage. In fact, the high prevalence of actinic damage among sailors prompted the use of the term *sailor's skin* to describe the typical dry, wrinkled, inelastic, leathery skin of those who have spent years out in the midday sun. Unfortunately, these skin changes are irreversible, so prevention is absolutely essential.

Ultraviolet Radiation

The sun continually emits a broad spectrum of radiation, ranging from gamma rays to radio-frequency waves. Fortunately for humans, only a tiny portion of this spectrum, *ultraviolet (UV) radiation*, is injurious (Figure 5.1).[1]

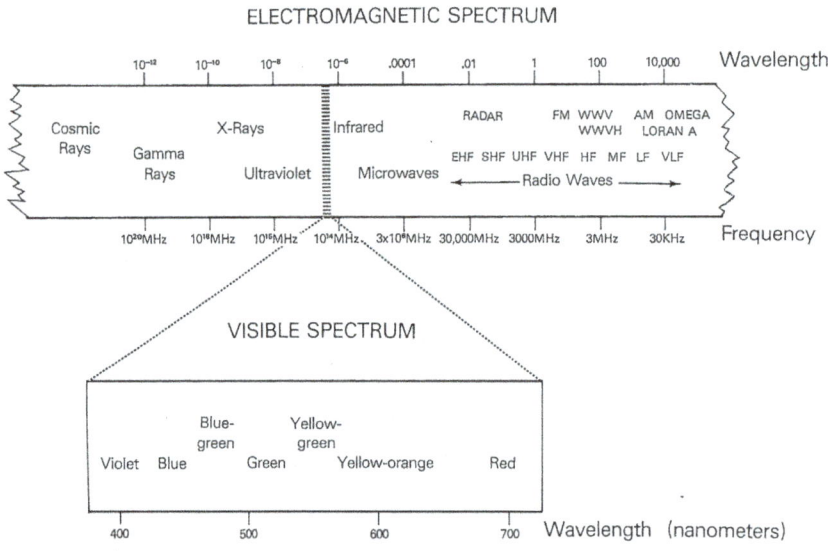

Figure 5.1 The electromagnetic spectrum

The longer wavelengths, such as the visible and infrared, produce light and heat but have no adverse effect on the skin. The atmosphere, with its protective layer of ozone, filters out the shorter gamma rays, X-rays, and some of the UV rays—all exceedingly dangerous to humans.

For convenience, UV radiation has been divided into three bands: UVC (200 to 290 nanometers), UVB (290 to 320 nanometers), and UVA (320 to 400 nanometers). UVC, although potentially dangerous, is of no concern to us since it is completely absorbed by the ozone layer and is not detectable at sea level. UVB and UVA do penetrate the atmosphere to varying degrees and are responsible for both sunburns and suntans, as well as actinic damage and skin cancer.

The effect of UV on the sailor's skin depends on two factors: (1) the cumulative dose of UV and (2) the individual's skin type (see Table 5.1).

UV Exposure

First, let us look at what determines the amount of UV that actually reaches the boater. This information is important, for the sailor must anticipate when he or she is likely to be exposed to significant UV. Only then can the sailor take steps to protect him- or herself. Once the skin is sunburned it is too late, because he or she has already sustained radiation damage. If the immediate sunburn was the only concern, there would be no need for alarm. A sunburn, after all, heals. However, both actinic damage and skin cancer result from the cumulative dosage of UV radiation *over a lifetime*. Every episode of exposure to the sun has, in a sense, left its radiational footprints in the sailor's epidermis.[2]

Unlike sunlight and infrared radiation, which can be seen and felt, UV radiation is entirely insensible. We can judge its presence only retrospectively by the degree of burn it leaves behind. Usually, UV traverses the atmosphere together with light and heat, which alert us to the danger. Sometimes, however, this warning system breaks down. Boaters are particularly vulnerable to a breakdown in the warning system since a moving boat generates a cooling breeze. It is easy in such circumstances to underestimate UV exposure. The warning system also breaks down on cloudy days when more UV penetrates the atmosphere than either light or heat.

How much UV penetrates to sea level depends primarily upon the particles present in the atmosphere. They filter out all radiation below 280 nanometers, including UVC, as well as much of the UVB and UVA. The degree of obliquity with which the UV strikes the atmosphere also determines the amount of UV penetration. The greater the obliquity, the longer the course; the longer the course, the greater the opportunity the UV has to be absorbed or scattered (Figure 5.2). The ozone layer, located in the stratosphere 9 to 22 miles (15 to 35 kilometers) above the surface of the earth, plays a vital supporting role in the absorption of UV.

The most dangerous period for UV exposure is midday between the hours of 10 a.m. and 2 p.m. standard time (or, more precisely, local time). During these four hours, approximately 66 percent of the daily UV radiation reaches the surface of the earth, and between 9 a.m. and 3 p.m., over 80 percent. During the midday hours, the sun is highest in the sky, and the UV rays travel a more direct, less oblique course through the atmosphere.

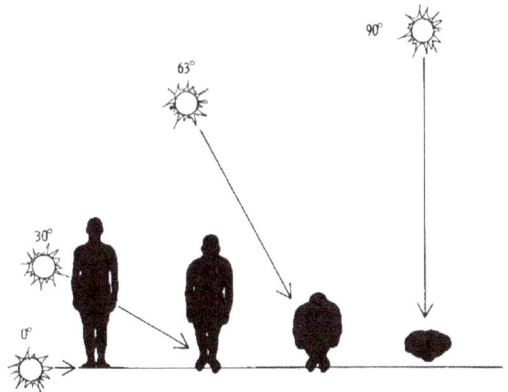

Figure 5.2 Direct versus oblique light

Increased UV radiation in the summer and in equatorial regions has a similar explanation. The summer sun is higher in the sky (more nearly overhead) than is the winter sun. In equatorial regions, the sun is more directly overhead at midday than it is at higher latitudes. In addition, the ozone layer is not distributed uniformly around the earth. It tends to be thinner at the equator than at the poles. This alone increases the UV load by about 15 percent.

Probably the most neglected source of UV is the sky. The sky appears blue because the shorter blue wavelengths of light are more scattered than are the longer red and green wavelengths. After bouncing around the atmosphere, the blue rays are eventually reflected back to earth. Similarly, much of the UV reaches the earth after being scattered throughout the sky. (This makes sense since UV is immediately adjacent to the blue portion of the electromagnetic spectrum.) This indirect "sky radiation" accounts for almost *50 percent of the total UV* that reaches the earth on a clear day. As a result, one can obtain a nasty sunburn even when standing in a shadow! The sailor invariably overlooks sky radiation, although it undoubtedly contributes to a sailor's above-average exposure. On the water, the expanse of open sky comprises a full 360 degrees—all of it radiating UV. The situation is obviously much different than in an urban setting where buildings and trees block out much of the sky radiation. In short, turning a back to the sun is not the answer.

The amount of UV radiated on a cloudy day is often underestimated as well. Because of its shorter wavelength, UV penetrates moderate cloud cover at a time when light and heat cannot. Up to 80 percent of UV transmission can occur with complete cloud cover. Under exceptional circumstances (high, towering clouds), the amount of UV may actually be greater—due to increased backscatter—than that radiated from a cloudless sky.

Contrary to popular belief, water is a poor reflector of UV. At midday, only about 5 to 10 percent is reflected from the surface. The percentage increases only slightly when the sun is lower in the sky. Although this benefits the sailor while sailing (otherwise the UV load would be even greater), when taking to the water to swim or snorkel, the sailor must consider that he or she will absorb UV while in the water. Such a situation can be extremely deceiving since the relative coolness of the water engenders a sense of security. When high UV radiation is anticipated, as in the Caribbean at midday, clothing and sunscreens are required while swimming or snorkeling. The sailor should be aware of thinly woven materials such as nylon, which may allow 25 percent or more UV transmission (see the ultraviolet protection factor clothing discussion later in this chapter). At higher altitudes, the thinner atmosphere absorbs less UV radiation.

Finally, the best available evidence indicates that high temperature, high humidity, and high wind velocity all augment UV damage. Extra precaution should be taken in these conditions.[3]

Sunburn

Sensitivity to UV varies considerably from individual to individual and depends on the amount of pigment, or melanin, in the superficial layers of the skin.[4] Melanin absorbs and scatters the UV, preventing its transmission to the deeper layers of the skin. In dark-complexioned individuals, melanin is present in the skin in large quantities even in the absence of sun exposure. In medium-complexioned individuals, little melanin is stored in the skin, but in response to UV, melanin is produced, a process referred to as tanning. In people with very fair skins, not only is there little or no melanin stored in the skin, but the ability to produce it is either poor or absent. About 15 percent of people are entirely incapable of developing a suntan. These people are the most sensitive to the adverse effects of solar radiation.

Type	Also Called	Sunburning	Tanning Behavior
I	Light, pale white	Always	Never
II	White, fair	Usually	Minimally
III	Medium, white to light brown	Sometimes	Uniformly
IV	Olive, moderately brown	Rarely	Easily
V	Brown, dark brown	Very Rarely	Very Easily
VI	Very dark brown to black	Never	Never

Table 5.1 Six categories of skin type (Fitzpatrick scale)[5]

Human skin has been divided into six basic types based on the amount of melanin normally stored in the skin and on the skin's ability to produce it (Table 5.1, Figure 5.3). The amount of melanin naturally found in the skin (natural skin color) as well as the capacity to produce melanin (ability to tan) are genetically inherited traits, and nothing can be done to alter them. This applies to both the rate and the end result. Quick tanning, therefore, is a myth, pure and simple. Tanning proceeds at its own pace for any given individual and depends primarily on the amount of UV received in a specific period of time.[6]

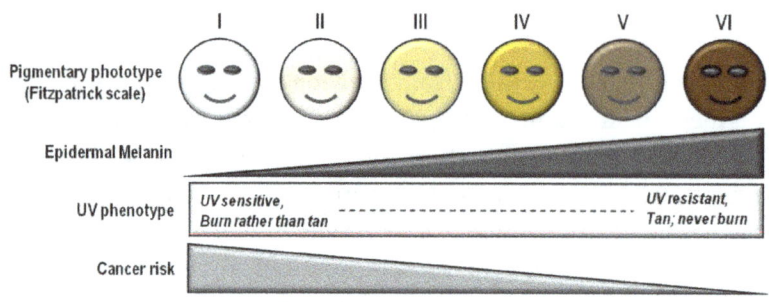

Figure 5.3 UV radiation and the skin[7]

The first evidence of UV exposure is a very faint redness, or erythema, of the skin that develops during the exposure and disappears almost immediately. Unfortunately, a latent period of two to four hours follows before the erythema appears, which we usually associate with sunburn. Because of this delay, the unwary boater may develop a severe burn before realizing that exposure has been excessive. This erythema reaches its peak at about twenty-four hours and begins to subside after seventy-two hours, although depending on the severity, it may persist for up to ten days. If the exposure is mild, erythema is faintly visible at twenty-four hours. The amount of radiation that produces this minimal erythema is known as the *minimal erythema dose* (MED). This dose varies from individual to individual depending on skin type. The time it takes to absorb 1 MED also depends on the time of day, season, and latitude, as discussed earlier. For example, a medium-complexioned, untanned individual exposed to midday, midsummer sun at 41 degrees north latitude (New York) receives 1 MED in about fifteen minutes. In an area of higher UV intensity, such as Florida, the same individual may absorb 1 MED in only ten minutes. The graphs in Figure 5.4 represent the time in which an average person receives 1 MED as a function of the time of day, season, and latitude.

Extrapolated from actual measurements of UV, these graphs should be used as rough guides rather than reliable, safe indicators of sun exposure. The only accurate way for a sailor to know the time it will take for him or her to receive 1 MED in a particular region is by trial and error. Usually, the sailor can estimate fairly accurately for the sailor's home port. For example, a medium-to-dark complexioned sailor may know that he or she normally requires thirty minutes of midday, midsummer Chesapeake sun to provoke a faint erythema 24 hours after the first exposure of the season.

Even though this estimated time to receive 1 MED is rough, it is important. What happens when it is exceeded? If exposure is extended so that the skin absorbs 2.5 MED, the result is a vivid and mildly painful erythema. A 5 MED, sunburn is not only red but decidedly painful, whereas a 10 MED exposure produces a severe sunburn with subsequent blistering. Exposures of this degree are usually followed within four to seven days by peeling of the epidermal layer. The area of peeling exposes pink, unprotected, supersensitive skin, which may be so damaged that it is not capable of producing any melanin for the next few months.

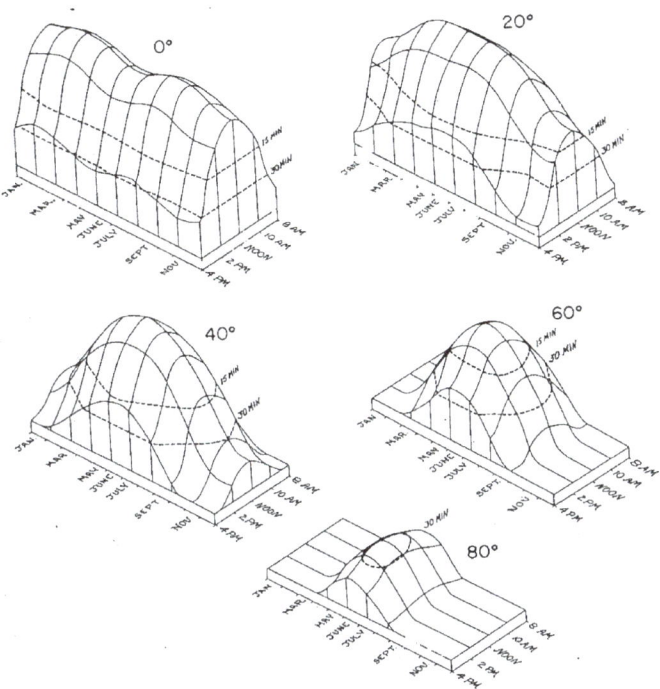

Figure 5.4 Minimal erythema dose (MED) in relationship to latitude, season, and time of day

UVB is the major culprit. It produces 90 percent of the sunburn damage, whereas UVA is only responsible for about 10 percent. (Actually, UVB is one thousand times as burning as UVA, but more UVA penetrates to sea level.) The most dangerous wavelength is 305 nanometers, right in the middle of the UVB band. Because of this, most of the earlier sunscreens were directed primarily or exclusively toward eliminating UVB wavelengths. *This approach is no longer acceptable for several reasons:*

First, very sensitive skins—especially type I—can still burn from pure UVA.

Second, it is becoming clear that UVA is linked to aging (actinic damage), wrinkling of the skin, and skin cancer. UVB is primarily responsible for sunburn (Figure 5.5). UV radiation is responsible for basal cell carcinomas, squamous cell carcinomas, and probably plays a role in the development of melanomas.

Third, a number of widely used medications sensitize the skin to UV radiation, a process called drug-induced photosensitivity. Table 5.2 lists some of the most common photosensitizing drugs. Most of the photosensitivity reactions are due to UVA, not UVB. It is important that the sailor select a sunscreen directed against both UVA and UVB (see discussion later in the chapter).

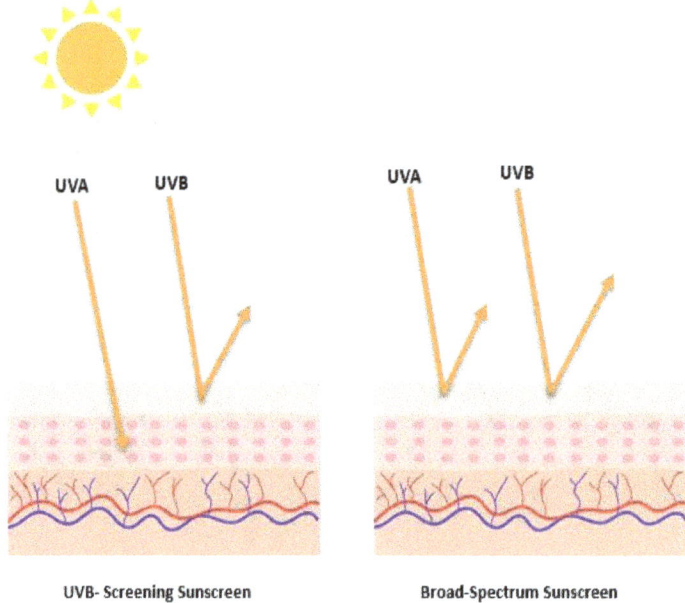

Figure 5.5 Penetration of UVA and UVB

Phototoxic skin reactions (Table 5.3 and Figure 5.6) occur minutes to hours after exposure and may appear as an exaggerated sunburn or, in severe cases, with blisters and bullae. The reaction is limited to sun-exposed skin. The skin may be itchy and occasionally change color (amiodarone, a heart medication, is associated with a blue-green pigmentation, for example). There is a second type of skin reaction (Table 5.3 and Figure 5.6) that can occur, referred to as photoallergic. Whereas in phototoxic reactions there is direct damage to tissue, in photoallergic reactions, the UV exposure changes the structure of the drug. The body's immune system views this altered drug as an invader (antigen) and sets up an allergic response—causing inflammation of the skin.

Drugs That May Produce Photosensitivity	
Antibiotics	ciprofloxacin, doxycycline, levofloxacin, ofloxacin, tetracycline, trimethoprim
Non-steroidal anti-inflammatory	ibuprofen, naproxen, celecoxib, piroxicam, ketoprofen
Cholesterol lowering	simvastatin, atorvastatin, lovastatin, pravastatin
Antihistamines	cetirizine, diphenhydramine, loratadine, promethazine, cyproheptadine
Diuretics	thiazide diuretics: hydrochlorothiazide, chlorthalidone, bumetanide chlorothiazide.; other diuretics: furosemide and triamterene
Phenothiazines	tranquilizers, anti-emetics: examples, chlorpromazine, fluphenazine, promethazine, thioridazine, prochlorperazine
Anti-fungals	flucytosine, griseofulvin, voriconazole
Sulfonamides	acetazolamide, sulfadiazine, sulfamethizole, sulfamethoxazole, sulfapyridine, sulfasalazine, sulfasoxazole
Sulfonylureas type 2 diabetes	glipizide, glyburide
Retinoids	Isotretinoin, acitretin
Other drugs	amiodarone, diltiazem, quinine, quinidine, hydroxychloroquine, enalapril, dapsone, voriconazole

Table 5.2 Drugs that may produce photosensitivity

Phototoxic versus Photoallergic reactions		
	Phototoxic	Photoallergy
Incidence	High	Low
Agent	Dose related	Small amount
Exposure	Single	More than one
Distribution	Sun exposed areas only	All areas
Onset	Minutes to hours	24-72 hours
Clinical characteristics	Sunburn, red, swelling, blisters	Eczematous, itchy lesions
Immunological	No	Yes

Table 5.3 Phototoxic versus photoallergenic reactions

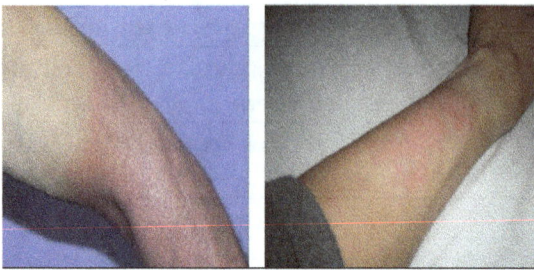

Figure 5.6 Phototoxic (A) versus photoallergic reactions (B)[8]

Tanning

In many cultures, people actively avoid the sun. The same was true in the western world for quite some time; pallid skin was a mark of the leisure class and darker tanned skin was evidence of working outside, probably in the fields. That remained true until early in the twentieth century when it was discovered that vitamin D deficiency was a cause of rickets. Then, in the 1920s, the fashionista Coco Chanel returned from a vacation looking tanned and it became popularized as a fashion statement. We still haven't completely gotten over that.

As sailors, no matter what we do, we are going to get sufficient sun to prevent vitamin D deficiency—that is not an issue. So we need to completely banish the concept of purposeful tanning and concentrate solely on protection. Sailors with Type I and II skin (see Table 5.1) need the most protection, as they are at high risk for sunburn, as well as skin damage and skin cancer. Types V and VI have a fair amount of built-in protection but must not become complacent (they can still develop skin damage and skin cancer). Types III and IV are the ones who need the most reeducation about concentrating only on protection, and not tanning.

In fact, we should banish the active verb "tanning" from the sailing vocabulary faster than we can banish the tanning salons that are still around despite the fact that we know for certain that they increase the risk of skin cancer. As sailors, if we spend any time on the sea, we are going to develop a tan whether we like it or not.

Both sunburns and suntans result from UV that has been transmitted through the layers of the skin. But whereas sunburn causes only damage (both immediate and cumulative), tanning serves a useful purpose. A well-developed tan provides some protection from future UV radiation. Unfortunately, to obtain a tan, a person must first suffer at least a mild burn. For those who are able to tan, the goal should always be to minimize this unavoidable burn.

Most people envisage the tanning process as a simple photochemical reaction; sunlight strikes the skin and somehow produces the darkening of skin pigment. Actually, the process is slightly more complex and far more interesting.

The skin is composed of two parts, the epidermis and the dermis. Tanning is confined exclusively to the epidermis. At the base of the epidermis are specialized cells called melanocytes, which manufacture melanin in response to UV (Figure 5.7). Of course, if the melanin is to diminish UV transmission through the skin, it must somehow be transferred to the surface. Nature accomplishes this by an ingenious method. The melanin is packaged into disklike structures called melanosomes. These melanosomes are then distributed to the other cells of the epidermis called keratinocytes, via processes known as dendrites due to their resemblance to nerve cell terminals.[9] In the human epidermis, each melanocyte is associated with about thirty-six keratinocytes. Together the melanocyte and its thirty-six keratinocytes constitute the epidermal melanin unit. Human skin contains a very large number of these units—one thousand to two thousand per square millimeter.

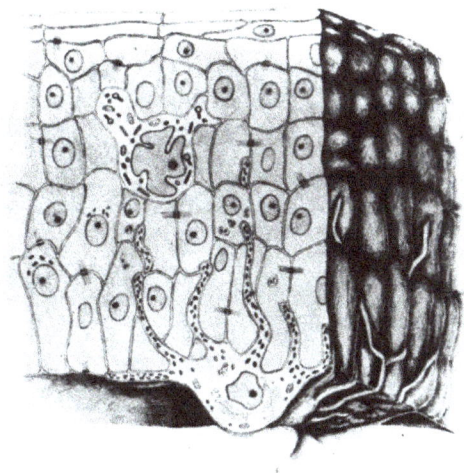

Figure 5.7 The epidermal melanin unit. The octopus-like melanocyte is transferring its melanosomes to the keratinocytes.

Once the melanosome is transferred to the keratinocyte, it remains within and travels with the keratinocyte to the skin surface during the normal process of skin regeneration. When the keratinocyte reaches the surface, it and the melanin within it are shed.

When sufficient UV penetrates the skin, two distinct phenomena occur. Under the influence of UVA there is immediate pigment darkening, which is a photochemical response of the melanin already present in the skin. Immediate pigment darkening lasts only a few hours, although faint traces may persist for one to two days. Under the influence of UVB primarily, the skin undergoes both burning (erythema) and true tanning. UVB excites the melanocyte to produce the melanosomes. The initial step involves a small amount of UVB-induced radiation damage to the DNA within the melanocyte.

The process of true tanning requires time: time for the production of the melanosomes, time for the transfer of the melanosomes to the keratinocytes, and time for the keratinocytes to ascend to the skin surface. This explains the three- to six-day latent period for true tanning; that is, for the first three to six days, the only noticeable change in the color of the skin is due to erythema, not tanning! And if during this period the skin is burned severely enough to produce peeling, the entire process must begin anew.

All sunscreens protect the skin by either absorbing or reflecting UV. Although there is considerable interest in the development of an oral sunscreen, to date all sunscreen agents must be applied directly to the skin.[10] In choosing a sunscreen, several factors should be taken into consideration: (1) the individual's skin type (Table 5.1); (2) the degree of protection provided—known as the sun protection factor (SPF); (3) the absorption spectrum—UVB, UVA, or both; (4) the cost, which varies widely; and (5) the particular disadvantages of specific preparations.

Individual sensitivity determines not only a person's choice of a particular sunscreen but also his or her entire attitude toward the sun! Sailors with type I and probably type II skin should forget about tanning and concentrate entirely on protection. These sailors should choose sunscreen agents with a high SPF (up to 50) and the broadest spectrum across both UVB and UVA. They should wear wide-brimmed hats and employ other forms of physical protection whenever possible. The helmsman, during the midday period, might consider a pair of light gloves. Because of humans' upright posture, certain areas receive more than average UV amounts and require above-average protection. These areas are: the nose, the tops of the ears, the lower lip, the upper back, and the area where the chest meets the neck. Also, don't forget the back of the neck, behind the knees, and the insteps.

At the other extreme, individuals with types V and VI skin require little protection. Nonetheless, they should not become complacent. There is no reason to court later skin damage and skin cancer (both of which are less likely to occur with these skin types) when protection is readily available. It certainly seems prudent to seek protection, at least during periods of high UV exposure. Skin types III and IV present the greatest challenge. These people do have something to gain from controlled UV exposure (the partial protection of a well-developed tan) as well as something to lose (actinic damage and cancer).

In order to facilitate the selection of an appropriate sunscreen, the U.S. Food and Drug Administration (FDA) has mandated that each sunscreen be identified by its SPF. SPF is a measure of the effectiveness of the sunscreen, regardless of the specific active ingredient, or, simply stated, a ratio of the MED with and without the sunscreen:

$$SPF = MED \text{ with sunscreen} \div MED \text{ without sunscreen}$$

For example, let us return to the sailor who usually requires 30 minutes of midday, midsummer Chesapeake sun to receive 1 MED. If the sailor applied a sunscreen with an SPF of 10, it would now take 300 minutes of exposure to produce a minimal erythema (1 MED). The sunscreen has increased by ten times the amount of time the sailor can remain in the sun and still only receive 1 MED. If, however, we take the same sailor and expose him or her to a midday equatorial sun, the MED time might drop to only 10 minutes. In this case, a sunscreen preparation with an SPF of 10 would produce 1 MED in only 100 minutes. If the sailor was exposed to four hours (240 minutes) of midday sun, he or she would end up with 2.4 MED (240 minutes in the sun divided by 100 minutes per MED) and a vivid erythema. (SPF numbers were kept low to assist those of you who are math-challenged!)

Once the sailor estimates the time it takes to develop 1 MED and the probable length of their exposure, they can choose a sunscreen with an appropriate SPF. Near the equator, for example, an SPF of 15 would allow an average sailor to stay out in the midday sun for 150 minutes before developing 1 MED. If planning to stay out for all four peak hours (10 a.m. to 2 p.m.), expect to receive about 1.6 MED (240 minutes divided by 150 minutes per MED). Obviously, these calculations are only rough approximations.

It turns out that the fastest (but not necessarily the safest) way to achieve a tan is to receive 2 MED per day. Even at this rate, it still takes about fourteen days to develop a full tan. Increasing the MED does not hasten the process. It increases only the risk of damage and may produce enough of a burn to promote peeling. Sailors who are chronically exposed to UV should not be interested in achieving the fastest tan anyway. Their major concern should be to reduce the amount of damage. Consequently, they should limit exposure to less than 2 MED per day.

Sunscreens

Sunscreen technology has been evolving very rapidly in the United States and around the world. An ideal sunscreen should be safe, chemically inert, nontoxic to humans and the environment, photostable, and nonirritating. There are two major issues that must be balanced as with all medication—safety and efficacy.

Let us look at efficacy first. The SPF number that we have been discussing applies to UVB. Most of the FDA-approved sunscreens listed below are effective primarily against UVB.

Padimate O	UVB	Avobenzone	UVA
Cinoxate	UVB	Oxybenzone	UVA and UVB
Homosalate	UVB	Aminobenzoic acid	UVB
Meridamate (coverage +/-)	UVA	Trolamine salicylate	UVB
Octinoxate	UVB	Dioxybenzone	UVB and +/- UVA
Octisalate	UVB	Octocrylene	UVB
Ecamsule(L'Oréal)low dose	UVA	**Zinc oxide**	UVB and UVA
Sulisobenzone	UVB	**Titanium dioxide**	UVB and UVA

Table 5.4 The most common chemical and mineral (bold) sunscreen agents

The major organic (chemical) agents that are active against UVA are oxybenzone and avobenzone, and there are problems with both. Oxybenzone, which until very recently had become one of the most popular agents, has been found to have *potential* health (hormone disruption in children and adults) and environmental issues. And despite its efficacy, avobenzone is relatively photo-unstable; that is, it often breaks down when exposed to light—not a stellar characteristic in a sunscreen. It is effective when mixed with stabilizing agents that mitigate the breakdown. Other agents listed above are not as effective against the full spectrum of UVA.

There are a number of effective agents approved elsewhere, but the FDA has insisted on additional testing before they can be approved in the United States. Tinosorb M and Tinosorb S have been approved in Europe, Australia, and Japan. Eucerin is one product line that incorporates Tinosorb S in some its products. Two other agents Mexoryl SX and Mexoryl XL also appear to be more effective than avobenzone and more stable. Mexoryl SX is the only one of these agents that has FDA approval and (as of 2019) only in a single L'Oréal product in low dose.

The United States also has a different approach to measuring UVA efficacy. It insists on protection at a critical wavelength of 370 nanometers as its standard for acceptance as broad-spectrum UVA protection. If it blocks up to 370 nanometers, then it can be marketed as broad-spectrum protection. Other regions such as Asia and Europe have adopted a different approach to UVA testing.[11] The European UVA attenuation must be at least one-third of the SPF. In other words, in Europe if a product is advertised as broad-spectrum SPF 30, its UVA protection must be at least ten. Developed in Asia, there are in vivo testing methods—persistent pigment darkening test (PPD) and a variation known as protection factor in UVA (PFA). (In vivo means they are tested on actual humans.) Because the standards for broad-spectrum UVA protection is stricter, many of the products sold in the United States would not pass muster in Europe. The chemical company BASF evaluated UVA protection of four agents from the United States and four from Europe, each of which had an SPF value of 50 or more. On average, the U.S. agents allowed three times more UVA than the European products, which had the more modern UVA filters. The U.S. FDA is still waiting for additional safety data.

Let's look at some of the labels (Figures 5.8 and 5.9). The first thing you will notice is that only the United States requires manufacturers to list the specific ingredients with their percentages. Score one for the United States in terms of transparency.

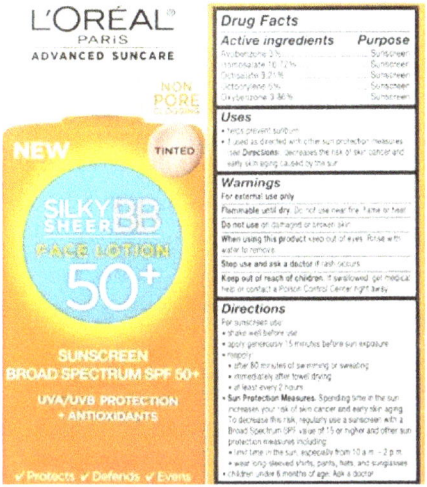

Figure 5.8 L'Oreal Silky Sheer BB: full labeling consistent with FDA requirements, for sale in United States

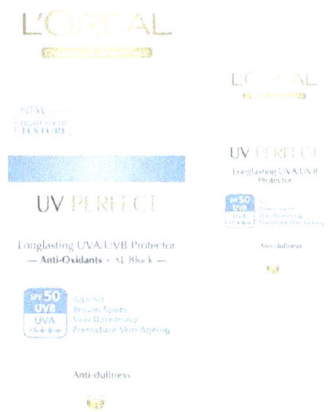

Figure 5.9 L'Oreal's UV Perfect without full labeling and not FDA approved. It contains Mexoryl, a superior UVA blocker. Note the use of the Japanese system for grading UVA (PA+++). See endnote 11 for more information on the Japanese system.

But wait. So far, we have only considered organic/chemical products. The other major class is mineral sunscreens—zinc oxide and titanium dioxide. From 2007 to 2018, there was a 40 percent increase in the use of mineral sunscreen in the United States.[12] Sunscreens using these two agents offer excellent protection from *both* UVB and UVA, are stable, don't contain harmful additives, and don't penetrate the skin. Zinc had been used for decades as a sunscreen for small exposed areas such as the iconic "lifeguard's nose." More recently, the particle size has been reduced and so the products are now relatively clear (transparent zinc oxide) without that white telltale sign. The smallest particles are *nano-sized*, a somewhat "literary" use of the term since there may be a mixture of sizes and not all are technically nanometers in diameter. The larger the particle the greater the protection by physically blocking the radiation, but the whiter the product the less it is useful for whole body protection. Figures 5.10 and 5.11 shows two products: EltaMD, which is pure zinc oxide (with an additional UVB filter, octinoxate) and Neutrogena, which features a combination of zinc oxide and titanium dioxide. In general, zinc is superior to titanium in blocking UVA, although there is nothing wrong with the combination. Compare the labels:

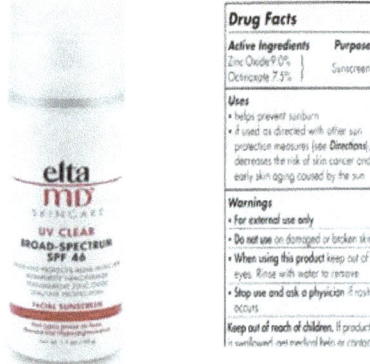

Figure 5.10 EltaMD, which contains zinc and octinoxate

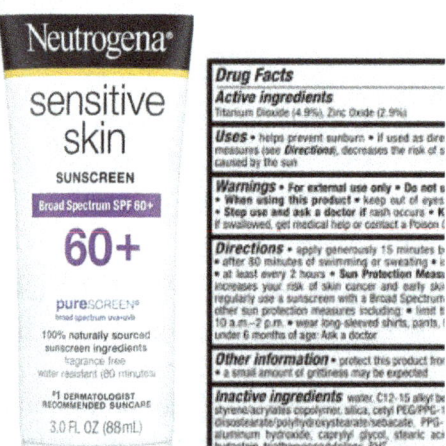

Figure 5.11 Neutrogena, a mixture of titanium and zinc

Tips for Staying Safe in the Sun

1. Use sunscreen regularly/daily.
2. Reapply often.
3. Apply sufficient sunscreen. Most people apply only 25 to 50 percent of the amount that they need. If you are covering the whole body, you need a "shot glass" full of sunscreen.
4. Plan around the sun. No midday sun! Avoid sun exposure between 11 a.m. and 3 p.m.
5. Find shade if possible—this is difficult on the water.
6. Think of using sun protective textiles: shirts, hats, shorts and pants that are ultraviolet protected factor certified (see below) provide the best protection from UV rays.
7. Use a hat and sunglasses (see Chapter 8 "Sailing Vision").
8. Avoid sprays, as they may get into the lungs, especially in children.
9. Do not rely on "waterproof sunscreen." There is no such thing, although it may be water resistant.
10. Pay attention to the expiration date on the bottle.
11. Be aware that any SPF rating higher than 50-plus is unnecessary and may tempt you to stay out longer. Remember that SPF ratings are not linear—SPF 30 provides 97 percent protection and SPF 50 provides 98 percent protection, an improvement but higher levels offer less and less advantage.

Ultraviolet Protection Factor Clothing

Ultraviolet protection factor (UPF) clothing is clothing that has been designed to provide UV protection for those areas of the body not amenable to chemical or mineral sunscreens. You will still need to apply sunscreen to the face, neck, and hands at the very least, but choosing clothing with a good UPF rating means that those areas are covered and do not need sunscreen. Most clothing manufacturers produce garments with a UPF rating of 50-plus. I would not settle for less. The UPF rating system for apparel is similar to the SPF rating system for sunscreens (see Table 5.5). However, UPF gauges the clothing's effectiveness against both UVB and UVA. That is very important. Unlike SPF, which typically uses human sunburn testing in a lab environment, UPF measures UV transmission using a spectroradiometer. Originally developed in Australia in 1994, the United States adopted the standards in 1998 and further refined them. The number of manufacturers creating UPF clothing is increasing exponentially, and the product lines are full so that you will have no difficulty finding clothing with a UPF tag that is also stylish.

Fabrics rated less than 15 are not considered protective. As an example, a typical white cotton T-shirt offers a UPF of about 5, which translates into a score of 80 percent UV radiation blocked. Sun protection as measured by UPF is due to the following factors, which the clothing manufacturer has used to reduce transmission:

UPF Rating	Protection	% UV radiation blocked
UPF 15-24	Good	93.3-95.9
UPF 25-39	Very Good	96.0-97.4
UPF 40-50+	Excellent	97.5-99+

Table 5.5 UPF ratings

- Fiber treatment: dyes and chemicals that absorb UV radiation
- Fiber type: polyester and nylon are excellent, wool and silk are moderate, and cotton, rayon, and hemp are fair to poor
- Fiber color: dark and vibrant colors generally absorb more UV than lighter colors
- Fiber construction: thick, tight, and dense fiber construction all minimize UV transmission

On the other hand, wetness, stretching, and wear will impair the clothing's inherent effectiveness.

Prickly Heat

Prickly heat, officially known as miliaria, might appear to be too trivial for the sailor's consideration, but it is not. Although minor individual attacks are inconsequential, repeated or extensive episodes can leave the sailor in jeopardy. Prickly heat occurs when it is hot and humid, and when sweating has been prolonged and copious. The skin lesions, which always appear at the sweat pores, may be crystal clear or opaque like gooseflesh, but most commonly they resemble tiny blood blisters. They may sting, itch, or burn. Portions of the skin that are covered are most vulnerable, especially when the clothing creates friction. The palms and soles are never involved, the face only rarely.

The rash erupts whenever the free flow of sweat is impeded. For reasons not entirely clear, keratin from the outermost layer of the epidermis plugs the sweat duct, blocking further sweat flow to the surface (Figure 5.12). In the absence of sweat, the eruption fades in a couple of days. If sweating begins again, the rash promptly recurs, and each recurrence tends to involve more sweat glands.

The major concern for the sailor is that extensive prickly heat predisposes to heatstroke (see Chapter 4). But even in the absence of heatstroke, repeated episodes impair sweating efficiency and reduce exercise tolerance. Prickly heat can be prevented. Clothing should be loose and well ventilated. A high salt intake can occasionally precipitate and sometimes aggravate it. The best preventive is to avoid the heat. Spending between four and six hours per day in a cool environment appears to be sufficient to prevent the disorder.

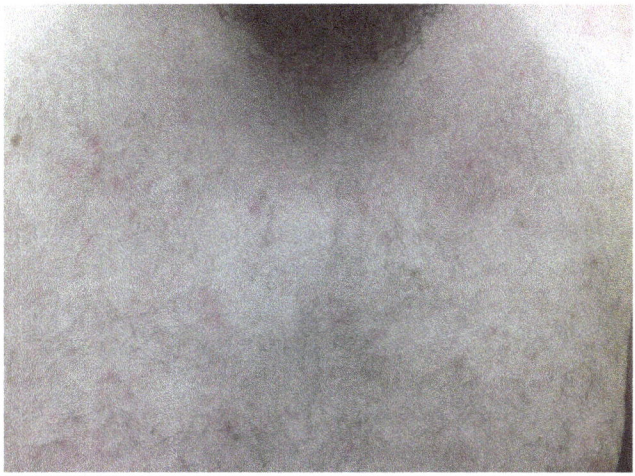

Figure 5.12 Prickly heat[13]

Seawater Boils

Seawater boils result from a bacterial infection of the hair follicles (Figure 5.1). The bacteria (Staphylococcus) are normally harmless inhabitants of the skin. However, when exposed to constant wetness, which is often unavoidable at sea, these bacteria grow, resulting in infection. Anything that irritates the skin, such as the friction of clothing, hastens the process. Bob Griffith discusses the problem the cruising sailor faces in *Blue Water*. He refers to the condition as helmsman's rear end, which is the most common location for seawater boils (you will have to use mental imagery for this illustration):

> This is the term we coined for the small sea boils or pustules located in the gluteal region that so commonly afflict small-boat sailors at sea. It is best prevented and best treated by keeping dry, and to this end I advise everyone not to wear underpants. While outer pants wet with saltwater dry in the air, underwear stays damp and the skin remains soft and irritated by salt and the pressure of sitting. Helmsman's Rear End results when bacteria infect the hair follicles or pores of the skin. In warm weather, when one isn't always careful about remaining dry on watch or working on the foredeck, Helmsman's Rear End sometimes is so bad that we have a daily clinic. The pustules are opened, drained, and dotted with dilute (1 to 100) formalin, tincture of iodine or other antiseptic, which is followed by a 20-minute sun treatment of the affected area.
>
> Saltwater boils on wrists and calves where cuffs and boots rub are a related affliction but worse because they inhibit a sailor's movements and are likely to be reopened in the course of deck work. They yield to essentially the same treatment but may require oral antibiotics. And they must be protected from abrasion from the cuff or boot that caused them.[14]

Swimmer's Itch

Swimmer's itch (also known as clam-digger's itch and swamp itch) is caused by the infestation of the skin with tiny parasites, the flukes. Of the numerous species of flukes, some are capable of parasitizing man, causing schistosomiasis, a serious disease prevalent in many parts of the world. These species are exclusively freshwater inhabitants, and for this reason caution is necessary when swimming in unfamiliar lakes, ponds, and streams. The species that cause swimmer's itch are not capable of causing schistosomiasis, only a dermatitis. These species are widely distributed throughout the freshwater areas of the world as well as some brackish and coastal waters (including the Atlantic seaboard, the Gulf Coast, California, and Hawaii). The initial exposure to the parasites usually produces a mild prickling and itching sensation after a person emerges from the water. As the film of water evaporates, the parasites penetrate the skin. Small skin lesions follow but usually disappear in a few days in nonsensitized people (Figure 5.13). In a person sensitized by a previous exposure, however, the reaction is often worse and may persist for one to two weeks. Usually the skin lesions predominate on exposed areas of the body and less frequently on areas that clothing or a bathing suit covers. Treatment usually consists of medication to relieve the itching. There is evidence that drying the skin thoroughly, immediately after exposure, may prevent the penetration of many of the organisms.

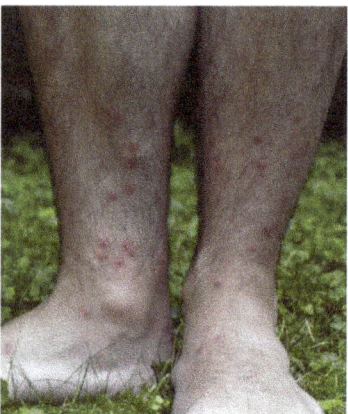

Figure 5.13 Swimmer's itch[15]

Notes

1. The term *ultraviolet light* is frequently used, although, strictly speaking, light refers only to radiation with a wavelength between 400 and 760 nanometers, making it visible to the human eye. (A nanometer is a billionth of a meter.)

2. The situation is analogous to that of X-ray exposure. The precise manner in which the X-rays are received is usually less important than the cumulative dosage over a lifetime. A lifetime of minor "insults" may be just as injurious as a lesser number of severe exposures.

3. D. W. Owens and J. M. Knox, "Influence of Heat, Wind, and Humidity on Ultraviolet Radiation Injury," *National Cancer Institute Monograph* 50 (1978): 161-167.

4. A few individuals are unusually sensitive to UV. They may experience welts, blisters, or skin lesions that look somewhat like juvenile acne. Since most of these conditions begin in childhood or adolescence, the sensitive individuals invariably are aware of their condition.

5. S. Eilers et al., "Accuracy of Self-Report in Assessing Fitzpatrick Skin Phototypes I Through VI," *Journal of the American Medical Association Dermatology* 149, no. 11 (2013): 1289-1294, doi:10.1001/jamadermatol.2013.6101.

6. An artificial carotene-based compound called canthaxanthin is available in the United States as a "tanning pill." It does not alter the body's melanin but is absorbed by and stains the skin, producing a brownish, orangish, or yellowish hue—simulating a tanned appearance. Canthaxanthin is approved by the Food and Drug Administration (FDA) as a food colorant but not as a sunless "tanning" aid. There have been side effects, and therefore DO NOT USE. There are safer alternatives if you desire tanner-looking skin. Bronzers are classified as cosmetics and are deemed safe by the FDA. They wash off with soap and water. Self-tanners or extenders are also topical and react with protein in the skin to produce a darker hue (the active ingredient is dihydroxyacetone [DHA]—also safe). Of course, artificial skin coloring by cosmetics of any type offers no protection whatsoever against solar radiation.

7. John D'Orazio et al., "UV Radiation and the Skin," *International Journal of Molecular Sciences* 14, no. 16 (2013): 12222-12248, doi:10.3390/ijms140612222; http://www.mdpi.com/1422-0067/14/6/12222/htm, CC BY 3.0; https://commons.wikimedia.org/w/ index. php?curid =49672997.

8. https://en.wikipedia.org/wiki/File:Sun_poisoning.JPG#/media/File:Sun_poisoning.JPG

9. The resemblance between the tanning process and central nervous system activity is by no means coincidental. During early human development, the melanocytes (or, more properly, their precursors, the melanoblasts) migrated to the skin from early central nervous system tissue. In other words, melanocytes are first cousins to the nerve cells in the brain. Many of the nutrients and enzymes are exactly the same. A prominent example is dopa. Dopa plays an important role in transmitting nerve impulses in the brain. Its absence in a specific region of the brain is associated with Parkinson's disease, and, of course, many of you are aware of its association with various impulse control disorders. It turns out that dopa is also the major ingredient in the production of melanin.

10. Para-aminobenzoic acid (PABA), which used to be an active ingredient in many sunscreen preparations, is no longer used for that purpose. We now have many better agents. It is still sold as a nutritional supplement in health-food stores and it has been used to treat a number of diseases, such as pemphigus, morphea, scleroderma, and Peyronie's disease. How effectively is another issue. Since it used to be used as a sunscreen, sailors should be advised that oral PABA provides no sunscreen protection whatsoever.

11. The Japanese use a system that you may see on sunscreens from Japan and Europe:
- PA+ = some UVA protection
- PA++ = moderate UVA protection
- PA+++ = high UVA protection
- PA++++ = extremely high UVA protection

There are drawbacks. First, not all countries agree with how the PA measurement values are achieved. The PA rating measures only how the sun's UVA rays cause the skin to become brown and stay brown, that is the persistent pigment darkening, or PPD. But not everyone's skin turns brown from being exposed to the sun, especially if only exposed to UVA. The color of different people's skin after UVA exposure is inconsistent.

12. www.fda.gov/Drugs/ResourcesForYou/Consumers/BuyingUsingMedicineSafely/Understanding Over-the-Counter Medicines/ucm239463.htm.

13. https://commons.wikimedia.org/w/index.php?curid=15788521.

14. Bob Griffith with Nancy Griffith, *Blue Water* (Boston: Sail Books, 1979), 184-185.

15. https://commons.wikimedia.org/w/index.php?curid=7322085.

Chapter 6

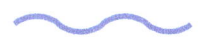

Hazardous Marine Life

"Sailors, with their built-in sense of order, service,
and discipline, should really be running the world."
—Nicholas Monsarrat

The widespread interest in marine life that could pose harm to human beings is of a relatively recent origin. It received its major impetus during World War II, when unprecedented numbers of men, casualties of downed aircraft or sunken ships, were forced to survive in the sea. This experience, coupled with subsequent biological research and our need to travel the globe, has provided us with an abundance of useful information. The problem, however, is extensive. It turns out that most, if not all, of the major groups of marine animals include at least one species that is potentially dangerous to man. From a human perspective, the assortment of venomous spines, stinging cells, rapacious jaws, and other unpleasantries seems frightening if not downright malicious! But, of course, each of these characteristics represents nothing more or less than the owner's evolutionary adaptation to its particular niche in the underwater world. Human motives such as malice simply don't apply. The jellyfish, for example, could never have endured for millions of years were it not for its vast array of stinging cells. These stinging cells developed long before humans were around to trespass upon the jellyfish's "turf."

The chance of coming into contact with potentially dangerous aquatic animals increase as boaters and sailors cruise to remote areas of the world and begin to explore the beauty and wonder beneath the sea. It is clearly in our best interest to become aware of the physical characteristics that make some of these species dangerous. *We can then avoid inadvertently triggering an instinctive, reflexive response that was not meant for us at all.* Approaching the sea in a cavalier fashion is equivalent to walking alone down a dark alley in a strange part of town—it's asking for trouble.

Animals That Sting

The Coral Reef

One of the most popular marine attractions is the coral reef. Because the reef supports such an exuberant diversity of flora and fauna, it has been compared to a tropical rain forest; like the rain forest, it harbors a great deal more than meets the eye. Although the lively and animated surface of the reef is readily apparent, there is a surprising amount of activity within the interior of the reef, out of view. In fact, many animals spend nearly their entire existence in the reef's honeycombed caves, crevices, and recesses.

Coral reefs occur in a belt of warm water found globally from 30 degrees north to 30 degrees south latitude. Because of ocean warming, coral reefs around the globe are struggling, and many are dying. Despite its beauty, the coral reef itself represents a hazard to the unwary visitor. The stony exterior belies the fact that it is an animal or, more correctly, a colony of animals known as *coral polyps*. Each coral polyp sits within its own tiny cup of limestone that it erects by gleaning chemicals from the sea. The tiny, jelly-like polyp retreats into its protective shell by day and hence is not visible. The brightly colored polyps can be seen only at night, when they emerge to feed, adding another chromatic dimension to the already multicolored reef.[1]

Coral cuts, lacerations, and abrasions are a major but generally avoidable nuisance. They usually result from careless swimming or snorkeling over shallow portions of the reef. Most people are simply unaware of the intrinsic sharpness of coral, as well as the increased vulnerability of wet human skin. Multiple factors determine the severity of coral cuts: (1) contact with the razor-sharp exoskeleton of the coral may cause a simple laceration; (2) microscopic pieces of the coral—calcium carbonate, sand, and other debris—retained within the abrasion or laceration may precipitate a "foreign body" reaction producing redness and inflammation; (3) bacteria, fostered by high temperature and high humidity, may infect the area; and (4) a weak venom that the polyp produces may cause swelling.

Since coral cuts may take months to heal (and frequently produce an unexpected scar), avoidance is the most prudent course. Never handle coral unnecessarily. Hands and feet should be well protected when swimming or diving on the reef. Divers should wear wet suits. If cuts, lacerations, or abrasions occur, they should be treated vigorously to prevent secondary infection and ulceration (the advice below also applies to barnacle cuts).

- ✓ Scrub the lesions with soap and water, using a soft brush or rough towel to remove any pieces of coral that may have become embedded in the wound.
- ✓ Flush the wound with fresh disinfected or clean drinking water.
- ✓ Apply a one-to-one solution of hydrogen peroxide/water and allow it to "foam" for several minutes.
- ✓ Rinse with water and then if available apply isopropyl (rubbing) alcohol.

- ✓ Rinse with water, dry, and apply antibiotic ointment (and cover with nonadherent bandage).
- ✓ Clean the wound twice a day.
- ✓ Begin an antibiotic such as ciprofloxacin (Cipro), cephalexin (Keflex), or levofloxacin (Levaquin) if there are any signs of infection.
- ✓ See a doctor to treat the wound surgically if it does not heal promptly.

Jellyfish (common varieties)

Jellyfish are only very remotely related to the bony, or vertebrate, fish. They are invertebrates of the Phylum Coelenterata, hence the expression "spineless as a jellyfish." Other members include true coral, false or fire coral, sea anemone, Portuguese man-of-war, and hydroids. The basic structure of all of the coelenterates is a saclike body cavity (-*coele*) that serves as the digestive system (*enteron*).

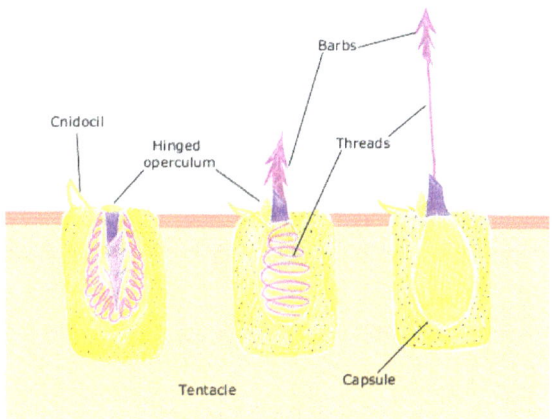

Figure 6.1 The nematocyst, or stinging cell[2]

In addition to the polypoid structure, coelenterates share another common feature, the *nematocyst*, or "stinging cell" (Figure 6.1). Each nematocyst consists of a minute capsule containing a coiled, hollow thread, bathed in a venomous fluid. A hairlike trigger known as a cnidocil projects from the capsule. When activated, the cnidocil opens the capsule and the thread springs forth. Both mechanical factors (such as friction) and chemical factors (such as fresh water) seem to play a role in activating the nematocyst. Once the point of the thread penetrates its victim, the venom is released—a kind of tiny "hypodermic" injection.[3]

In many cases, the jellyfish's reputation is worse than its sting. This is certainly true of most species of scalloped jellyfish, which periodically "bloom" during the warm summer months. The common species include the "moon" jellyfish (*Aurelia aurita*), the "hair" jellyfish (*Cyanea capillata*), and the sea nettle (*Chrysaora quinquecirrha*). Contact with the tentacles of these species usually results in nothing more than a prickly or stinging sensation. Common species of jellyfish occur worldwide.

Seawasp

In stark contrast is the deadly sea wasp, a member of the jellyfish family, and perhaps the most dangerous animal in the sea! There are three closely related and similarly appearing genera: *Chironex*, *Chiropsalmus*, and *Carybdea*. Contact typically occurs when the victim is wading, swimming, or diving in shallow waters. This venomous jellyfish may never be seen. Following contact, the sea wasp usually manages to tear itself away, but it leaves behind its calling card—a string of tentacles that resemble pink, purple, or grayish earthworms. The victim is usually in pain and attempts to struggle to shore. With extensive stings, the victim may lose consciousness and need to be dragged from the water. Deaths due to cardiac arrest have occurred within thirty to sixty seconds.

The sea wasp's shape readily distinguishes it from more benign species. In contrast to the scalloped hemisphere, the sea wasp is a cuboidal bell with flattened sides (Figure 6.2). Fortunately, its distribution is limited. The most dangerous species, *Chironex fleckeri*, is found almost exclusively in Australian waters, where most of the deaths have occurred. *Chiropsalmus quadrigatus* commonly inhabits the waters in and around the Philippines and has been responsible for a few deaths. The closely related *Chiropsalmus quadrumanus*, despite its wider range (including the tropical and subtropical Atlantic and Indo-Pacific), is much less toxic. Species of *Carybdea* are found worldwide but have not been responsible for any serious reactions.

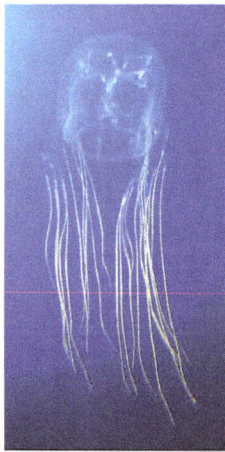

Figure 6.2 Sea wasp, or box jellyfish[4]

Jellyfish are feeble swimmers and are largely at the mercy of wind and wave. Incoming tides and storms are thus likely to bring the jellyfish closer to shore and increase the possibility of contact. Bathers should be forewarned that jellyfish washed up on shore are still capable of inflicting a serious sting. Even their detached tentacles have "live" nematocysts that can retain their stinging capabilities for up to three months.

Portuguese Man-of-War

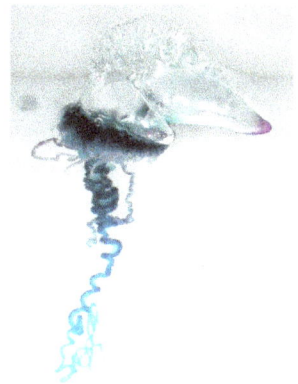

Figure 6.3 Portuguese man-of-war[5]

Many people consider the Portuguese man-of-war a jellyfish, but it is a very different kind of animal. Unlike the jellyfish, the Portuguese man-of-war is a floating colony of different, specialized coelenterate polyps performing different jobs for the good of the aggregate (a true "socialist"). One type of polyp produces the bright blue (or sometimes red or green) float that bobs over the surface, while others lie beneath the float hanging head down, trailing long tentacles (Figure 6.3). The tentacles are armed with batteries of nematocysts similar to those of the jellyfish. The tangled mass of tentacles may reach 100 feet (30 meters) in length, thus, a swimmer can be stung even at a great distance. The Portuguese man-of-war has no control whatsoever over its own destiny. It rests upon the water, its float acting as a sail, and its tentacles as a sea anchor. There are two species: a larger Atlantic species (*Physalia physalis*) is found in the tropical Atlantic, throughout the West Indies, as far north as the Hebrides, and as far east as the Mediterranean, and the smaller IndoPacific species (*Physalia utriculus*) is found in Hawaii, Japan, and throughout the Indo-Pacific. The Portuguese man-of-war has an undeservedly bad reputation. Contact with its tentacles produces the same pain and welts as the jellyfish and on occasion systemic symptoms also, such as muscular cramps and a feeling of chest tightness. However, death by exposure to this creature is extremely rare and is most likely to occur in either children or older individuals who sustain massive contact. The treatment is the same as that for jellyfish stings.

Irukandji

Irukandji jellyfish (Figure 6.4) are any of the tiny extremely venomous species of box jellyfish (related to the sea wasp). The animal can be as small as a cubic centimeter (less than half an inch in size) but along with box jellyfish are one of the deadliest jellyfish in the world. They inhabit the waters of Northern Australia and Southeast Asia, and its venom sends between fifty to one hundred people to the hospital each year. The pain may be delayed for twenty to thirty minutes after the sting and generalized rather than local. There may be systemic effects, including agitation, confusion, increased heart rate and blood pressure, and, in a small percentage, cardiac arrest and respiratory failure.

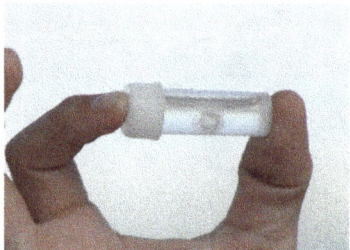

Figure 6.4 Irukandji jellyfish[6]

Treatment of Jellyfish Stings

This remains an area of confusing recommendations. First, let's debunk the old wives' tales. *Do not pee on the wound.* I know that sounds like a cool thing to do but unless your urine is so concentrated that you are dehydrated near death (see Chapter 4, "Heat and Dehydration") your urine is too dilute to be helpful. This brings up the next point: *fresh water is to be avoided as is scraping off the remaining tentacles with a knife or credit card.* Both fresh water and friction will in fact increase the amount of toxin released. And do not use drinking alcohol, rubbing alcohol, toilet water, cologne, perfume, or meat tenderizer; they'll all make things worse. Now to the controversial—vinegar. With little evidence to back up the recommendation, vinegar has frequently been recommended to treat most jellyfish stings. *For the most common jellyfish stings, vinegar is no longer recommended.* So, what to do?

We could do worse than follow the recommendations of Australian-based Berling and Isbister.[7] Australia has the most experience with both the common jellyfish and the other types discussed above. The sting severity is related to the number of stinging cells that fire (it can run into the many thousands) and the potency of the injected venom.

For most common jellyfish stings, producing local pain for one to two hours:

- Wash the site with seawater and carefully remove the tentacles (with tweezers or towel or gloved hands—try not to scrape).
- Immerse the affected area in hot water (45 degrees Celsius or 115 degrees Fahrenheit) for twenty minutes.
- Avoid vinegar as it may worsen pain.
- Use lidocaine if available or hydrocortisone cream and bandage for pain.
- Clean open sores two to three times a day and apply antibiotic ointment.
- Use ice for additional pain relief.

For major box jellyfish stings like those from a sea wasp, which can cause severe pain and (if extensive lines of tentacle contact) cardiovascular collapse and death:

- Apply vinegar and remove tentacles.
- Use analgesia medications (oral and intravenous).
- Begin CPR if unconscious.
- *Give antivenom if available.*[8]
- Transport to the hospital if possible.

For Irukandji, treatment is similar to that for box jellyfish except there may be no visible tentacles and the pain is generalized. Antivenom is *ineffective*, however.

Other Coelenterates

Since all coelenterates possess nematocysts, it is not surprising that quite a number of other species are capable of stinging people. Despite its appearance, fire coral (also known as false coral and stinging coral) is not a member of the true coral family. Rather, it is more closely related to the Portuguese man-of-war. Like true coral, however, it is widely distributed throughout the tropical seas of the Pacific, Indian Ocean, Red Sea, and Caribbean. The most dangerous of the fire coral is *Millepora alcicornis* (Figure 6.5), followed by *Millepora dichotoma*. Both are so elegant that it is often tempting to break off a piece, but these species will offer a swift retribution in the form of a searing, white-hot pain.

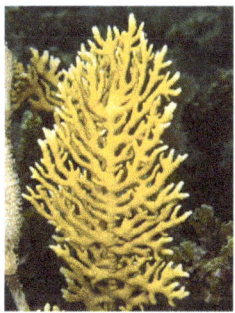

Figure 6.5 Branching fire coral (*Millepora alcicornis*)[9]

Feather hydroid *(Lytocarpus)* is fairly abundant in tropical and subtropical waters. Swimmers are most commonly affected while climbing onto offshore rafts or swimming around pilings. The feather hydroid venom produces one of two skin reactions: (1) weals that surface within minutes of contact or (2) a delayed chicken pox-like reaction four to twelve hours after contact.

Because of their variety of colors, sea anemones (Figure 6.6) are frequently mistaken for their botanical namesakes. Unfortunately, they are not as harmless. The severity of the sting varies greatly from species to species. Sometimes there is only a burning at the site of contact. With more severe stings, systemic symptoms may occur, such as headache, nausea, vomiting, fever, chills, and muscular spasms. Multiple abscesses, which are resistant to treatment, have also been reported. The sea anemone, like the fire coral, demands a "hands-off" policy!

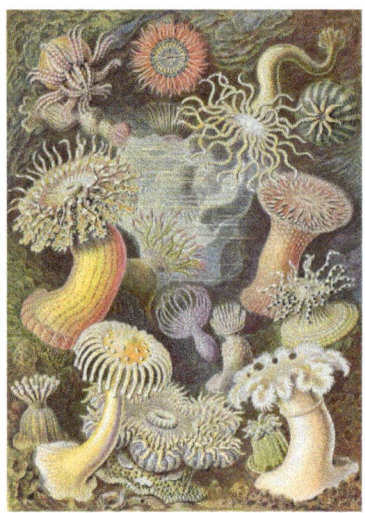

Figure 6.6 *Sea Anemones* by Ernst Haeckel[10]

Sea Urchins, Starfish, and Cucumbers

Nestling into nearly every nook and cranny in the reef is the ubiquitous sea urchin, aptly known as the living pincushion (Figure 6.7, top). Its body consists of a globular shell from which project calcareous spines. On the undersurface, in addition to the mouth, are short spines and tube feet, which allow slow locomotion across the ocean floor. There are numerous species of sea urchin, with great variability in the size and shape of the spines. Some species have blunt spines, whereas others have sharp, brittle spines up to a foot long resembling knitting needles. Most species are not venomous. Sea urchin spines enter human skin with ease and can also penetrate leather or canvas gloves, shoes, and flippers. In some species, a violet colored liquid, possibly a venom, is released into the wound. The intense pain and burning create the impression of having stepped on a red-hot spike. The pain may last for hours if the penetration is deep. Because of their extreme brittleness, once a spine penetrates the skin, there is a tendency for it to break off and become difficult to withdraw. If the spine cannot be removed, the body usually absorbs it in a few days. Occasionally, the spine must be removed surgically. Soaking in dilute acetic acid, boric acid, or even urine supposedly hastens absorption.

Closely related to the sea urchins are starfish (Figure 6.7, bottom). Most of the starfish species are relatively safe to handle. One species, however, the crown of thorns (*Acanthaster planci*), possesses large spines and is capable of inflicting a painful wound. The spines are also venomous, which accounts for the occasional reports of numbness and partial paralysis. The crown of thorns can be found throughout the Indo-Pacific region. This species periodically proliferates widely: in the 1960s, it laid waste vast portions of the Great Barrier Reef.

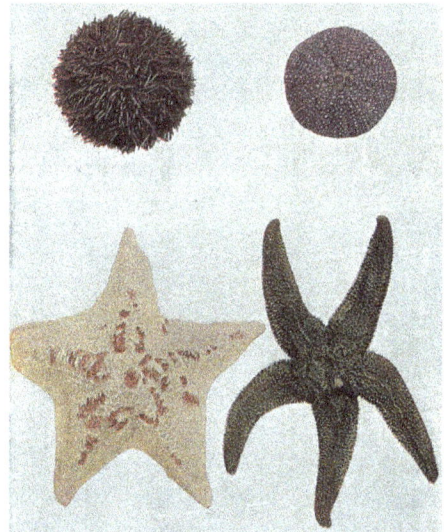

Figure 6.7 Sea urchins (top) and starfish (bottom)[11]

Cone Snails

Cone shells (Figure 6.8) rank among the most prized acquisitions of shell collectors. There are more than five hundred different multicolored predatory species, one of which, the "glory of the sea" (*Conus gloriamaris*), has commanded prices as high as several thousand dollars. However, the living cone snail (inside the shell) is as dangerous as its shell is attractive. At least a dozen people are known to have died and scores have been injured by its venom.[12] The cone snail surely possesses one of nature's most unique weapons (Figure 6.9). It stores tiny harpoon-like structures—known as radular teeth—in a sack, like arrows in a quiver.

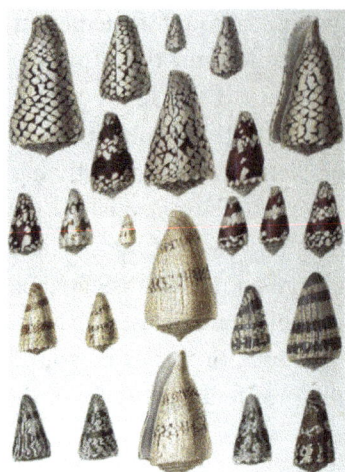

Figure 6.8: Cone shells[13]

These radular teeth are hollow and equipped with venom, which is stored in a separate venom bulb. When the cone shell prepares to strike, it transfers a radular tooth to the tip of the shell's muscular proboscis, which can extend several inches in all directions. It has been extrapolated that there is sufficient toxin in one cone snail to kill up to seven hundred people.

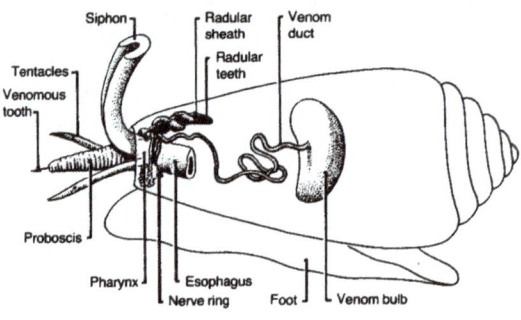

Figure 6.9 Cone shell locked and loaded

The victim experiences excruciating pain and numbness first in the area struck, but then over the entire body. Difficulty in speaking and swallowing and paralysis may follow. The cause of death is usually respiratory paralysis, cardiac failure, or some combination.

Although species vary in toxicity, all live cone shells should be treated with caution and handled only with thick gloves. Supposedly, it was thought to be safe to pick up the cone shell by the "big end," but not always. The proboscis is quite extensible and may reach all the way back from the "little end" to strike the hand of the holder.

Hazardous Marine Life

The most important intervention after cone snail envenomation is immediate hospitalization. En route to the hospital, the most important therapy is the pressure immobilization technique (PIT), developed by an Australian, Dr. Struan Sutherland (Figure 6.10).[14] It consists of bandaging the limb with an elastic bandage (if available), starting below the bite and wrapping up toward the axial joint and then back down again. It should be tight but not to the point of curtailing the circulation or being painful, because it is vital that the victim does not move (splint if possible).

- Apply a broad pressure bandage over the site as soon as possible
- The bandage should be 10-15cm wide
- Wind the bandage firmly around bitten limb |
- Start from the site of the bite **1**
- Bandage the distal leg or arm first **2**
- Then proceed to bandage up the arm or leg **3**
- Apply a splint to prevent limb movement (arm or leg) **4**
- Apply a second bandage over splint to hold it in place

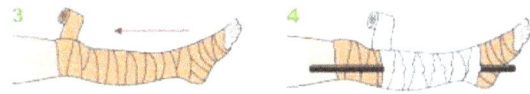

Figure 6.10 Pressure immobilization technique (PIT)[15]

Octopus

Victor Hugo deserves much of the blame for the maligned reputation of the octopus. In his book *Toilers of the Sea*, he describes the octopus as "a disease embodied in monstrosity." Actually, most species (including the large Pacific octopus, which has an arm spread of 30 feet [10 meters] and weighs more than 100 pounds [45 kilograms]) are not aggressive toward man. Ironically, the most dangerous species of octopus is the smallest—the blue-ringed octopus (*Octopus lunulatus*; Figure 6.11).

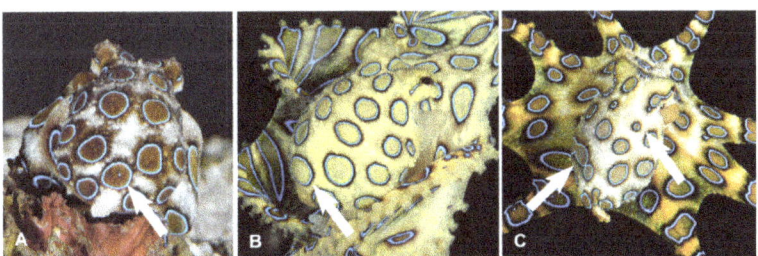

Figure 6.11 Unique body color patterns in blue-ringed octopus[16]

All octopi have a sharp parrotlike beak, which they use to attack prey. Connected to the beak are two salivary glands that produce venom. In most cases, the venom is not particularly toxic to humans although the toxin—tetrodotoxin—is the same toxin that occurs in puffer fish envenomation. In severe cases, there may be generalized paralysis with respiratory failure (similar to puffer fish poisoning). Usually, however, the victim of an octopus bite feels mild pain and a burning or stinging sensation. In some cases, a spreading numbness occurs, along with partial paralysis. There have, however, been a small number of fatalities due to octopus bites. Although there are a few closely related species inhabiting the waters around Australia, Japan, and the Indian Ocean, all of the fatalities, so far, have occurred in waters off Australia. The species responsible is small enough to be held in the hand. The speckled rings of blue often attract bathers, who have been known to pick them up and play with them! In fact, the wounds inflicted are so small that the two tiny puncture marks are sometimes overlooked. The venom must be extremely potent since, despite the small size of both creature and wound, death from respiratory paralysis may occur within two hours. The immediate treatment is similar to that of cone shell envenomization (see the PIT in Figure 6.10).

Stingray

Stingrays cause more injuries to humans than any other venomous fish. It has been estimated that there are at least 1500 victims per year in the United States alone. The many different species of ray are common inshore inhabitants of nearly all tropical, subtropical, and warm temperate seas. An additional reason for the large number of human injuries is the fact that stingrays are predominantly shallow-water animals. They frequently burrow into the sandy or muddy bottom, making themselves almost impossible to identify and a hazard to anyone wading through the water.

Although the stingray has a sinister appearance, there is no evidence of aggression toward people. In fact, quite the opposite is true. Virtually every attack is prompted by unintentional aggression on the part of humans.[17] In a typical scenario, the victim wades through the water and steps upon the stingray, often pinning it down. The creature's only defense is its venomous spine, or sting, located at the base of the tail. The tail whips forward, usually contacting the victim's foot (Figure 6.12), although any portion of the human anatomy may be affected. The injury is due primarily to tissue trauma rather than intoxication. Pain is the first symptom, usually developing immediately or within five to ten minutes. It increases in severity during the next thirty minutes and may spread to involve the entire leg. The pain is most severe by two hours and gradually subsides over the next two days. If the wound is deep and a substantial amount of venom has been introduced, systemic symptoms may occur, such as vomiting, diarrhea, sweating, shock, paralysis, and, rarely, death. The major problem is usually the wound itself and not the toxin. There is apt to be significant tissue damage, since the sting has backward pointing teeth, which make its withdrawal a "nonsurgical" proposition.

Hazardous Marine Life

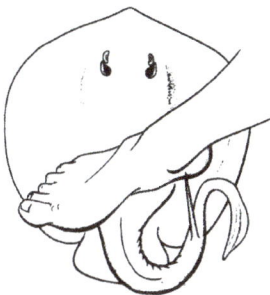

Figure 6.12 Stingray injury

The ensuing tissue damage increases the absorption of the venom, which is contained along the side of the sting and covered by a sheath. When the sheath is stripped away during penetration, the venom is exposed. A sting that has been used repeatedly and not yet replaced may be so traumatized that little of either sheath or venom is left. In that case, only the wound needs to be dealt with.

Treatment should be prompt. The wound should be irrigated with cold seawater to constrict the blood vessels of the skin and reduce further absorption of venom. Next, the wound must be explored carefully for pieces of the sting that should be removed. Once the wound has been cleaned, it should be soaked in hot water (45 degrees Celsius or 114 degrees Fahrenheit) for up to ninety minutes or so. Local anesthetics may be needed during the debridement. Antibiotics may be given and, when feasible, a health care professional should conduct an X-ray or ultrasound to exclude retained fragments of the spine. You should obtain a surgical referral if there are retained fragments.

Prevention is obviously the key. The chief danger, stepping on the animal, can be largely eliminated by either shuffling one's feet along the bottom of the sea or probing the area with a stick.

Sea Snakes

Sea snakes—all of which are venomous—are members of the family Hydrophidae. With one exception, they are confined to the western Pacific and Indian oceans. The exception is the yellow-bellied sea snake (*Pelamis platurus*), which is widely distributed from the east coast of Africa to the west coast of South America. This species reaches the western coast of Central America and Mexico in considerable numbers (Figure 6.13). Sea snakes have a distinct preference for sheltered coastal waters and especially river mouths. Since they are air breathers, they are usually found in shallow water.

Their disposition has long been a matter of dispute. There is now general agreement that most species are usually docile, although if provoked they may be aggressive toward humans.

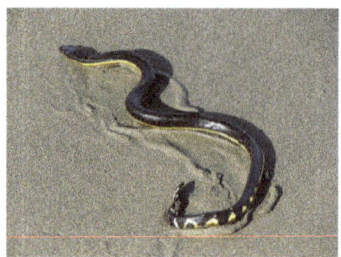

Figure 6.13 Yellow-bellied sea snake[18]

Fishermen frequently are bitten while handling nets or sorting fish. Bathers may be bitten if they accidentally step upon the snake.

Immediate treatment consists of PIT (Figure 6.10). A sea snake antivenin has been developed and should be given if available. It can be obtained from Seqires, the same company that developed the sea wasp antivenin. It is recommended for anyone contemplating extended cruising in the Indo-Pacific.

Scorpionfish (the *Femme Fatale* of Fish)

Although a great variety of vertebrate fish have spines, only a small percentage possess a true envenomization apparatus. The most dangerous of these is the family of scorpionfish, which includes several hundred species. For convenience, we will discuss three main groups: the stonefish (*Synanceia*); the zebrafish (*Pterois*), also called the turkeyfish or lionfish; and the true scorpionfish (*Scorpaena*). Despite some obvious differences in appearance, these species all have approximately thirteen venomous dorsal spines in addition to an assortment of others. The venomous glands lie within grooves along both sides of the dorsal spines. In the stonefish, the glandular tissue forms two discrete, more highly developed glands, each with its own venom duct. It has caused numerous deaths and countless injuries. The stonefish has a habit of lying completely motionless under rocks, in coral crevices, or beneath a layer of sand or mud. To abet its camouflage, it has developed the most incredible appearance (Figure 6.14).

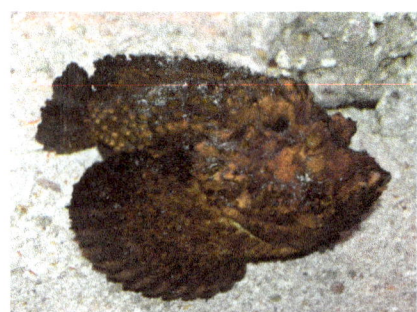

Figure 6.14 Stonefish: The most toxic fish in the world[19]

Its skin, which has a wartlike texture to begin with, becomes encrusted with bits of coral debris, mud, and even algae from continual burying in the sand. It looks like a piece of weathered coral or a chunk of stone, whence came the name. When stepped upon, the pressure forces the venom from the bulb along the duct into the wound, much like a hypodermic injection. The spines are sharp and strong enough to puncture even a thick rubber sole.

Pain spreads rapidly from the wound to involve the entire limb. In severe cases, the localized symptoms rapidly yield to nausea, vomiting, profuse sweating, delirium, convulsions, difficulty breathing, and sometimes death.

Treatment consists of alleviating the pain, combating the effects of the venom, and preventing secondary infection. The wound should be cleaned with the gentle removal of any obviously protruding spines. Heat treatment is widely recommended, and the limb should be immersed in water up to 45 degrees Celsius or 114 degrees Fahrenheit for at least thirty minutes. As with other toxins discussed above, this may denature the toxin and help with pain control. Wound management requires removal of spines straight out with tweezers or forceps so that they are intact.[20] The development of a specific antivenin has made a profound difference in the outcome of stonefish stings. For example, on the South Pacific island of Rarotonga, where stonefish stings are common, victims used to require hospitalization for several days. Since the introduction of the antivenin, hospitalization has usually been unnecessary. Stonefish inhabit waters of the Indo-Pacific, Australia, China, India, and as far west as the Red Sea and the East African coast.

The lionfish is as beautiful as the stonefish is ugly (Figure 6.15).

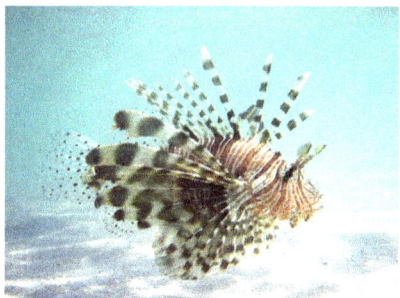

Figure 6.15 Lionfish[21]

This rather small fish, usually 3 to 10 inches (8 to 25 centimeters) long, is found adorning coral reefs throughout the tropics. It is sometimes called zebrafish or turkeyfish because of its habit of spreading its fanlike pectorals and lacy dorsal fins, like a strutting turkey gobbler. This fish is truly fearless! If approached, it rotates its body to confront the intruder with erect dorsal spines. People are often tempted to grab this beautiful creature, especially when it lies motionless in the water. Invariably they receive more than they bargained for. There is immediate local pain. The tissues near the wound site become red and swollen as in a stonefish sting. In severe cases (usually the victim has received several stings), the pain is followed by nausea, vomiting, delirium, convulsions, respiratory paralysis, and sometimes death. The treatment is the same as for stonefish stings.

The scorpionfish family comprise a more heterogeneous group, widely distributed throughout all temperate and tropical waters, a few species even extending into polar regions. Unlike stonefish and lionfish, some of the species of scorpionfish that inhabit temperate waters are of considerable commercial value as food fishes. For the most part, these species are bottom fish, preferring the rocky coastal regions—hence the term *rockfish*. The most common injury from these fish is to the hands of fishermen. The intensity of the sting varies from species to species, but generally there is at least an intense throbbing pain. The treatment is the same as for stonefish stings.

Weeverfish

The weeverfish are a group of small marine fish confined to the east Atlantic and the Mediterranean. European fishermen have been aware of the venomous nature of these species since ancient times, long before most of the other venomous fishes were recognized. The weevers primarily inhabit flat, muddy, or sandy bays. They bury themselves in the soft mud or sand with only their heads exposed, intermittently darting out to capture their prey. Weevers each have approximately seven dorsal spines (plus a few other spines). Weevers' wounds produce instantaneous pain, usually described as burning, stabbing, or crushing. It is initially confined to the area of the wound but soon spreads to involve the entire limb. The pain usually subsides within two to twenty-four hours. The treatment of weeverfish stings is similar to that of stingray wounds.

Animals That Bite

Shark

> "How strange, the tiger of the sea;
> He runs from you and dines on me."
>
> —*U.S. Navy,* Shark Sense, *1959*

Without a doubt, the most feared adversary in the sea is the shark. Is this fear justified? Well, yes and no! Certainly, unprovoked shark attacks do occur, causing mutilation and death. In fact, it is difficult to imagine a more horrible way to depart this vale of tears than by being eaten alive by a shark. But from a statistical point of view, the likelihood of such a death is quite small.[22] The International Shark Attack File investigated 130 incidents of alleged shark-human interaction occurring worldwide in 2018. Of these, there were only sixty-six confirmed *unprovoked* shark attacks globally; the remainder consisted of provoked attacks, boat attacks, doubtful cases, and so forth. This total of sixty-six was actually lower than the average of eighty-four incidents annually over the most recent five-year period recorded (2013-2017). Of the sixty-six attacks, the vast majority were in the United States (thirty-two) and Australia (twenty).

These numbers, however, represent *unprovoked attacks*. *Encounters* are much more numerous, as any seasoned diver can attest. Most of the time, a shark or sharks come over to investigate and, having satisfied their "curiosity," eventually depart.

Contrary to what you might expect, most shark victims live to tell the tale. Less than a third of shark attacks result in death. The likelihood of being killed by a shark is of the same order of magnitude as the chance of being struck and killed by lightning.

We are only now beginning to understand what makes a shark tick. That shouldn't be surprising, because when we are face-to-face with a shark, we are really looking back across an abyss of time. The shark is a product of the late Mesozoic era and has changed but little in the intervening three hundred million years.[23]

Of the 250 species of shark, only about twenty-five (or 10 percent) have been implicated in attacks on humans. Except for the hammerhead, the name of which well characterizes its appearance, most sharks look very much alike to the untrained eye. The distinguishing features scarcely impress most swimmers and divers who encounter them in the water. Sharks range in size, at maturity, from 6 inches (15 centimeters) to more than 50 feet (15 meters). Interestingly, the largest species, such as the 50-foot (15-meter) whale shark or the 45-foot (14-meter) basking shark, are inoffensive plankton strainers, harmless to humans. At the other extreme, many species are too small to cause any serious harm to people. Most of the species potentially dangerous to humans are 7 to 20 feet (2 to 6 meters) in length, although it is a good general rule that *any* shark more than 3 feet (1 meter) in length *may* be dangerous, especially if there is food or blood in the water. Most shark attacks occur between 45 degrees north and 45 degrees south latitude. The highest incidence is in tropical and warm temperate waters above 68 degrees Fahrenheit (20 degrees Celsius), partially because more people swim and dive in warm water. It is a myth, however, that sharks need warm water to attack. The most frequent period of the day for attacks is late afternoon and at night, which is sharks' most active feeding time; however, attacks may occur at any time. Generally, sharks attack people in one of the following situations: while they are swimming or surfing, while they are diving, or after they survive a sea or air disaster.[24]

While Swimming or Surfing

(1) Know the area. Ask locals or preferably a lifeguard if any sharks have been spotted.

(2) Stay out of water that sharks are known to frequent. A swimmer or surfer is in the most vulnerable situation since he or she has neither warning nor defense.

(3) When possible, swim with a buddy or a group.

(4) Never wade if you can swim, even in shallow water. Swim with even strokes, as splashing may look like fish movement.

(5) Avoid swimming in water when the underwater visibility is poor, or at dusk or at night.

(6) Avoid wearing bright colors, especially yellow. Do not wear jewelry.

(7) Do not swim in the vicinity of garbage dumps. They are shark hangouts.

(8) Avoid river mouths that meet the ocean. Bull sharks may be there.

(9) Do not swim with seals or sea lions.

(10) Before you enter and exit the water, first look around. Then move rapidly. The swimmer is most vulnerable at the surface of the water.

(11) Never enter or remain in the water with a bleeding wound.

(12) If a shark is encountered, begin to leave the area with slow, purposeful movements, rather than erratic, panicky splashing. Sharks are especially sensitive to low-frequency, irregular movements indicative of distress. If possible, face the shark at all times while making your exit.

While Diving

(1) Never dive alone.

(2) Always have assistance available. If you dive in known shark-infested areas, carry something to fend off an attack.

(3) Wear dark clothing; bright, shining objects and contrasting shades tend to attract sharks.

(4) If the group is threatened, form a tight circle and face the shark. Try to move steadily toward the boat or shore but stay submerged until the last moment. If there are only two of you, stand back-to-back. If you find yourself alone, try to maneuver against a rock to protect your rear.

(5) If attack is inevitable, the following maneuvers have occasionally worked: releasing bubbles, shouting underwater, charging, clubbing the shark on the snout. For clubbing, use any object that is available, but use bare hands only as a last resort, since shark skin is quite rough and capable of inflicting severe abrasions—the last thing needed, since blood will attract other sharks and perhaps prompt a feeding frenzy.

For Survivors

(1) Do not abandon any clothing, as it can afford some protection against the abrasive skin of the shark.

(2) Remove wounded survivors from the water as soon as possible.

(3) Remain quiet and conserve energy.

(4) Do not dangle arms or legs over the side of the raft. You should assume that there are sharks in the immediate area—and there usually are. They are attracted to the raft by the fish that take up residence beneath it.

(5) Do not fish when sharks are visible, and abandon a hooked fish if sharks congregate. Do not jettison garbage willy-nilly. Rather, save it on board in a container, if possible.

(6) Employ whatever shark chaser you have.

Finally, it is worth remembering that there are innumerable shark encounters for every shark attack. The odds are overwhelmingly in your favor.

If you are an avid swimmer, surfer, or diver and frequent areas of shark attacks (see www.trackingsharks.com for the latest information), you should consider the purchase one of the many recently developed shark repellents—but do your research, caveat emptor. These technologies include:

- Magnetic shark repellent
- Electropositive shark repellent
- Electrical shark repellent
- Acoustic shark repellent
- Semiochemical shark repellent

Barracuda

There are about twenty different species of barracuda, which differ markedly in their aggressiveness toward humans. This fact partially explains the conflicting accounts of the danger the fish presents. All barracuda are members of the family Sphyraenidae, and all are voracious carnivores, but the only species ever implicated in human attacks is the great barracuda (*Sphyraena barracuda*). Smaller species, which tend to travel in large schools, have never been known to attack people.

The larger specimens of *Sphyraena barracuda*, which look like large pikes, grow 6 to 8 feet (2 to 3 meters) long, weigh more than 100 pounds (45 kilograms), and possess enormous knifelike canine teeth. They are found in tropical and subtropical waters around the globe. Like all barracuda, they are swift creatures and hunt largely by sight. Unlike sharks, barracuda usually make only a single attack, which in most instances is not fatal to humans. Mutilation and amputation are not uncommon, however.

Actually, there are only about three dozen documented attacks on humans by *Sphyraena barracuda*. Some have occurred when divers have towed dead fish behind them through the water, a practice to be avoided since it attracts both shark and barracuda. Some appear to be legitimate cases of mistaken identity, where the barracuda mistook the victim, or something he or she was wearing, for a more usual prey. Flashy metallic or multicolored clothes or gear may simulate the underbelly of a food fish. These attacks have usually occurred when turbid water impaired the fish's vision. In clear water, humans arouse little more than the barracuda's curiosity.

Moray Eel

Of the twenty or so species of moray eel (Figure 6.16), most inhabit tropical or subtropical regions, although a few range as far north as Europe. Larger species may attain a length of 10 feet (3 meters) and weigh as much as 100 pounds (45 kilograms). The moray is primarily a nocturnal creature. During the daytime, it spends most of its time peering out from rock and coral crevices or pieces of wreckage waiting to grab prey that stray close by. Occasionally, one is seen undulating across the ocean floor. At night, it squirms out of its hiding place to hunt fish and octopus. Whether by day or night, the moray eel almost never attacks humans unless provoked. Invariably, an inadvertent poking of a hand or foot into the moray's lair or a direct assault upon the animal precedes an attack. Grasping or walking on a coral reef (not a good idea anyway) or feeling about inside submerged wreckage is an invitation for a vicious bite. In the open water, however, when the moray does not feel threatened, it prefers to flee.

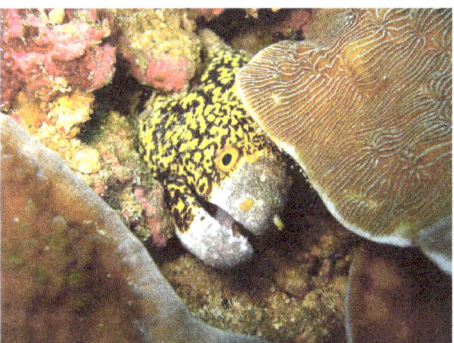

Figure 6.16 Moray eel waiting[25]

The moray is a notoriously powerful biter and can inflict severe lacerations with its narrow, muscular jaws, which are armed with strong, knifelike teeth. The wound is jagged and torn and readily becomes infected.

Manta (Giant Devil) Ray

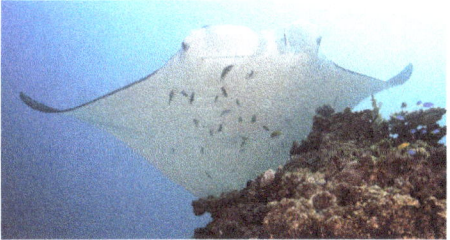

Figure 6.17 Manta ray[26]

The manta, or giant devil, ray (Figure 6.17) dwarfs the rest of the ray family. Specimens may attain a wingspan of more than 20 feet (6 meters) and weigh more than 3,500 pounds (1,575 kilograms). Mantas are generally found cruising or basking near the surface of the water. Inexplicably, they suddenly leap from the water and belly flop onto the surface, producing quite a splash. The manta is not at all aggressive toward humans.

Unlike its relatives, it does not possess a caudal stinging apparatus. It is dangerous only because of its huge size.

Needlefish

Needlefish are members of the family Belonidae. They have a svelte body that tapers into two elongated jaws filled with sharp teeth. Larger needlefish may be as long as 6 feet (2 meters). Human fatalities and serious injuries from needlefish are due to puncture wounds to the head, chest, and abdomen. These fish are frequently attracted to bright light at night and have been known to leap out of the water in its direction. Anyone standing in their flight path is liable to be punctured.

Needlefish primarily inhabit tropical waters. A person sailing or fishing at night with a bright light should be aware of this potential danger.

Giant Grouper

Giant grouper, or sea bass, as they are sometimes called, have occasionally caused problems for swimmers and divers. Some of the large species may be 12 feet (4 meters) in length and weigh more than 500 pounds (225 kilograms). They tend to hang out in caverns, old wrecks, and underwater caves. Although they are not truly aggressive toward humans, they sometimes pose a threat because of their huge size, curious attitude, and cavernous jaws. It has been suggested that Jonah must have been swallowed by a giant grouper, since whales cannot open their jaws wide enough to admit a person! The smaller specimens are as tame as puppies.

Orcas (Killer Whales)

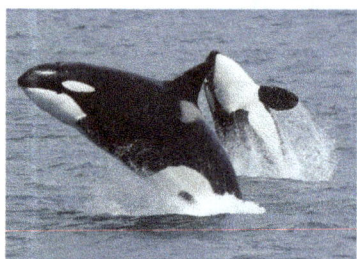

Figure 6.18 Orca (killer whale)[27]

The orca, or killer whale (*Orcinus orca*), has long been considered a ferocious and ruthless killer. It is about 30 feet (9 meters) when mature, swims fast, and has a formidable array of sharp teeth set within a powerful set of jaws. It usually travels in a pod of 30 to 40 individual orcas and preys on a wide variety of marine life, such as fish, birds, walrus, seals, and even some whales. It is quite capable of snapping a large sea mammal in half. But is it a man-eater?

Roger A. Caras, in his book *Dangerous to Man*, has thoroughly examined the evidence and comes away unconvinced.[28] He marshals an impressive array of marine experts who support his contention that the orca is usually not a threat to humans. If anything, the orca may be more of a threat to the boat than to a person (small comfort, perhaps, miles from land). Two sinkings due to orcas near the Galapagos Islands support this theory. Orcas probably rammed and sank the Robertson family's boat, although everything happened so fast it is difficult to ascertain who saw what.[29] The boat sank in a very brief period of time, yet the whales made no attempt to attack the survivors. An injured sperm whale, not an orca, likewise attacked the Baileys' boat, making no attempt to molest them.[30] It is not known why whales occasionally attack boats. The act of feeding does not seem to prompt these attacks. Perhaps it is a case of mistaken identity (breeding rather than feeding!) or simply an example of cetacean psychopathic behavior.

Giant Tridacna Clam

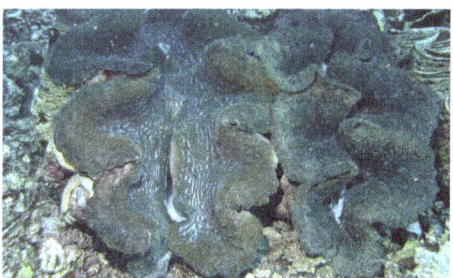

Figure 6.19 Giant tridacna clams[31]

The giant tridacna, or so-called killer, clam abounds in tropical waters. There are some claims that divers accidentally stepping into these clam's open valves have become trapped and have drowned, but these reports are not well documented. Since these clams close up tight with the slightest activity in the area, and close very slowly, many authorities doubt that it is possible that a human could ever become trapped. Dr. W. G. Van Dorn has stated, "Anyone so careless as to step into an open one while wading in the shallows along the Great Barrier Reef would probably deserve his untimely demise."[32]

Animals That Make Us Sick

"Give a man a fish and feed him for a day. Give a man a fishing lesson and he'll sit in a boat drinking beer every weekend."

—Alex Blackwell

Considering the number of fish that are caught and safely eaten each year, is there any reason for the cruising sailor to worry about eating his or her catch? From a strictly statistical point of view, there is probably not. But if you don't enjoy being a statistic, consider these two facts:

(1) Marine poisons are, on average, one hundred to one thousand times as potent as sodium cyanide.
(2) Many of the world's most idyllic cruising grounds are replete with poisonous fish.

Although there are numerous types of marine poisonings, most are rarely encountered by the cruising sailor. The sailor should be concerned about three major types of fish poisoning (ciguatera, puffer poisoning, and scombroid poisoning), shellfish poisoning, and a few others.

Ciguatera

The most common of the marine poisonings is *ciguatera*. The current frequency of ciguatera poisonings is estimated to be 10,000 to 50,000 people per year who live in or visit tropical and subtropical areas.[33] Although the syndrome was not described until 1787, it has presumably afflicted humans since antiquity. It almost prematurely ended the second Pacific expedition of the *HMS Resolution* under the command of Captain James Cook. The incident took place on July 23, 1774, at Malekula, New Hebrides. Cook and four crew members ate three fish ("red pargo"), which are now believed to have been red snapper (*Lutjanus bohar*), one of the most common causes of ciguatera.

Ciguatoxic species are tropical or subtropical reef fish that are either bottom dwellers or feed upon bottom dwellers. Ciguatera usually does not result from fish that are caught in the open ocean; however, if these oceanic species do happen to wander close to shore and feed upon reef fish, they too may become toxic. Ciguatera is confined to a circumglobal belt that extends from 35 degrees north to 35 degrees south latitude. The most dangerous areas by far are the reef islands. Tropical reefs that fringe continental shelves (such as those in Florida) are also dangerous. Even within this belt, the geographic distribution is spotty. Fish from one sector of an island may be safe, whereas those from another a short distance away may be toxic. A region that has supported abundant safe fishing for as long as anyone can remember may suddenly suffer mass outbreaks of poisoning from a harvest of the same, previously safe species. Later, these species may revert to their nontoxic state, although this process often takes months. The cause of these rapid shifts is unknown. Sometimes they are associated with catastrophes, either natural (hurricanes, earthquakes) or man-made (wrecks, dumping, explosions), but usually there is no obvious triggering event. The relative unpredictability is particularly frustrating. In many places, it virtually prohibits the establishment of shore fisheries.

The biogenesis of ciguatera is illustrated in Figure 6.20. There is unanimous agreement that the toxin—ciguatoxin—has its origin in the coral reef food chain of herbivorous bottom-dwelling fish. The origin of the toxin has been identified: it is the dinoflagellate *Gambierdiscus toxicus*. The dinoflagellates are single-celled organisms that are a major constituent of oceanic plankton. They straddle the plant and animal kingdoms, possessing functions of both and prompting the name "plant-animals". Herbivorous fish that eat the dinoflagellates acquire toxicity but are themselves unaffected. Carnivorous fish become toxic by feeding on the toxic herbivores and are likewise unaffected. As a rule of thumb, the larger carnivores tend to be the most toxic because they can rapidly acquire large quantities of the toxin already concentrated in the herbivore. It is well known that the larger the fish, the greater the amount of toxin per unit weight and the greater the chance of becoming poisoned if the fish is consumed.

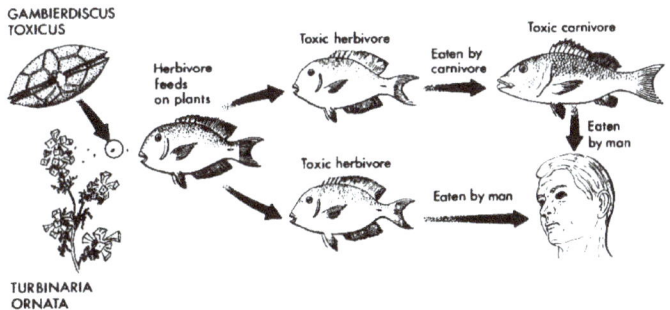

Figure 6.20 Ciguatera biogenesis

The food-chain theory is supported by the fact that the most toxic portion of the fish is usually the liver, followed by the intestines, ovaries, testes, and muscle. More than four hundred species of fish have been incriminated at one time or another. The most frequently poisonous species are: *moray eel, grouper, snapper, barracuda, jacks, kingfish, parrotfish, surgeonfish, triggerfish, hogfish, coral trout, and filefish*. The Florida Department of Health with the Florida Fish and Wildlife Conservation Commission prepared and distributed Figure 6.21 to educate people about this condition.

The victim of ciguatera is usually aware of intoxication within one to six hours, although signs may not appear for more than a day. There are two groups of symptoms: gastrointestinal and neurological. The initial symptoms are usually gastrointestinal (60 percent), consisting of nausea, vomiting, abdominal pain, and diarrhea. Some victims, however, report muscle aching, cramping, and weakness as their first reaction. The next symptoms are numbness and tingling in and around the mouth, in the throat, and subsequently over the rest of the body. There may be "sensory reversal," when cold feels hot, and vice versa. Later on, the victim may complain of headache or dizziness, or they may be confused. By the next day, the victim may have intense itching and a rash.

In severe cases, muscle weakness and incoordination become pronounced and are followed by convulsions, coma, and death due to paralysis of the muscles of respiration. Although the fatality rate of ciguatera intoxication had been as high as 12 percent in the past, most of the recent outbreaks have been milder. There is a treatment that appears to be quite effective—intravenous mannitol—but it is only available in the hospital. There is evidence that it is effective for both acute symptoms and in preventing the long-term neurologic consequences of the illness.

Except for some numbness, the symptoms in uncomplicated cases subside within twenty-four hours. Recovery from a severe ciguatera intoxication is typically slow, lasting weeks, months, and even years!

As of now, there are few effective treatments *other* than intravenous mannitol for ciguatera intoxication. Induced vomiting is suggested to remove any remaining unabsorbed toxin from the stomach. Bedrest and painkillers are helpful. Severe cases should involve hospitalization, but it is often not feasible because of remoteness.

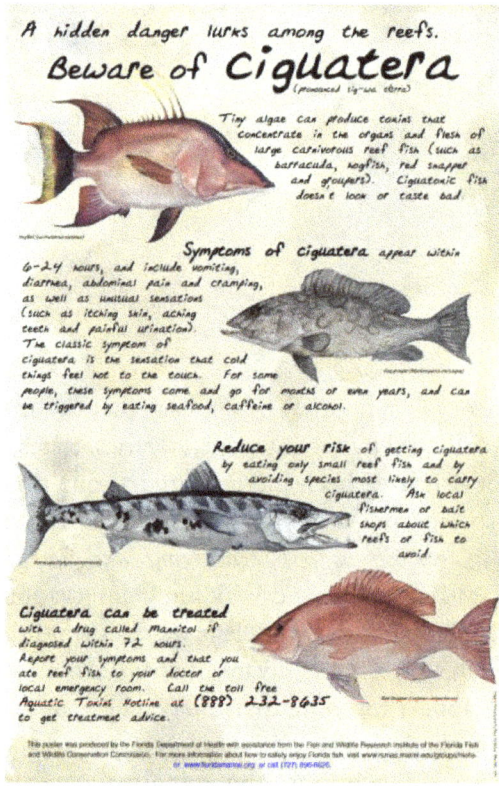

Figure 6.21 Ciguatera poster

Therefore, prevention becomes crucial. Obviously, avoid all species listed previously, unless you have good evidence that they are safe. In fact, the circumspect sailor should be wary of any species caught near shore in the ciguatera belt, since open-water species occasionally approach land and feast upon the indigenous reef species. Local knowledge is most helpful, but by no means foolproof. Natives actually make up a large percentage of all poisoning cases!

Despite numerous native folk practices, there is no reliable way to detect the presence of the toxin short of witnessing its effect on a living animal. The appearance, smell, and taste of the fish are entirely normal. Ordinary cooking techniques, such as frying, broiling, boiling, baking, and steaming, have no effect on the toxin. Since the liver, intestines, testes, and ovaries have a higher concentration of toxin, discard these parts of the fish.[34]

Pufferfish Poisoning

Pufferfish poisoning is one of the most violent biotoxications. In contrast to ciguatera, however, it is a much more manageable threat to the sailor since all of the species implicated are members of a single order, Tetraodontiformes, which includes the puffers (globefish, blowfish, balloonfish, toadfish, and swellfish), the porcupine fish, and the ocean sunfish. These fish are all characterized by their remarkable ability to inflate themselves like a balloon by gulping down large quantities of water or air (Figure 6.22).

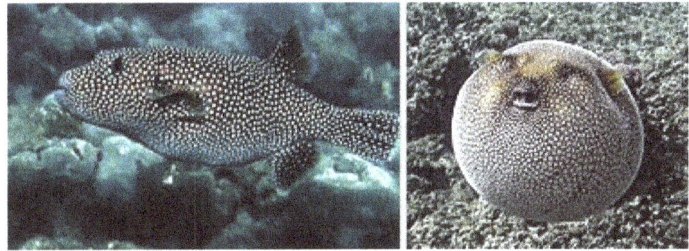

Figure 6.22 Guineafowl puffer—unpuffed and puffed[35]

The geographic distribution of the Tetraodontiformes is extensive, from 47 degrees north to 47 degrees south latitude. Some of the species primarily inhabit tropical or subtropical reefs, whereas others, such as the sunfish, are open-water fish.

The problem of puffer poisoning is certainly not new. Egyptian tombs of the Fifth Dynasty (circa 2700 BC) depict the pufferfish *Tetraodon stellatus*. The accompanying hieroglyphics indicate that it was considered poisonous then as now. One of the Mosaic dietary laws (Deut. 14:9-10) was likewise directed at eliminating pufferfish from the diet of the Israelites: "These ye shall eat of all that are in the water; all that have fins and scales shall ye eat; and whatsoever hath not fins and scales ye may not eat; it is unclean unto you." This would effectively eliminate all varieties of pufferfish as well as the oft-deadly moray eel, which causes ciguatera. It has been pointed out that essentially the same admonition was given to U.S. troops during World War II, three millennia later:

> All of the important fish with poisonous flesh belong to one large group, the Plectognathi [the former name for Tetraodontiformes], of which there are many kinds in the tropics. All these fish lack the ordinary scales such as occur on bass, grouper, sea trout. Instead these poisonous fish are covered with bristles or spiny scales, strong sharp thorns, or spines, or are encased in a bony boxlike covering. Some of them have naked skin, that is, no spines or scales. Never eat a fish that blows itself up like a balloon.[36]

As with ciguatera, the toxicity is unpredictable. The toxin, tetrodotoxin, has been well studied and is now unequivocally produced by a variety of symbiotic bacteria including Actinomyces, Aeromonas, Alteromonas, Bacillus, Pseudomonas, and Vibrio (for you microbio nerds)[37] The most toxic portions of the fish are the skin, liver, ovaries, and intestines. In contrast to ciguatera, where toxicity is related to size, small puffers are capable of packing a lethal wallop. The toxin is also found in the blue-ringed octopus, rough-skinned newt, and moon snail.

Tetrodotoxin is a neurotoxin (a sodium channel blocker); gastrointestinal symptoms are usually absent. Within ten to forty-five minutes of ingestion, the sailor notices malaise, pallor, dizziness, and oral tingling that soon spreads to involve the entire body. Weakness and paralysis of the muscles of respiration follow. Death may occur in fifteen to twenty minutes, and there is absolutely no treatment. If death occurs (and the fatality rate is 60 percent), it usually takes place within the first twenty-four hours of ingestion.[38]

If these fish have been identified readily since biblical times, why does puffer poisoning present any challenge at all? The sailor who eliminates all scaleless fish from his or her diet will never come into contact with the poisoning. Most cultures in fact consider all of the Tetraodontiformes to be "trash fish." But just to prove that "one man's fish is another man's poison," the Japanese (and to a lesser extent the Koreans and Chinese) consider pufferfish, which they call *fugu*, a delicacy! Because of the frequent outbreaks of poisoning—the fish are the cause of more deaths by poisoning in Japan than any other food—the government strictly regulates the sale and preparation of fugu. Fugu chefs are licensed, and there is even a cookbook on the safe preparation of the fish. It takes ten years to become a licensed fugu chef in Tokyo. However, as Halstead points out, it is "disconcerting to note that even the finest puffer cooks occasionally succumb to their own cooking."[39]

In survival situations, the fish should be immediately eviscerated and only the muscle eaten. Small pieces of the muscle should be soaked in water for three to four hours, during which the fish should be kneaded and the water frequently replaced. Since the toxin is water soluble, much of it can be leached out. Cooking has no effect on the toxin.

Since James Cook nearly lost his life to ciguatera (see earlier in the chapter), one would assume that he would be more circumspect in his choice of fish dinners. Nevertheless, on September 7 (only forty-six days after his bout with ciguatera), he very nearly succumbed to puffer poisoning! On this occasion in New Caledonia, Cook and two of his scientific staff sat down to a meal containing a small amount of the liver and roe of a large puffer fish. All three men became severely ill and transiently paralyzed.

Scombroid Poisoning

Scombroid poisoning is the third type of fish poisoning of interest to the sailor. The name refers to the suborder Scombroidei. Susceptible fish include albacore, amberjack, anchovy, Australian salmon, bluefish, bonito, kahawai, herring, mackerel, mahi-mahi, needlefish, sardine, skipjack, wahoo, and yellowfin tuna. Scombroid poisoning, unlike ciguatera or pufferfish poisoning, is a product of spoilage and subsequent bacterial contamination. The poisoning is not due to bacterial toxins per se. Rather, in the absence of adequate handling and refrigeration, several strains of marine bacteria interact with the fish flesh to produce histamine, which is responsible for the symptoms.[40]

Histamine usually does not change the appearance or the smell of the fish, which may appear to be normal although there may be a sharp or peppery taste as well. Symptoms develop within minutes and consist of intense headache, dizziness, abdominal pain, nausea, vomiting, dryness, burning of the throat, and difficulty in swallowing. Shortly thereafter (or before) comes flushing of the skin, itching, and hives. The face becomes swollen, the eyes red and watery, and the nose runny. In severe cases, an allergic, asthmalike condition develops. Although deaths have occurred, the symptoms are usually transient, lasting less than a day.

Treatment consists of induced vomiting and the administration of antihistamines such as diphenhydramine (Benadryl) 25 to 50 milligrams every six hours and ranitidine (Zantac) twice a day. In severe cases, epinephrine and steroids may be necessary. Scombroid poisoning may be prevented by avoiding all tuna and other species not freshly caught or adequately refrigerated.

Paralytic Shellfish Poisoning

The biblical account in Exodus (7:19-21) of the Egyptian water turning into blood is probably the earliest record of what is now referred to as the red tide. This phenomenon results from the periodic proliferation, or "blooming," of dinoflagellates.[41]

The process of paralytic shellfish poisoning begins when these toxic dinoflagellates proliferate and are ingested in large quantities by one or more of the filtering bivalve mollusks—clams, mussels, oysters, or scallops. The mollusk concentrates the toxin in its tissues but remains unaffected. Humans complete the process when eating the contaminated mollusk. The toxin in paralytic shellfish poisoning has been identified and labeled saxitoxin, after the clam *Saxidomus giganteus*, from which it has been isolated.

Within thirty minutes of ingestion, there is a tingling or burning sensation of the mouth, lips, face, arms, and legs. In severe cases, tightness of the throat, difficulty in speaking and swallowing, dizziness, headache, prostration, muscle weakness, and incoordination follow. In the terminal phase, the muscle paralysis becomes more severe, and the victim has difficulty in breathing (the usual cause of death). The prognosis is favorable if the individual survives the first twelve hours. Among 409 cases in one series of paralytic shellfish poisonings, the fatality rate was 8.5 percent, although recent cases reported to the U.S. Center for Disease Control were without fatalities. Two of these fifty-five cases did require respiratory support for a time.

Outbreaks of paralytic shellfish poisoning have occurred in various locations around the world. The dinoflagellates tend to bloom in waters above 30 degrees north and below 30 degrees south latitude. Most outbreaks in the Northern Hemisphere occur between May and October, when the temperature of the water is the highest. Thus, the adage that cautions against eating shellfish during the months without an "r" has some truth to it, although September and October are also dangerous months.

There is no specific treatment (obviously supportive care) except to induce vomiting. Thus, prevention is the key. Despite folk tales to the contrary, it is not possible to distinguish toxic from edible mollusks. As with fish poisoning, cooking does not inactivate the toxin.

It is important to differentiate paralytic shellfish poisoning from two other types of shellfish disease. Bacterial shellfish poisoning is a nonspecific food poisoning due to spoilage. The symptoms are due to the bacteria, not to the shellfish, so they are precisely the same as those of bacterial food poisoning acquired from other foods. Erythematous shellfish poisoning is an allergic reaction to the high iodine content of the shellfish. Within a few hours there is redness (erythema), swelling, and blotches over the face and neck, sometimes spreading to the rest of the body, and itching may be intense.

Additional Caveats

In addition to the common fish poisons listed above, some species of fish have toxic blood, others toxic roe, and still others have poisonous livers. As a general rule, never eat the viscera (internal organs) of any fish.

Bacterial food poisoning is caused by numerous bacteria and generally occurs either by infection or by toxins the bacteria produce. Salmonella is the most common example of an infection. Any food, especially meat, poultry, and dairy products, may transmit salmonella, or the foods may be contaminated by food handlers. After an incubation period of eight to forty-eight hours, the victim experiences nausea, abdominal pain, and loose, watery diarrhea. Symptoms usually subside in two to five days. Antibiotics are usually not necessary. Although salmonella is relatively resistant to heat, thorough cooking kills most strains. Inadequate refrigeration of contaminated foods allows the organisms to multiply. Therefore, thorough cooking and prompt refrigeration diminish the chances. Avoid milk that has not been pasteurized. Staphylococcal (staph) food poisoning is due to contamination by food handlers. Pastries, custards, dairy products, and meats subjected to improper refrigeration are the common offenders. Symptoms typically appear one to six hours after ingestion due to a toxin the staph has already produced. The onset is abrupt, with severe nausea, vomiting, abdominal pain, and diarrhea. The symptoms last less than twenty-four hours, and no treatment is necessary. Cooking has no effect on the toxin once it is produced.

One other annoyance of which the cruising sailor should beware regards parasitic diseases. These diseases are especially prevalent in the developing areas of the world, which include many of our most idyllic cruising grounds. Freshwater fish are capable of transmitting both liverflukes and fish tapeworm. Beef is liable to harbor the beef tapeworm, and pork remains a hazard for both pork tapeworm and trichinosis. Fortunately, thorough cooking destroys all of these organisms. Smoking or marinating does not offer any guarantee of safety. Therefore, no matter how the sailor prefers his or her food at home, in foreign countries he or she should eat all freshwater fish, beef, and pork well cooked.

Notes

1. It is a great temptation to break off a piece of coral to take home as a souvenir. Don't! Not only will you irreparably mar the beauty of the reef, but you will also find that coral transports very poorly. After all, within the calcium-carbonate matrix there is living organic matter that will putrefy. The only coral that is proper souvenir material is dead coral washed up on shore. It can be recognized by the bone-white color, which signifies the absence of living polyps.

2. https://commons.wikimedia.org/w/index.php?curid=2909974.

3. A number of factors determine the degree of hazard for man. In many species, the nematocyst is incapable of penetrating human skin, whereas in others it can penetrate with a vengeance. The toxicity also varies. True coral, as we have seen, does possess nematocysts, but they are not dangerous, producing at most a mild burning sensation. At the other extreme is the deadly sea wasp, *Chironex fleckeri*, which is capable of killing a person in less than thirty seconds. The amount of venom and the length of contact are also important. Although each nematocyst contains only a tiny amount of venom, contact with one or two tentacles of a jellyfish or a Portuguese man-of-war can easily activate thousands or hundreds of thousands of nematocysts—a formidable venom apparatus!

4. https://commons.wikimedia.org/wiki/File:Avispa_marina_cropped.png.

5. https://en.wikipedia.org/wiki/Portuguese_man_o%27_war#/media/File:Portuguese_Man-O-War_(Physalia_physalis).jpg.

6. https://commons.wikimedia.org/w/index.php?curid=5652099.

7. I. Berling and G. Isbister, "Marine Envenomations," *Australian Family Physician* 44, no. 1-2 (2015): 28-32.

8. Seqires, a CSL company formerly The Commonwealth Serum Laboratories, in Melbourne, Australia, manufactures the antivenin for sea wasp stings. Anyone contemplating an extended cruise of Australian waters would be well advised to obtain the antivenom in advance.

9. https: //en. wikipedia.org/wiki/Fire_coral#/media/File:Millepora_alcicornis_ (Branching Fire_Coral).jpg.

10. From Ernst Haeckel, *Kunstformen der Natur* [Art Forms in Nature] (Leipzig, Germany: Verlag des Bibliographisches Institut, 1904). If you are intrigued by the beautiful illustration by

Ernst Haeckel, you can view additional illustrations by visiting the website https://publicdomain-review.org.

11. https://commons.wikimedia.org/wiki/File:NSRW_Sea_Urchins_and_Star_Fish.jpg.

12. A case from a few years ago is typical. A man was diving in Guam when he picked up a cone shell and put it in his shirt sleeve. He continued diving, never realizing that he had been stung. After an hour he felt numb and weak and was immediately taken to a hospital, but he died en route.

13. https://en.m.wikipedia.org/wiki/File:Cone_shells_by_Chenu.png.

14. Struan and John Sutherland, *Venomous Creatures of Australia: A Field Guide with Notes on First Aid*, 5th ed. (Oxford: Oxford University Press, 2006).

15. Picture redrawn from the work of Dr. Struan Sutherland.

16. https://commons.wikimedia.org/wiki/File:Variable_ring_patterns on mantles of the blue-ringed_octopus_Hapalochlaena_lunulata.png.

17. Steve Irwin, the famed naturalist and conservationist, was killed in a freak accident by a stingray that was swimming beneath him and attacked him unprovoked. He presumably was mistaken for a predator. The tail barb penetrated his chest, and he presumably died instantly from massive chest trauma rather than anything to do with envenomation. All injuries to the trunk (chest or abdomen) require urgent hospitalization.

18. https://en.wikipedia.org/wiki/Yellow-bellied_sea_snake#/media/File:Pelamis_platura, Costa Rica.jpg.

19. http://en.wikipedia.org/wiki/Stone_fish.

20. Scott Gallagher, "Lionfish and Stonefish Envenomation Treatment and Management," Medscape, January 13, 2017, https://emedicine.medscape.com/article/770764-treatment.

21. https://commons.wikimedia.org/w/index.php?curid=52713408.

22. International Shark Attack File, "Yearly Worldwide Shark Attack Summary," *Florida Museum*, February 15, 2019, https://www.floridamuseum.ufl.edu/shark-attacks/yearly-worldwide-summary/.

23. Sharks have been described as "beasts without a bone in their bodies or a brain in their heads," a statement not far from the truth. The skeleton of sharks (as well as of the closely related rays and skates) is composed entirely of cartilage without any true bones, a primitive but fuel-efficient arrangement. And although the shark brain is exceedingly small—and two-thirds of that is devoted entirely to the sense of smell—the shark more than compensates for any "intellectual deficiencies" with an exceptional ability to analyze and synthesize environmental stimuli.

24. For distances up to about 50 feet (15 meters), vision is the primary sensory organ. Ridiculous claims have been made in the past that the shark has poor vision, due in part to the myth that the shark has to be led to its prey by pilot fish. Pure nonsense. There is nothing to suggest that most, if not all, of the potentially dangerous species have anything less than excellent vision. Of course, individual sharks may be farsighted or nearsighted, just as some humans have less than perfect eyesight. In addition to its vision, the shark's sense of smell is acute. It allows the detection of food or blood in the water at levels as dilute as a few parts per billion or less! Sharks are also endowed with taste buds and chemical skin receptors to analyze changes in the chemical composition of the water. For distances greater than 50 feet, the shark depends on its acute sense of smell, its hearing apparatus, and a group of low-frequency vibration detectors, which are sensitive to vibrations that a struggling fish or a person swimming might make in the water from as far away as a third of a mile or more.

There are two different types of feeding patterns common to most species. The first is the normal feeding pattern. Sometimes the movements are slow and determined, whereas at other times they are rapid and erratic. The final attack varies with the species and the circumstances. Frequently, a circling pattern around the victim presages the final attack, but this may be absent. When there is a sudden large quantity of food or a catastrophic event, such as an explosion, plane crash, or vessel sinking, a feeding frenzy—the second feeding pattern—may develop. Numerous sharks congregate and their movement becomes absolutely manic! They snap at everything in sight; cannibalism is frequent under these circumstances. The chances of a human surviving in the midst of a feeding frenzy are remote.

25. https://en.wikipedia.org/wiki/Morayeel#/media/File:Spottedmoray_eel.jpg.

26. https://en.wikipedia.org/wiki/Manta_ray#/media/File:Manta_alfredi_at_a_%E2%80%98cleaningstation%E2%80%99-journal.pone.0046170.g002B.jpg.

27. https://upload.wikimedia.org/wikipedia/commons/thumb/3/37/Killerwhales_jumping.jpg/1024px-Killerwhales_jumping.jpg.

28. R. A. Caras, *Dangerous to Man* (New York: Holt, Rinehart, and Winston, 1975).

29. D. Robertson, *Survive the Savage Sea* (New York: Praeger, 1973).

30. M. Bailey and M. Bailey, *Staying Alive* (New York: McKay, 1974).

31. https://upload.wikimedia.org/wikipedia/commons/thumb/5/52/Giant_Clam_%28Tridacna_gigas%29_%286058446919%29.jpg/1024px-Giant_Clam_%28Tridacna_gigas%29_%286058446919%29.jpg.

32. W. Van Dorn, *Oceanography and Seamanship* (New York: Dodd, Mead, 1974).

33. M.A. Friedman, L.E. Fleming, M. Fernandez, et al. "Ciguatera Fish Poisoning: Treatment, Prevention and Management. Mar. Drugs 2008, 6, 456-479; DOI: 10.3390/md20080022

34. Some tribes feed a portion of the fish in question to a pet cat or dog, and if the animal does not show signs of toxicity in a few hours (or better yet, overnight), they eat the fish. A variation of this technique could be called "trial by swallow" or perhaps "potluck." Since the degree of toxicity is related to the amount of fish consumed, one person can eat a small portion of the fish and wait several hours or overnight to see what happens. In the absence of any ciguatera symptoms, the fish is probably safe to eat. This is most certainly NOT recommended by the author!

35. https://en.wikipedia.org/wiki/Tetraodontidae#/media/File:Arothron_meleagris_byNPS.jpg.

36. B. W. Halstead, *Poisonous and Venomous Marine Animals of the World* (Princeton: Darwin, 1978).

37. https://en.wikipedia.org/wiki/Tetrodotoxin.

38. V Bane, "Tetrodotoxin: Chemistry, Toxicity, Source, Distribution and Detection," *Toxins* 6 (2014): 693-755, doi:10.3990/toxins6020693.

39. Halstead, *Poisonous and Venomous Marine Animals*.

40. P. Stratta and G. Baldino, "Scombroid Poisoning," *Canadian Medical Association Journal*, 184, no. 6 (2012): 674, doi:10.1503/cmaj.111031.

41. Although red is the most common discoloration, plankton blooms may be yellow, green, brown, black, or milky-white.

Chapter 7

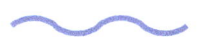

Voyaging and the "Sea Diseases"

"For the number of seamen in time of war who die of shipwreck, capture, famine, fire or sword are but inconsiderable in respect of such as are destroyed by the ship diseases, and by the usual maladies of intemperate climate."
—*Scottish Naval Surgeon James Lind (1716-1794)*

"The pessimist complains about the wind; the optimist expects it to change; the realist adjusts the sails."
—William Arthur Ward

Historians of seafaring nations and peoples have unflaggingly chronicled the heroic adventures and brave deeds of the nautical community. But for the common sailor, the perils of battle, storm, or shipwreck were minor compared to the danger of the *sea diseases*. Until recent times, the sea diseases, or *ship diseases*, as they were also known, routinely decimated the sailing ranks. During the eighteenth century, for example, one in seven sailors stationed in the Caribbean died annually of these diseases, and one in fifteen was constantly on the sick list.

What were the sea diseases? The three major categories were *scurvy*, the *fevers*, and the *fluxes*. With the exception of scurvy, however, these disorders were not strictly associated with the sea. Even the early observers recognized that many were due to a "noxious land breeze." Today, most of these diseases would be classified as *tropical diseases*. Of course, until last century, the only way to get to the tropics was by sea.

Scurvy, a vitamin-C deficiency that afflicted sailors for hundreds of years, is discussed at length in Chapter 9. By the end of the eighteenth century, the Royal Navy had successfully mandated the routine use of lemon juice as an antiscorbutic.

The *fevers* included a number of communicable diseases that were not always readily differentiated from one another and so were grouped together. One of the most devastating of these fevers was *typhus*. It killed two thousand men of the first English fleet sent to America in 1756. We now recognize that body lice transmit the disease. The eighteenth-century naval custom of sending out press-gangs to "recruit" the more unfortunate members of society guaranteed a constant supply of vermin-infested clothing, and the hideous overcrowding of ships assured the spread of lice among crew members.[1] Although typhus still exists (primarily in mountainous regions in the developing world), the risk for sailors is now minuscule. In fact, no American traveler has contracted typhus since 1950. The other fevers that posed a threat, and continue to threaten us, include *malaria* (previously known as the "ague"), *yellow fever* (or the "black vomit"), and *typhoid fever*.

The *fluxes*, or diarrhea, usually afflicted men debilitated after long periods at sea or convalescing from one of the fevers or another illness. The outbreaks, which often reached epidemic proportions, were due to a variety of causes, including *cholera*, *amebic* and *bacillary dysentery* (shigellosis), *viral enteritis*, *salmonella*, and even *staphylococcal* food poisoning. Although the fluxes had a lower mortality rate than the fevers, they could be devastating. Soon after the defeat of the Spanish Armada, the English crews were so affected by acute enteritis that "many of the ships have hardly enough men to waie [weigh] their anchors."[2] Had the post-Armada epidemic occurred somewhat earlier, this book might have been written in Spanish!

Today, the risk of acquiring illness generally depends on geography. Travelers in developing countries are at greater risk of contracting an illness than those traveling in developed areas. In most developed countries, the risk is no greater than that incurred while traveling throughout the United States. Canada, Australia, New Zealand, Japan, and Western Europe are considered to be in that category. In Africa, Asia, South and Central America, the South Pacific, the Middle East, and the Far East, living conditions and standards of sanitation and hygiene vary considerably. Travel to major tourist areas entails less exposure to food and water of questionable quality and consequently poses a smaller risk for contracting an unwanted illness. As sailors, we frequently venture into smaller cities, towns, and ports for provisioning, which may be off the usual tourist beat. Therefore, additional vigilance is often in order. This chapter contains recommendations regarding vaccination and prophylaxis for sailors traveling to various parts of the world. One key concept when thinking about these diseases is *risk*. Ask yourself: Who is at risk? How great is the risk? Who is going to bear the risk?

Quarantinable Diseases

From another point of view, all of the sea diseases (or tropical diseases) fall into two groups, depending on *whose interests are being protected*. The first group consists of quarantinable diseases; the second, and much larger group, are nonquarantinable. Quarantinable diseases are those from which *various countries are trying to protect themselves*.

The word *quarantine* comes from the seventeenth-century Venetian for *quaranta giorni*, which means forty days. Because of fear of the plague, ships arriving in Venice from infected ports were required to sit at anchor for forty days before crew and passengers could disembark. In the United States, outbreaks of yellow fever prompted Congress to pass federal quarantine legislation in 1878. We still have active quarantine laws and regulations in the United States. The Secretary of Health and Human Services is "authorized to take measures to prevent the entry and spread of communicable diseases from foreign countries into the United States." The authority for carrying out these functions has been delegated to the Centers for Disease Control and Prevention (CDC). Isolation and quarantine help protect the public:[3]

- *Isolation* separates sick people with a contagious disease from people who are not sick.
- *Quarantine* separates and restricts the movement of people who were exposed to a contagious disease in order to see if they become sick.

Federal isolation and quarantine are authorized for the following communicable diseases: cholera, diphtheria, infectious tuberculosis, plague, smallpox, yellow fever, viral hemorrhagic fevers (like Ebola), severe acute respiratory syndrome, and influenza that could cause a pandemic.

Although the concept of quarantine is less common around the world, it affects the nautical community in two ways.

First, a number of countries have strict rules concerning people who have been in countries where there might be exposure to yellow fever. If travelers have been in a country that is known to have outbreaks of yellow fever, then they must be able to present evidence of vaccination, documented and stamped on a page in the International Certificate of Vaccination.[4] This even applies to travelers who have transited through a yellow fever country without leaving the airport. The traveler may be barred entry or have to undergo a period of quarantine—perhaps a week—before entering the country. So, we need to know our most likely itinerary *in advance* in order to obtain necessary immunizations to avoid refusal or quarantine.[5]

A second issue pertains to animals carried on board. Many boaters carry pets on board, and those planning to take an animal to a foreign country must meet the entry requirements of the destination country (as well as the transportation guidelines of the airline). Any animal may be restricted from entry into the United States if there is reasonable knowledge that there is a risk to human health. There are specific CDC restrictions for dogs, cats, turtles, nonhuman primates, African rodents, civets, and bats as well as products made from them. The main issue is with dogs. A rabies vaccination is required for all dogs entering the United States from a country where rabies is present. Dogs must be accompanied by a current, valid rabies vaccination certificate. Countries around the world are designated in the following categories:

- Rabies-Free Countries
- Rabies-Controlled (Third) Countries
- High-Rabies Countries

For a further discussion of pet movement from one of the above designated categories to one of the others (and it is rather involved), visit the PetTravel.com website (http://www.pettravel.com/).

From a practical point of view, the sailor is not likely to contract and carry any of the quarantinable diseases! The major reason for being vaccinated against them is to facilitate entry into a country. Without a valid vaccination certificate, you may be denied entry or be quarantined (and you might not want to be quarantined in any country that would quarantine you).

International Nautical Travel

The previous section on quarantine dealt with a country attempting to limit the risk to its citizens from infected people (and other animals) bringing infections with them on entry. The country limits its risk by forcing the entering party to provide proof (e.g., an International Certificate of Vaccination) that they are not bringing in "trouble."

This section focuses on the need to decide the risk *you* are willing to take if you sail into foreign waters, or if you need to mitigate that risk with prior treatment or vaccination. Estimating the risk depends on having the most up-to-date information about which diseases you are likely to encounter. There are basically two approaches that make the most sense to me: either you and your physician go online to the CDC website (which has an online-accessible and interactive version of the *CDC Yellow Book* maintained with input from the Massachusetts General Hospital staff) or you make an appointment with a local travel clinic (which will base its recommendations—at least in part—on the information in the *CDC Yellow Book*, print or online version). The print edition has a great deal of additional information, although the online version may be more current.

Cholera

Just about the only identifiable "flux" that we share with sailors of yore is cholera, an acute bacterial infection of the intestines caused by some strains of *Vibrio Cholerae*. These bacteria are found in fresh and brackish water; cholera infections are most commonly acquired from drinking water. Cholera is endemic in Africa and Asia, although isolated epidemics, such as that which occurred in Haiti in 2010, will appear from time to time. From 2010 through 2014, 75 percent of cases returning to the United States were associated with travel to the Caribbean. Cholera most commonly manifests as watery diarrhea and is usually mild or asymptomatic unless dehydration occurs. The treatment is rehydration unless severe, in which case antibiotics are required. Doxycycline is often the first-line antibiotic for adults. Frequent handwashing and safe food and water precautions will limit the risk, and unless traveling to a known cholera region, vaccination is not necessary.

Traveler's Diarrhea

If cholera represents a relatively insignificant risk, the same cannot be said about traveler's diarrhea (TD). TD is the most common and predictable travel-related illness, with attack rates according to the CDC ranging from 30 percent to 70 percent of travelers depending on the season and destination. Most commonly, it is due to strains of bacteria with which the sailor's gastrointestinal (GI) tract is not familiar. These strains are indigenous to a particular area, and the local inhabitants have adapted to them. In Mexico, for example, certain strains of the common bacteria *E. coli* (different from those that normally colonize your GI tract) most often cause TD. In other ports of call, different foreign strains are responsible. What is common to all of these bacteria is that they elaborate a toxin similar in its effect to the toxin that cholera produces (although not as powerful). This toxin causes a loss of water and electrolytes (sodium, chloride, potassium, and bicarbonate) from the GI tract, resulting in diarrhea.

As mentioned, *bacteria* are the most common cause, especially strains of *E. coli* (enterotoxigenic strains), although other bacterial culprits include salmonella, shigella, campylobacter, and vibrio. *Viral* agents include the Norwalk virus (norovirus—of cruise ship fame), rotavirus, and enteroviruses. *Protozoa* causing TD include giardia, *Entamoeba histolytica*, and *Cryptosporidium parvum*.

The most important determinant of the risk is the destination, generally divided into three zones or levels:

Low-risk: United States, Canada, Northern and Western Europe, Australia, New Zealand, and Japan

Intermediate-risk: Caribbean islands, Eastern and Southern Europe, and South Africa

High-risk: Mexico, Central and South America, most of Asia, Africa, and the Middle East

TD symptoms range from looser watery stools, abdominal cramps, bloating, and nausea to severe abdominal pain, fever, vomiting, and bloody stools.

Bacterial toxins generally produce symptoms within a few hours. The incubation period for bacterial and viral organisms is six to seventy-two hours. Protozoa such as giardia have an incubation period of one to two weeks. Untreated bacterial diarrhea usually lasts three to seven days while viral lasts two to three days. Protozoal diarrhea may persist for weeks to months.

Minimizing the risk of TD includes careful food and beverage selection, scrupulous handwashing with soap, and the use of alcohol-based hand sanitizers, such as Purell, when soap and water are not available.

Healthy Boating & Sailing

Food and beverage selection are critical. Observe the following food recommendations.

- Avoid salads and raw leafy vegetables
- Avoid undercooked meat, fish, and shellfish
- Avoid raw food, especially seafood
- Avoid unpasteurized fruit juices and dairy products
- Avoid raw fruits that are eaten unpeeled (e.g., strawberries)
- Peal your own fruits
- Consider whether your unpeeled fruits have been injected with water to plump them up—and beware
- Eat fully cooked food (including eggs) when served hot, for maximum safety
- Fully reheat stored, cooked food
- Refrigerate perishable cooked food within one hour

Liquids can be just as risky and can contain the same TD-causing agents as discussed above, including bacteria, viruses, and parasites. Therefore, tap water in some places will be unsafe for drinking, cooking, making ice, preparing food, and even brushing your teeth. The following beverage precautions should be followed:

- Only use commercially bottled water or beverages from a sealed container
- Do not "purify" liquid with alcohol; only straight alcohol is fine
- Consider whether bottled beverages are sterilized, which may be impossible to ascertain—unopened, factory-sealed bottles or cans, fruit drinks, and pasteurized drinks may or may not be safe
- Wipe liquid outside a bottle or can before drinking from it
- Do not drink fountain drinks or anything else with ice
- Assume that hot coffee or tea are fine to drink

Small quantities of water may be sanitized by either boiling, adding chemicals, or filtering. Betadine (10 percent povidone-iodine), iodine tablets, and bleach (sodium hypochlorite) can be moderately effective in a pinch and in limited quantities.[6] However, if you are boating in "interesting" waters, you should have a watermaker (see also the discussion in Chapter 4). Watermakers are now very affordable and come in units varying from manual operation, through portable generator-run units, all the way to installed units of a size and complexity to meet the needs of your vessel and crew. One major advantage of a watermaker is that the semipermeable membrane that is at the heart of the unit will produce clear, safe drinkable water free of particulate matter, bacteria, viruses, and parasites.[7] It functions by "reverse osmosis"—the opposite of typical osmosis—by transferring water molecules from a higher concentration to a lower concentration.

Finally, avoid recreational water in medium- or high-risk areas since the same organisms are present in pools, water playgrounds, and saunas.

Prevention/Prophylaxis

The agent that has been used the longest is bismuth subsalicylate, contained in Pepto-Bismol and Kaopectate. It may provide some protection (up to 50 percent in one study in Mexico), but there are side effects—blackening of the tongue and stools, nausea, constipation, and tinnitus (because, like aspirin, it is a salicylate). In general, prophylactic antibiotics are not recommended.[8]

Signs and symptoms of dehydration

Moderate Dehydration	Severe Dehydration
Restlessness / irritable	Lethargy / unconscious
Sunken eyes	Weak or absent pulse
Dry mouth and tongue	Very dry mouth and tongue
Increased thirst	Low blood pressure
Skin goes back slowly when pinched	Skin goes back very slowly
Decreased urination and decreased tears	Minimal to no urine

Table 7.1 Signs and symptoms of dehydration (CDC)

Signs of Adequate Rehydration

- Pinched skin returns to normal
- Thirst subsides
- Urine flows
- Pulse strengthens

Treatment

(1) *Oral rehydration*. With mild cases, fluid replacement will make the sailor feel better. Sports drinks can be substituted, as these will partially replace electrolytes that are lost in the diarrhea. In moderate and more severe cases, oral rehydration is critical and sports drinks (those with high glucose levels) should not be used.

The easiest and most reliable method for rehydration is oral rehydration therapy. The most ubiquitous form comes in packets of oral rehydration salts, sold around the world (see Figure 7.1). These are rapidly dissolved powders that contain the correct amount of electrolytes and sugar (again, not too much) to rehydrate both children and adults. Since they are individually packaged, take up little space, and have a relatively long shelf life, they should be aboard every vessel that leaves the harbor for points unknown. The proper amount of water is listed on the package. The water in all of these recipes must be pure. If uncertain, it should first be boiled and then left to cool.

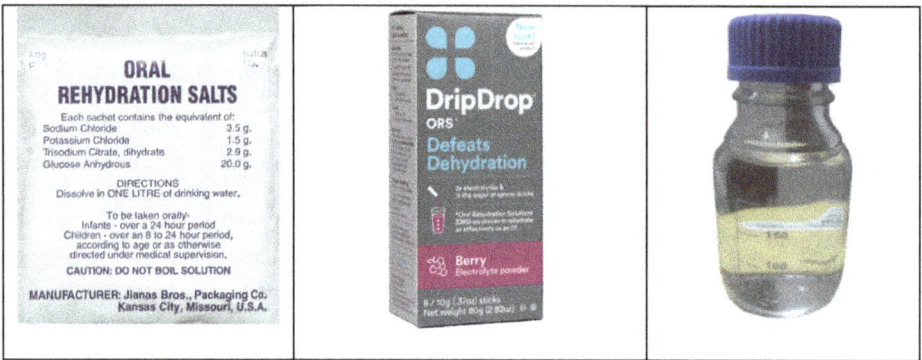

Figure 7.1 Packets, powders, and simple mixtures of oral rehydration salts

Another approach is the two-glass method:

(1) Prepare two separate glasses with the ingredients listed in Table 7.2.
(2) Drink alternately from each glass. Water, tea, or carbonated beverages can supplement, but most of the replacement fluids should be from these two glasses.

Glass No. 1	
Fruit juice (e.g. orange or apple)	8 ounces (1/4 L)
This is rich in potassium→	
Honey or corn syrup	½ teaspoon (2.5mL)
Glucose, essential for absorption (not too much) →	
Table salt	1 pinch
Table salt is sodium chloride →	

Glass No. 2	
Water (carbonated or boiled)	8 ounces (1/4 L)
Baking Soda (sodium bicarbonate)	¼teaspoon 1.25mL)

Table 7.2 Ingredients for two-glass oral rehydration

Alternatively, the World Health Organization has recommended a simple approach with water, salt, and sugar. Simply add 1/2 teaspoon of table salt (sodium chloride) and 6 teaspoons of granulated sugar to 1 liter (5 cups @ 200 milliliters) of clean water. Stir well until all is dissolved. Be careful to mix the correct amounts. Making the solution a little too diluted is not harmful.

Moderately dehydrated adults should drink 4 liters (quarts) or more in the first four to six hours. Children should be given a cup or so of whatever oral rehydration salts are available every hour.

(2) *Antimotility drugs.* These provide symptomatic relief and include loperidine (Imodium) and diphenoxylate (Lomotil). Previously it was felt that if the purging process could be controlled, the patient would quickly recover. A more recent approach holds that diarrhea is nature's way of ridding the body of both the toxin(s) and the bacteria that produce it; as a result, diarrhea should be allowed to continue, *provided the fluid can be replaced.* If antidiarrhea agents are used, they should be used with caution and never for more than two to three days. Using these agents with an antibiotic makes the most sense.

(3) *Antibiotics.* Yes, for severe cases, antibiotics are recommended, especially if there is fever, pus, or blood in the stool. These include fluoroquinolones, azithromycin, and rifaximin.[9]

Prevention and Vaccinations

In order to prepare for international travel, the boater needs to consider the following:

- Where you are traveling (your itinerary)
- Your age and state of health (hopefully fine)
- Your vaccination history (hopefully up to date)

Before considering recommendations for vaccinations for specific locations, you need to be certain your *routine vaccinations* are up to date. For example, what is your status regarding measles? *Measles, you ask?* That is a childhood disease, is it not? Well, yes many of us *mature* individuals have had measles in childhood. But, as I write this chapter, there are measles outbreaks in the United States, England, France, Greece, Italy, Israel, Columbia, and Brazil, among others. *The point is, you need to take care of your routine vaccinations before worrying about the "tropical diseases."* Let's review the basics one by one:

(1) Measles, mumps, rubella vaccine (MMR). If you were born before 1957, you are presumed to have lifelong immunity. Why? Because there were so many outbreaks before the advent of vaccines that everyone of that age is presumed to have immunity (of course if you were born before 1957 you may not remember!). If born after 1957, you should have had, as an adult, two doses of MMR. Evidence of immunity includes written documentation of immunization, laboratory evidence of immunity, or laboratory confirmation of the measles virus. Preteens should seek advice from their pediatrician.

(2) Shingles vaccine (Shingrix). This vaccine has, for the most part, replaced the older Zostavax. If you are over fifty, you should have two doses of Shingrix two to six months apart. The second dose imparts long-term immunity. Shingrix offers 90 percent protection from shingles and Zostavax only 51 percent. I have spent my career as a neurologist treating patients with post-shingles pain (postherpetic neuralgia). Trust me, you don't want that to ruin your trip, or your life. Please discuss with your provider.

(3) Tetanus, diphtheria, pertussis vaccine (Tdap or Td; there are a number of varieties and some without pertussis, or whooping cough). Adults should obtain Tdap or Td every ten years (if you are around newborns, get the vaccine with pertussis). Infants, preteens, and teens should consult their pediatrician.

(4) Hepatitis A vaccine. This is a viral disease where the virus is excreted in the stool and transmitted from person to person: therefore, the same precautions for traveler's diarrhea apply to Hepatitis A. Hepatitis A is a usually a self-limited disease lasting up to a few months, although relapses of hepatitis may occur for up to nine months. It is found throughout the world except for in Northern Europe and North America. One dose of the vaccine offers protection. Should you obtain it if you are traveling beyond Europe or North America? It is among the common vaccine-preventable travel-related diseases, so it's something to consider. It's one of those conundrums to discuss with your provider.

(5) Flu and pneumococcal vaccines. Flu is worldwide, so it makes sense to obtain a flu shot when available. And if you are sixty-five or older, the pneumococcal vaccine is a must.

Now let's get down to the hardcore nuts and bolts of travel medicine. As nautical types, we fall into at least three categories with different needs: those whose boating is restricted to low-risk areas such as Northern Europe or the United States/Canada; those whose boating is local or regional in whatever risk area; and finally those whose sailing takes them to distant shores (and this would include some folks on cruise ships). The first group need not worry so much about extra vaccinations, but they should still follow through with their routine vaccinations. The second group usually is familiar with the local and regional risks, but the third group is the one that needs to pay the most attention, and who would benefit the most from a travel medicine clinic.

The two diseases that are a concern worldwide are yellow fever and malaria.

Yellow Fever

Yellow fever is a viral disease transmitted by mosquitoes to humans, with humans (and primates in Africa) then serving as hosts. The disease is spread when a mosquito bites a human, transmitting the virus, which then multiplies in the human, causing disease. When that infected human with viremia (lots of virus particles) is bitten by a second mosquito, the virus is spread when that infected mosquito bites a second individual. So, there is human-to mosquito-to-human spread. For people infected, they develop symptoms after three to six days. Initially it appears to be a nonspecific illness with headache, fever, chills, nausea, vomiting, and myalgia. Most patients will improve, but about 15 percent progress to the serious form with jaundice, multisystem organ failure, shock, and death. The mortality rate for those who progress is 20 to 50 percent, according to the CDC.

Yellow fever occurs mostly in sub-Saharan Africa and tropical South America (see Figures 7.2 and 7.3). Realistically, not many sailors will be travelling to the sub-Saharan African coasts. (Those who do—good luck and Godspeed to you—should first attend a travel medicine clinic.)

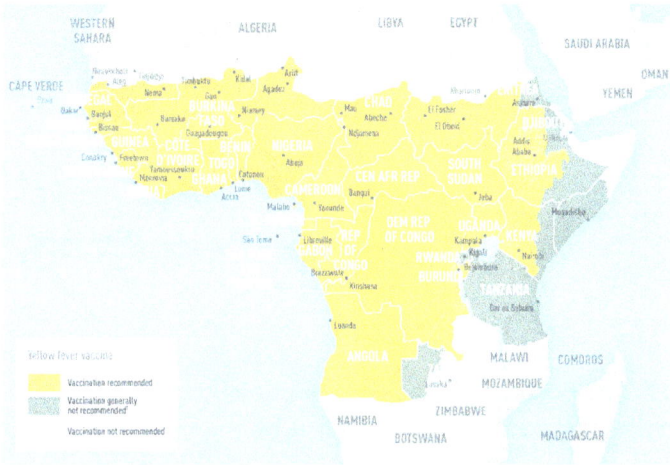

Figure 7.2 Yellow fever in Sub-Saharan Africa

The same is not true of Central and South America. Countries with a risk of yellow fever include Argentina, Bolivia, Brazil, Columbia, Ecuador, French Guiana, Guyana, Panama, Paraguay, Peru, Suriname, Trinidad and Tobago, and Venezuela (only a portion of these countries may be affected as opposed to the entire country). Figure 7.3 demonstrates precisely why you need to obtain not only the latest edition of the CDC's *Yellow Book* but also the most up-to-date, online information possible. Let's look at the coast of Brazil. Until an outbreak in 2017, the coast of Brazil was free of yellow fever. In fact, on the 2018 map, the peach-colored area along the shore is light gray—an area designated "vaccination not recommended." Fast-forward to today and you will find that it is currently "vaccination recommended."

The yellow fever vaccine consists of one dose and is both safe and effective. However, prevention is still critical. All steps need to be taken to protect against mosquito bites:

- Be aware of peak exposure times and places
- Wear long-sleeved shirts, pants, and socks
- If possible, wear clothing treated with permethrin (wash separately)
- Use bed nets if sleeping area is not screened or air conditioned
- Apply one of the following repellents to exposed skin

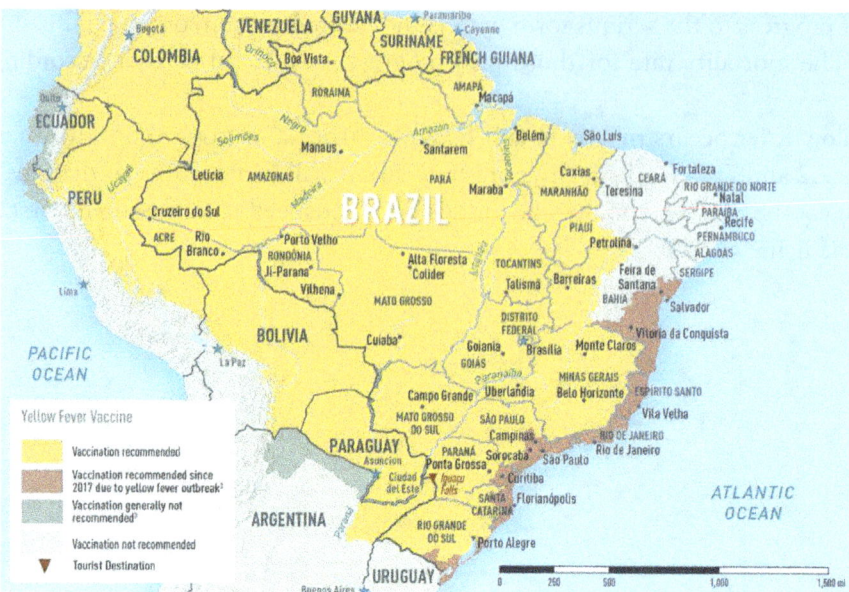

Figure 7.3 Yellow fever in Brazil

1. DEET: The possibility of adverse reactions can be minimized if the following precautions are taken as recommended by the CDC: apply repellent sparingly only to exposed skin or clothing; avoid applying high-concentration products to the skin, particularly on children; do not inhale or ingest repellents or get them into the eyes; avoid applying repellents to portions of children's hands that are likely to have contact with eyes or mouth; never use repellents on wounds or irritated skin; wash repellent-treated skin after coming indoors; and if a suspected reaction to insect repellent occurs, wash treated skin and seek medical attention.
2. Picaridin
3. Oil of lemon eucalyptus (OLE or PMD)
4. IR3535
5. 2-undecanone

Malaria

Malaria is another mosquito-born disease, and the same precautions listed for yellow fever are relevant for malaria prevention. Malaria is widespread, and although the overall prevalence has been slowly declining worldwide, the number of affected travelers has been relatively steady. It is caused by several species of *Plasmodium*, a parasite that infects red blood cells. It is usually transmitted to humans through the bite of an infected anopheles mosquito. Headache, malaise, fever, chills, and sweats, which may occur at intervals, are symptoms of the disease. There may be anemia and jaundice, and in the case of one malarial species, *Plasmodium falciparum*, even heart or kidney failure, coma, and death. Deaths due to malaria are preventable. Symptoms may appear as early as seven days after initial exposure, although usually after fourteen days. Suspected cases represent a medical emergency requiring urgent intervention especially with cases involving *Plasmodium falciparum*. Everyone, regardless of age, who enters an area where the risk exists for malaria transmission should take prophylactic medication, even for visits as brief as one night. The anopheles mosquito is mainly out feeding in the evening and night, so take maximum protection from dusk through dawn. If possible, anchor offshore and use netting and all possible mosquito protection. Clothing should be loose, and cover the entire body, including the extremities. See the section on yellow fever for personal mosquito repellents.

In 2013, there were more than 1,700 cases of malaria diagnosed in the United States and documented by the CDC, resulting in ten deaths. Of these cases, 82 percent were acquired in Africa; 11 percent of the cases resulted from exposure in Asia; 6 percent in the Caribbean, Central America, and South America; and 1 percent in Oceania (Polynesia, Micronesia, and Melanesia). See Figures 7.4 and 7.5 from the CDC for more detail. The risk of acquiring disease is not uniform from country to country or even within countries, and it frequently changes from year to year. It depends on local conditions, such as mosquito density, prevalence of infection, weather, and altitude. Since the pattern of malaria changes frequently, available information should be used with caution. Seek the most up-to-date information from the CDC or your local travel medicine center.

You may consider choosing a medication for malaria prophylaxis. There are a number of factors that need to be considered in selecting a chemoprophylactic regimen, including:

- Whether the travel itinerary will place the sailor at risk of acquiring malaria, especially the more serious *Plasmodium falciparum* form
- What the underlying health of the boater is and what medications they take for other conditions (which could interfere with the malarial medications)
- Whether there has been a prior allergic or other reaction to antimalarial drugs
- Whether or not medical care will be readily accessible during voyage

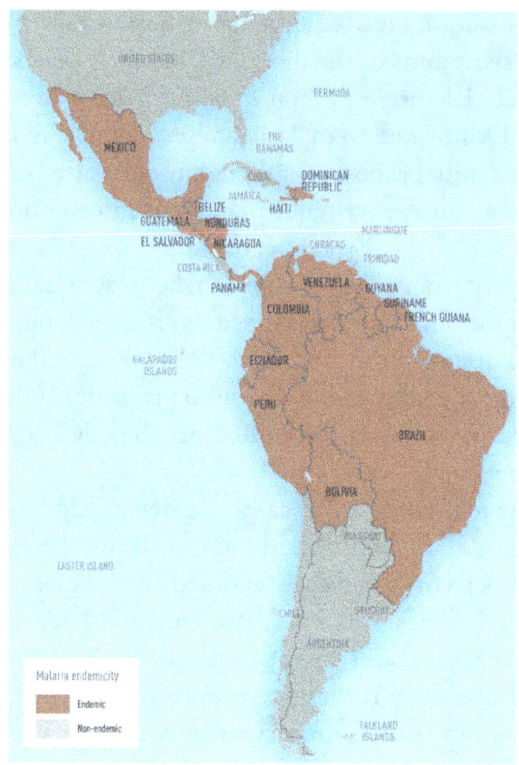

Figure 7.4 Malaria in Central America and South America

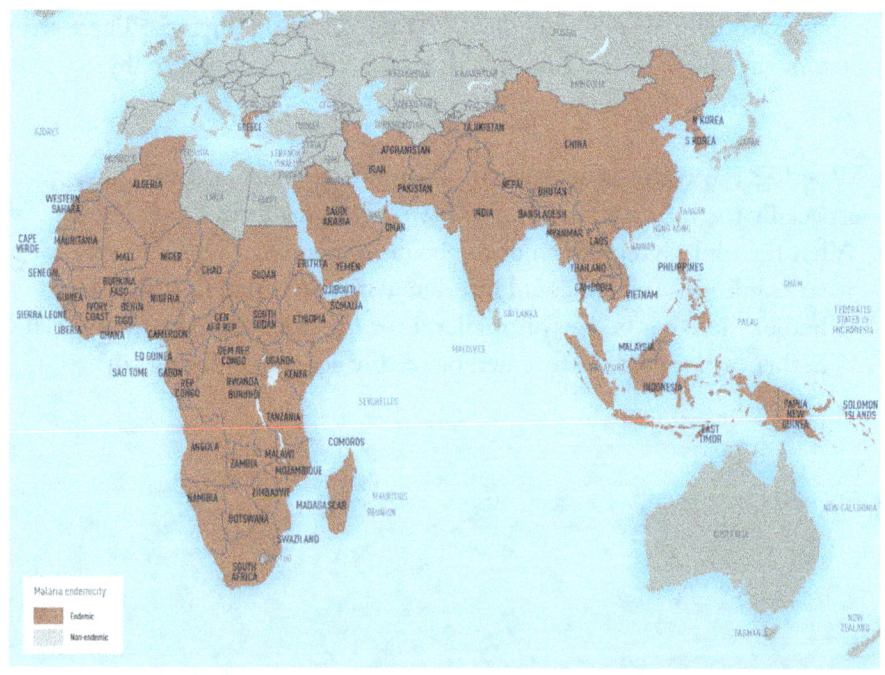

Figure 7.5 Malaria in Africa and Asia

Chloroquine was one of the initial recommendations for malaria prophylaxis but, alas, resistance has developed and there are fewer places in the world (certain locations in Central America, the Caribbean, and the Middle East) where it is still effective. Other medications that are now available and effective include:

- Mefloquine
- Doxycycline
- Proguanil
- Malarone

Because some of these medications, such as mefloquine, must be started weeks before weighing anchor, you must plan ahead. Personally, I believe that if you are planning on travelling to any of these areas you should make an appointment and follow the advice of a travel medicine clinic. You need a detailed plan for both yourself and your crew.

Final Thoughts

Risk. Of course, all life is risk. And as boaters we are used to assessing risk on a daily basis. To mitigate risk, we check the weather forecast, we top off our tanks before departure, and we file a float plan, among other things. But nevertheless, risk is always there. Dr. David R. Shlim has a thoughtful perspective entitled "Travelers' Perception of Risk" in the *Yellow Book 2018* print edition.[10] He notes that there is a great deal of subjectivity involved in the perception of risk even when it has been calculated and is known precisely. As he states: "15 per 100,000 means it's dangerous" to some people whereas to others "it may be 15 per 100,000, but it's worth it." In addition, as Daniel Kahneman has pointed out, we often don't even bother to take the time and the mental effort to estimate or calculate our risk ("thinking slow"); we just proceed with our gut reaction ("thinking fast").[11]

I believe that the perception of risk problem Dr. Shlim refers to is hardwired into our central nervous system. (Hardwired doesn't mean it can't be rewired.) For example, skydiving is way too risky for me but an exciting, not-overly-risky experience for my son—which he of course shared only after he did it.

But the mental laziness of thinking "fast," which is often equivalent to not thinking at all, is something we can fix. We need to arm ourselves with the best available information and then take the time to make the best estimation or calculation of our risk.

Only then, with the relevant information in hand from your travel medicine center or the CDC, can you begin to deal with the subjective perception of risk. As a captain of the vessel, it is your responsibility to think "slow" and calculate the risk, realizing that others, for example your passengers or crew, may perceive the same risk very differently, indeed.

Notes

1. There was a perverse logic in the once-common practice of packing and overcrowding the ship. Sea diseases routinely decimated the crew, but there were already extra bodies so the loss to disease didn't make much difference. It was not realized until much later that overcrowding actually hastened the spread of these diseases.

2. L. H. Roddis, *A Short History of Nautical Medicine* (New York: Hoeber, 1941), 125.

3. *CDC Yellow Book 2018: Health Information for International Travel* (New York: Oxford University Press, 2017).

4. International Certificate of Vaccination or Prophylaxis

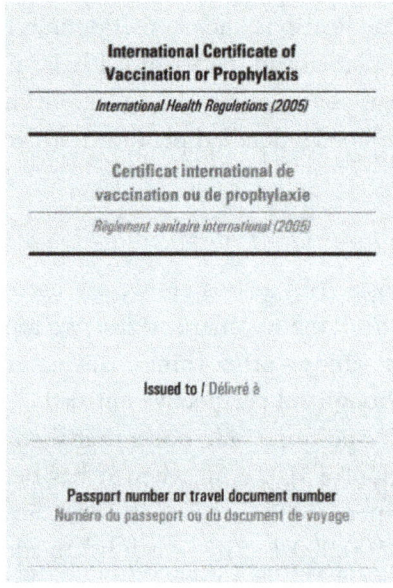

5. Travelers must realize that the entire journey determines what documentation and immunization are required for the trip. The site is most effective if you have the entire itinerary already planned out.

6. The excellent text by E. A. Weiss and M. E. Jacobs entitled *Marine Medicine: A Comprehensive Guide* (Seattle: The Mountaineers Books, 2012) contains tables concerning the use of iodine liquid and tablets as well as the use of bleach (sodium hypochlorite). Highly recommended as a nautical first aid text.

7. It is recommended that the unit preferentially operate away from polluted waters, as some of the oil residue in the water may damage the membrane. It will operate virtually anywhere, however.

8. *CDC Yellow Book 2018*, p. 51.

9. *CDC Yellow Book 2018*, p. 53, Table 2-6.

10. *CDC Yellow Book 2018*, p. 25.

11. D. Kahneman, *Thinking, Fast and Slow* (New York: Farrar, Straus, and Giroux, 2011).

Chapter 8

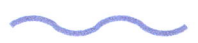

Sailing Vision

*"The sea never changes, and its works,
for all the talk of men, are wrapped in mystery."*
—*Joseph Conrad,* Typhoon, *1902*

*"I must go down to the sea again, to the lonely sea and the sky.
And all I ask is a tall ship and a star to steer her by."*
—John Masefield

Imagine yourself in a pea-soup fog on a moonless night off a lee shore. What is your response to this situation? Well, depending on your experience, it falls somewhere between anxiety and terror! We can never feel entirely at ease on the water when deprived of our most valuable sense—vision. It doesn't matter how much we surround ourselves with modern electronic gadgetry; we are never comfortable until we can *see* the lighted buoy that marks the shoal or channel. This example serves to highlight the pre-eminence of vision in the day-to-day life of every mariner, be they boater or sailor, racer or cruiser, weekender or circumnavigator. From spotting a cat's paw or a buoy to finding the entrance to a coral reef, sailing is first and foremost a visual activity.

Despite the preeminence of vision, few sailors are familiar with anything but the rudiments of the human body's visual system. This is doubly unfortunate. First, the system is both sensitive and sophisticated, and the better we understand it, the more of its untapped resources we can use. Second, since it is sophisticated, we must be on guard lest we misunderstand what it is telling us. These misunderstandings or visual illusions are particularly common on the water.

The Grand Spectrum

Although we don't usually think about it, light has a precise definition. Light is energy from a specific portion of the electromagnetic spectrum that can stimulate the retina of the human eye.[1] To be precise, the human eye is only sensitive to radiation with wavelengths between about 400 and 700 nanometers (a nanometer is one-billionth of a meter.) Radiation of longer wavelengths comprises the infrared band, whereas shorter wavelengths produce ultraviolet (UV) radiation (see Figure 8.1). There is no a priori reason why the human eye should be limited to this narrow band—infrared, UV, and even X-ray vision are within nature's technical capabilities. There is, however, a simple evolutionary explanation: the wavelengths we perceive as light are *maximally transmissible through water*; shorter and longer wavelengths simply do not travel through water very well. Since our oceanic "ancestors" were not exposed to much infrared or UV radiation, there was no reason to develop receptors that were sensitive to either. Although the spectrum has shifted slightly since we came ashore and "dried out," by and large we respond to the same range of wavelengths as fish do.

Let us look more closely at the structure of light. If we could stop a wave of light for an instant, it would look something like Figure 8.1.

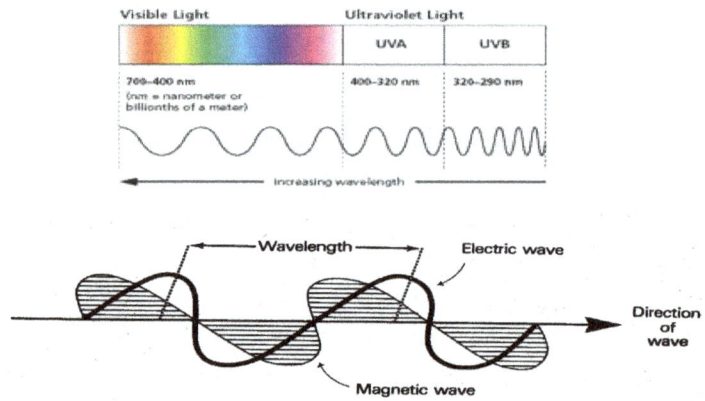

Figure 8.1 Electromagnetic wave from the visible light and UV spectrum

The wave is moving in the direction of the arrowhead, and perpendicular to it are the planes of the electric and magnetic fields. (The magnetic field is of no consequence for our purposes and can be ignored.) The direction of the electric field is important, for upon it depends the phenomenon of *polarization*. Figure 8.2 shows an end-on view of the electric fields in a beam of light.

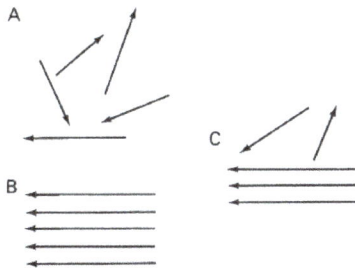

Figure 8.2 Polarized Light (A) unpolarized, (B) polarized, (C) partially polarized

The light in Figure 8.2A is *unpolarized*. All the waves of light are coming toward the observer (out of the plane of the paper), but the directions of the electric fields are random. In comparison, Figure 8.2B represents *polarized* light, and Figure 8.2C *partially polarized* light. Polarized and partially polarized light are produced in several circumstances. When sunlight is reflected from a regular surface such as water, it may be completely or partially polarized depending on the angle at which the light strikes the water; that is, the surface of the water acts to rearrange the electric fields of the light. For most surfaces, such as water or glass, the light becomes horizontally polarized as in Figure 8.2B.

Glare

While sailing, we are never confronted with completely polarized light because the reflecting surface is never perfectly smooth. But enough of the sunlight is polarized to interfere with the identification of objects. Before we consider how polarized light impedes visual discrimination, let us look at the larger problem of glare. The term *glare* is used to describe the effect of excessive light. This excessive light enters the eye and tends to wash out the contrast of what we are looking at, making it difficult or impossible to identify fine detail. Everyone is familiar with the need to pull down the shade when viewing a monitor or a television screen. In fact, during periods of glare, the eyes are receiving 10 to 100 times the amount of light they need to function optimally. Sometimes glare is solely the result of intense sunlight, but often light reflected from surfaces such as water makes a major contribution.

There are several practical responses to glare that interfere with vision. First, the pupils of the eyes constrict, automatically and almost instantaneously. Unfortunately, this response is not very effective. Even when the pupils are reduced to a tiny dot, they cannot eliminate much of the excess light. The next response is to eliminate some of the light by squinting. But there are problems with squinting. It is rather ineffectual, and if boaters squint for a prolonged period, they are likely to develop a headache. Rather than squinting, the sailor should wear a wide-brimmed hat or a visor. Of course, the most effective mechanism is to filter out some of the unnecessary light with sunglasses.

Sunglasses Technology

Sunglasses *technology*? Yes, the days of buying a pair of sunglasses based solely on how "cool" they look are long gone. And if you think all you have to worry about are UV light and polarization, think again. The more time you are on the water, the greater your need to take advantage of all of the technological advances that can now be *built into* your sunglasses. Since your vision is critical in everything you do on the water, and since sunlight will cause both acute and chronic changes to your vision, you need to pay attention; in fact, the earlier you pay attention the better, so that hopefully you do not end up with vision problems later in life.

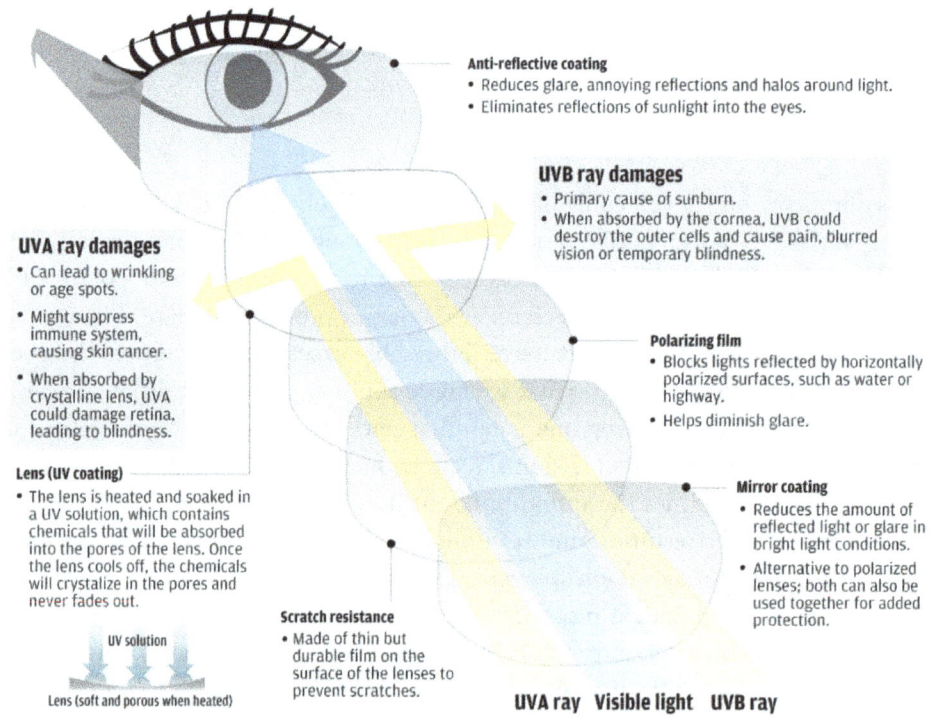

Figure 8.3 How sunglasses work[2]

Sunglasses technology components that you should consider include the following:

- Tinting
- Mirroring
- Polarization
- UV coating
- Scratch-resistant coating
- Anti-reflection coating

Light Transmission and Lens Color

All sunglasses operate by filtering out or reflecting away a certain percentage of the light rays that were otherwise destined to reach the eye. The darkness of the tint will determine the *light transmission factor*, or LTF. For example, an LTF of 15 percent (which is about average for most nonprescription sunglasses) will allow approximately 15 percent of the light through the lens and is ideal for most sunny conditions. This pertains to *visible* light. As we will see, all reasonably priced sunglasses should eliminate essentially 100 percent of the UV light.

Neutral lenses are always various shades of gray because they filter out a certain percentage of all light rays that reach them. The darker the gray, the less light transmitted. For example, a lens that has a transmission of 20 percent filters out 80 percent of the light (i.e., eight of every ten light rays that strike the sunglasses do not reach the eye). Note that neutral sunglasses affect all portions of the light spectrum equally—just as much blue, green, or red is filtered through the lenses. Because of this, there is no color distortion, an important characteristic for boaters and sailors. Many manufacturers use an older technique, known as *constant density*, which involves mixing the color into the glass or polycarbonate, producing a uniformly tinted color throughout the lens.

Colored or *tinted lenses* selectively affect the transmission of certain portions of the light spectrum more than others (see Table 8.1). Green sunglasses, for example, appear green because more of the green and less of the rest of the spectrum is transmitted. The overall transmission may be the same (e.g., 20 percent) as neutral lenses. Table 8.1 describes the technology behind colors (these are general guidelines, and your sensitivity may vary).

Reflecting or Mirror Lenses

Reflecting or *mirror lenses* act like partially silvered mirrors, and reflect light away from the eye. Their popularity among police officers in the United States earned them the name "cop shades." They are a very effective means of reflecting light away from the eyes, and acting as one-way mirrors. When the mirror coating is applied in a thick manner on the outer surface of the lens, it acts as the major component decreasing light transmission. However, more recent advances in the application of mirroring to lenses allows

Gray	Gray: a neutral all-purpose color which reduces glare while avoiding color distortion. This is ideal for both water and land.
Amber/brown	Brown and Amber: increases contrast in most conditions especially on cloudy days and filtering high frequency near-UV light. Preferentially blocks blue light and will distort colors like yellow but increases clarity. This is a good choice for all water sports.
Yellow/orange	Yellow and Orange heightens contrast especially in haze and is ideal for seeing details on overcast days; but yellow tint distorts colors.
Green	Green: filters some blue light and enhances visual acuity especially for fishing but is often worn for everyday use.
Purple/red	Purple and Red: heightens visual acuity and enhances color especially objects against a blue or green background. Better for fishing then boating.

Table 8.1 Lens colors[3]

for the coating to be thin enough to be only one component—sometimes referred to as half-silvering. At the molecular level, there are only about half as many molecules, so it is not totally reflective, as with fully mirrored lenses. It may be applied in a gradient fashion, gradually changing shades from top to bottom or bottom to top—that is, the underlying tinting and mirror coating may be customized, effectively acting together to decrease light transmission. For example, for variable light conditions, you could consider a copper base to enhance contrast and a blue mirror to divert blue light. If you don't want a color shift, you could consider a neutral gray base and a blue mirror coating (see Figure 8.3).

Polarizing Lenses

Polarizing lenses are very discriminating in their appetite for light rays. The polarizing material consists of a chemical film applied to glass or plastic, in which the molecules align in parallel and create a microscopic filter absorbing any light rays that match their alignment. Nearly all polarized glasses are oriented *horizontally* to block the horizontally polarized light that is reflected from a horizontal surface, such as the ocean. Only vertically aligned light rays can get through. In practice, some of the light polarized in other directions is also absorbed, producing a further reduction in glare.[4]

In certain circumstances—when avoiding coral reefs, for example—the difference between nonpolarized sunglasses and polarized ones can be crucial. Figure 8.4 illustrates a boat approaching a coral reef. Because of the glare from light reflected from water

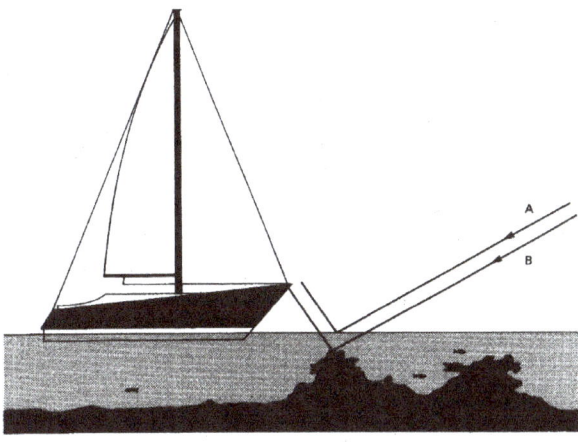

Figure 8.4 Boat approaches a coral reef in glare. Polarized sunglasses can eliminate light ray A, which is polarized horizontally. Without interference from light ray A, light ray B reflecting from the coral is visible.

(surface A), the ability of the eye to perceive light reflected from the reef (surface B) is diminished. Ordinary sunglasses would be of little value since they would diminish both light rays. Polarized glasses, however, would preferentially eliminate light ray A since it most likely would be polarized horizontally. This would allow light ray B to be better appreciated. Frequently, the effect is dramatic—like possessing X-ray vision.

Of course, this effect would not occur unless conditions were right for light ray B to be transmissible: that is, the water would need to be clear and relatively free of particulate matter and any surface disturbance that might scatter light ray B before it could reach the eye. Also, excessive light would have to be available so that we could discard some of it and still have enough left over to stimulate the eye (i.e. time of day is a factor). Polarized lenses would in no way augment the transmission of light ray B from the reef. Rather, they would reduce the glare from the polarized light ray A. In places that are "reef-strewn," such as the Caribbean, polarized glasses are invaluable.

Photochromatic Lenses

Photochromic lenses have been around for decades, initially only available in glass. The lenses automatically adjust from light to dark and back again, depending on the ambient light. The earliest glass lenses depended on silver halide or chloride reacting to UV light, but most of the current photochromic lenses use specific dyes which undergo chemical change when exposed to UV rays. As with everything, there are advantages and disadvantages. The major disadvantages are that the degree of darkening and lightening is brand specific, and some take longer to change than others. And they do not darken inside of cars (since the windshield eliminates most UV).

UV Radiation

Both plastic and glass lenses absorb some UV light, but typically the lens is heated and soaked in a UV solution that allows the chemicals to be permanently absorbed in the pores of the lens. *Only purchase sunglasses that block 100 percent of all UV light.* This is equivalent to absorbing all UV light up to 400 nanometers.

Scratch Resistant

While glass is scratch resistant, most plastic is not. Scratch resistance is achieved via the application of a thin film on the surface of the lens to reduce or prevent scratching. Films are made of diamond-like carbon, or polycrystalline diamond.

Antireflective Coating

Antireflective coating is applied to the backside of the lens (nearest the eye). It prevents glare from ricocheting off the backside of the lens into your eye. Similar to scratch-resistant coating, anti-reflective coating is a hard, thin layer (which may also be applied to the front in prescription lenses).

Lens Material

Glass is the traditional lens material. It offers excellent optical clarity and remains very scratch resistant. Newer technology has allowed the glass to be thinner, but it tends to be twice the weight of plastic or polycarbonate.

Plastic (most commonly CR39) has good optical quality, is lightweight, and is shatter resistant, but tends to scratch easily. You should look for scratch-resistant film to compensate for that.

Polycarbonate lenses have exceptional strength, being ten times more impact resistant than other lenses. They are thin, lightweight, and block 100 percent of UV rays without needing a special coating. They do, however, require scratch-resistant coating.

Trivex and *SR-91* are newer materials, which are said to be superior to the other materials in every way. But they are more expensive (you probably saw that coming), and some of their inherent superiority may be reduced by applying the coatings discussed above.

Lens Shape and Frame Style

There are a number of lens and frame styles on the market, including aviator, cat-eye, fisherman, double-bridge, shield, and wraparound. The latter are highly curved and have both disadvantages and advantages.

From an optical point of view, the flatter the lens the less distortion. Curved lenses (as occur in wraparound glasses) tend to bend or refract the light rays (see section "Bending Light Rays" below). Therefore, light doesn't travel in a direct line to your eye. However, there is lens technology known as *prismatics* (tiny prisms built into the lens) that can correct the distortion before the light rays reach your eye. Why even purchase a curved lens? Because the shape of the lens and the frame may contribute to blocking out light that enters from the side. As long as the inside layer of the curved lens has an antireflective coating, the side protection can contribute a great deal to reducing the amount of light reaching your eye. It also reduces the drying effect on your eyes caused by air and wind.

Lens Prescription

Many of the higher-end brands currently on the market can be manufactured with a personal refractive prescription embedded in the lens. If you require prescription glasses for normal activities, you should consider investing in a pair of prescription sunglasses. Alternatively, most regular glasses will accept clip-ons. Although they add weight to the glasses, they have the distinct advantage that when covered with spray they can be removed and cleaned without losing the visual correction—just be certain that they filter out 100 percent UV and are polarized.

Contact Lenses

What about contact lenses at sea? Some sailors swear by them since they don't fog up, or become streaked with spray or rain. The only real problem with contact lenses at sea (aside from the need to bring along additional sunglasses as well as contact lens paraphernalia) is the increased risk of corneal abrasion and ulceration. The constant wind at sea tends to dry out the eyes. If the eyeball's natural tear film, on which all contact lenses rest, should evaporate, the eye is at increased risk. *If you wear contact lenses, you must still wear some type of glasses to lessen tear evaporation due to the wind.* Sunglasses are fine if it is bright, but for overcast days or nighttime sailing, a pair of clear glasses should be purchased. The contact lens wearer must remember to avoid *overwear* due to long watches or irregular schedules. If anything, wearing time tends to be *shorter* than normal. The sailor must have lubricating drops in case of miscalculation. Finally, all sailors, whether they are planning to wear contact lenses or glasses, should bring along an extra pair of glasses. And the sailor should, without fail, wear a safety band with his or her glasses. If the sailor doesn't, he or she deserves to lose them overboard (harsh, I know).

Bending Light Rays

As sailors, we spend our time at the interface of two very different fluid states, sailing through one by harnessing the power of the other. In addition to its own properties, both states have a third set of properties that exists only at the interface. I am referring to light which behaves differently at the interface of the two than it does in either air or water separately.

The speed of light is approximately 3×10^8 meters per second, but this value is strictly true only in a vacuum. As soon as light enters the atmosphere, it slows down. The velocity of all electromagnetic radiation depends on the density of the medium through which it travels: the denser the medium, the slower the travel speed. One measure of the density of the medium is the index of refraction. The higher the index of refraction, the slower the light travels. The index of refraction of water, for example, is 1.333, so that light travels only 75 percent as fast in water as it does through air.

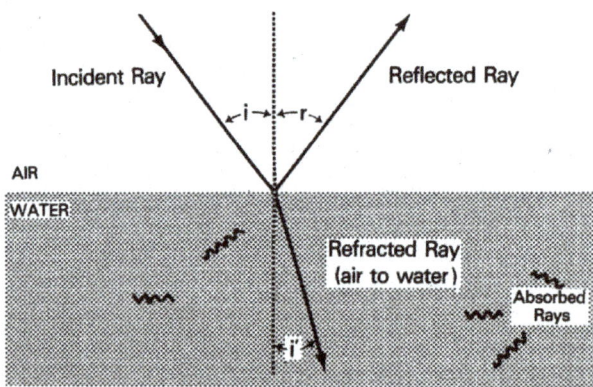

Figure 8.5 Light traveling from air to water: reflection, refraction, absorption

When light strikes a surface such as water, it may be *absorbed*, *reflected*, or *refracted* (Figure 8.5). The amount of light that the water absorbs (and converts to heat) depends on the angle of incidence, which is greater when the sun is at the zenith compared to when it is near the horizon. The degree of reflection varies with the smoothness of the surface. It is easy to see a reflection on a still lake but quite another matter on a wind-swept bay. Other rays enter the water and are bent or refracted.[5] Usually when light strikes the water at an angle, reflection and refraction occur simultaneously; some light rays are reflected, some refracted. The properties of the surface, especially its smoothness, determine the proportion.

So far, we have been concerned only with light passing from air into water, but in order to see an underwater object, this light must be reflected off the object and then traverse the surface a second time before reaching our eyes. During this second transit, light is again either absorbed, reflected, or refracted. If the light strikes the surface at too great an angle, however, it will not emerge from the water, producing a phenomenon called *total internal reflection* (Figure 8.6). If the light does escape the surface, our eyes and brain can never discern its precise origin. *All that we can perceive is the direction from*

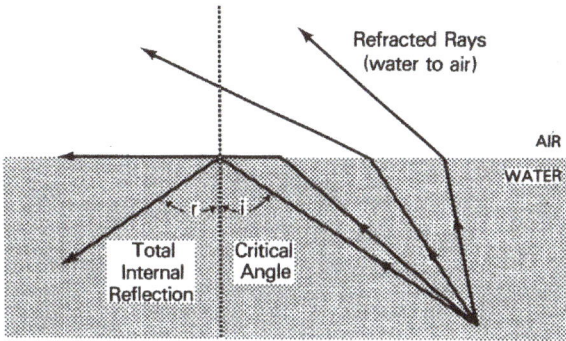

Figure 8.6 Light traveling from water to air: reflection, refraction, and absorption. Notice that if a reflected ray strikes the surface at or above a critical angle, there is total internal reflection. For this reason, the sun should be high in the sky when watching for subsurface impedimenta such as coral heads.

which light strikes the retina of the eye. After all, when we see ourselves reflected in a still lake or a mirror, it appears that we are *in* the water or *behind* the mirror because the light is coming from that direction. In other words, we note the direction from which the light arrives and *assume* that since light usually travels in a straight line the object must be at the end of that straight line. Figure 8.7 illustrates this illusion. Due to refraction, an underwater object appears shallower and larger than it really is. This concept of *image displacement* is crucial to understanding maritime optical illusions.

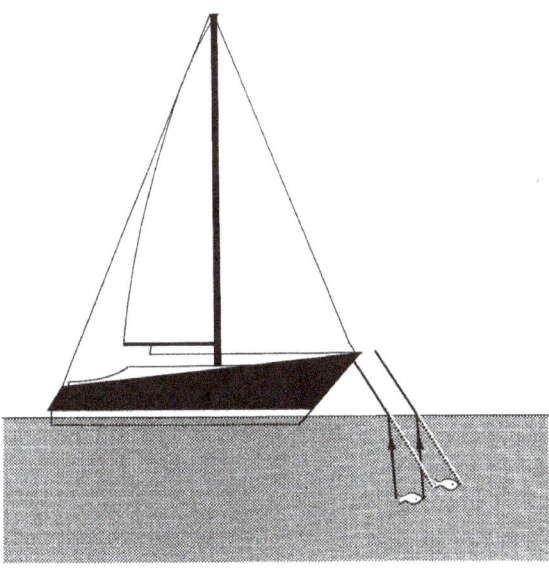

Figure 8.7 Image displacement

Nautical Ophthalmic Conditions

Acute Ophthalmic Conditions Due to Excessive Sunlight

Keratitis, or corneal sunburn, is due to excessive UV exposure. It is a condition wherein the cornea, the clear refracting surface that admits light to the retina, has literally been burned. There may be a latent period of six to twelve hours before the condition becomes apparent. Symptoms include:

- Redness of the eyes
- Eye pain
- Photophobia
- Gritty sensation
- Excessive tearing
- Blurred vision

Most often, the symptoms of photokeratitis improve on their own within twenty-four to forty-eight hours, however, even mild photophobia may last up to a week. Treatment consists of staying out of the sun, applying cool compresses, keeping eyes moist with preservative-free artificial tears, and using over-the-counter pain relievers. Avoid rubbing your eyes.

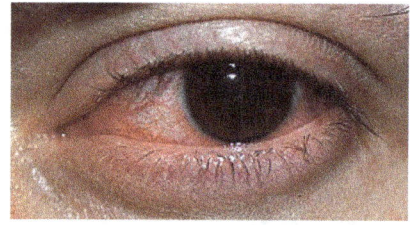

Figure 8.8 Ocular inflammation. The redness is in the conjunctiva (the white of the eye). The cornea, where the solar burn occurs, is the central clear portion.[6]

Long-Term Ophthalmic Conditions Due to Excessive Sunlight

Macular degeneration is one of the common causes of visual loss, especially in the elderly. One of the causes is thought to be sunlight damage that is cumulative over many years and due to UVA and high energy visual light—violet/blue light in the 400-450 nanometers visible spectrum. The macula is the center of our retina and responsible for fine visual discrimination, including reading. Since the damage to the macula is cumulative, you should start wearing sunglasses early and often!

Pinguecula (pin-GWEK-yoo-lah) is a yellowish, raised thickening of the conjunctiva (the white of the eye) close to the edge of the clear cornea. This condition causes noncancerous bumps and usually occurs near the middle of the eye (the part that is exposed most to the sun and is more common on the nasal side than the outer side). Pinguecula is benign but may cause dryness, itching, burning, and a foreign body sensation. The condition can be treated with anti-inflammatory drugs and eye drops (to treat the dry eye). Rarely, surgical removal is necessary.

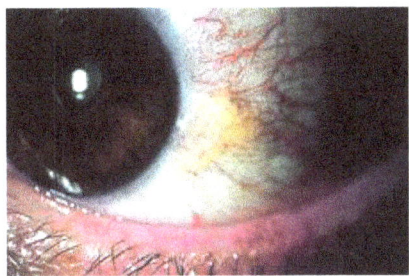

Figure 8.9 A pinguecula. See the yellowish bump.[7]

Pterygium (ter-rig-ee-uhm) is similar to pinguecula in that there is an elevated wedge-shaped bump on the eyeball; but unlike pinguecula, it can invade the cornea. It is referred to "surfer's eye," but you don't have to be a surfer to get one. Being in the bright sunlight on the water with constant wind increases your risk. These also develop more frequently on the side closer to the nose. The symptoms are similar to pinguecula, but because this condition can invade the cornea, it is more dangerous. Pterygium often become inflamed, causing red eye. Treatment consists of lubricants, steroid drops, additional medication, and surgery.

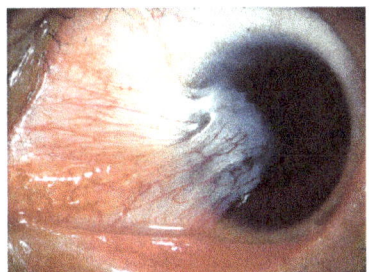

Figure 8.10 Pterygium invading the cornea[8]

Cataracts are caused by a progressive clouding and yellowing discoloration of the normally clear, crystalline lens. Approximately 10 percent of cataracts are directly attributable to excessive UV exposure.

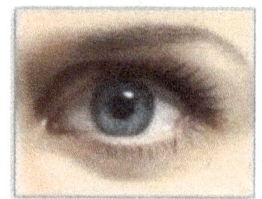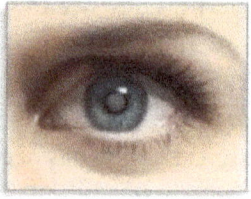

Figure 8.11 Lens clouded by cataract (white pupil on the right)

Eyelid cancers include basal cell carcinoma and squamous cell carcinoma. Both are associated with intense sun exposure. Melanoma, which can affect the eyelid and the eye itself, is even more highly associated with excess sun exposure.

Sailing Acuity

Although nature has produced a prodigious number of different kinds of eyes to meet the needs of its species, there have been two major lines of development. One line has produced a system of *high visual acuity*, which allows the animal to analyze fine visual detail. The culmination of this line of development occurs in the predatory birds, some of whom possess better visual acuity than humans. The only drawback to this system is that it requires a lot of light to function, so animals that depend on it to make their living are restricted, for the most part, to daytime activity.

The other major line has produced a system that sacrifices visual acuity for *visual sensitivity*. This type of eye is designed primarily for nocturnal active time. It makes maximal use of the meager amount of light available at night. The trade-off is that high visual sensitivity precludes high visual acuity. But a sailor searching for a buoy light or a freighter's running lights or an animal searching for its prey are not as interested in fine visual detail as they are in early detection.

The human visual system has borrowed from each of these systems. It is wrong, however, to consider the human eye as a compromise between these extremes. If it were a compromise, our vision would be best during periods of twilight. Rather, nature has incorporated elements of both systems into our sense of sight so that in a way we have four eyes and not just two.

Each system has its own specialized receptor (Figure 8.12). *Cones*, on the one hand, are light-sensitive receptors concentrated in the center of the retina and responsible for high visual acuity and color vision. *Rods*, on the other hand, are located primarily in the peripheral portions of the retina and are responsible for visual sensitivity (especially at night), peripheral vision, and motion detection. Since most of our active sailing is done in the daytime when there is adequate illumination, let us first examine our daytime visual system.

STRUCTURE OF THE RETINA

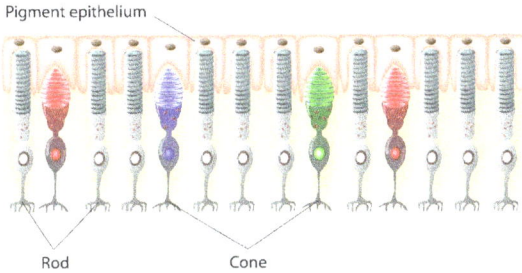

Figure 8.12 Rods and cones

Visual acuity is a measure of the ability of the eye to distinguish visual detail, stated in terms of *visual angle*. The visual angle is the angle that light rays coming from the outer limits of an object form at the eye. Figure 8.13A illustrates the visual angle that a distant sailboat creates in the retina of the eye. It is small and inverted. Figure 8.13B represents either a larger sailboat, or the same boat nearer the observer. Thus, the size of the visual angle depends upon the size of the object and its distance from the observer.

Figure 8.13C illustrates the most common means of quantifying visual acuity: the eye chart. In the figure, the "E" is one-third of an inch (0.85 centimeter) high, and at 20 feet (6 meters), the outer limits of the E extend under a visual angle of five minutes of arc. However, to recognize the E, the detail of the letter (the black bars and white gaps) must be appreciated. Since the bars and gaps represent one-fifth of the overall size of the letter, the minimum detail needed to recognize the letter subtends one minute of arc. This detection of detail is called *resolution*—the eye is said to have a *resolving power* of one minute of arc.[9]

It may surprise you to learn that a similar concept of visual acuity was appreciated in antiquity. Although the ancients did not have an eye chart (the Dutch ophthalmologist Snellen invented it in 1862), they took advantage of what was readily available—the sky. Figure 8.14 illustrates the stars of the Big Dipper or Plough (what it's called in the United Kingdom and Ireland), with the distances between the stars rendered in terms of visual angle, equivalent to the angle of a great circle on the celestial sphere.

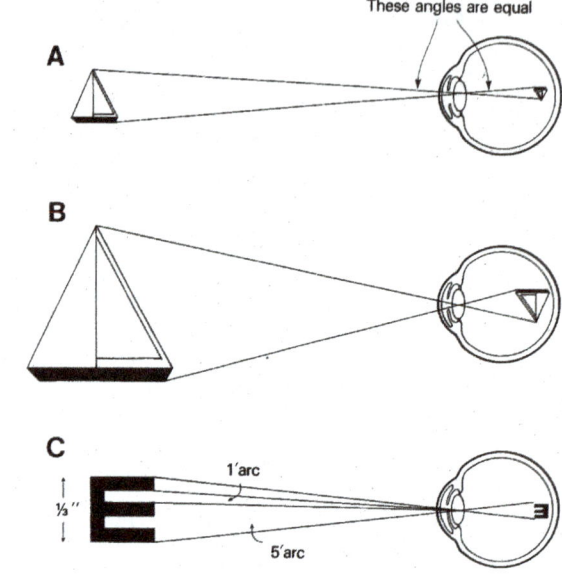

Figure 8.13 Visual acuity

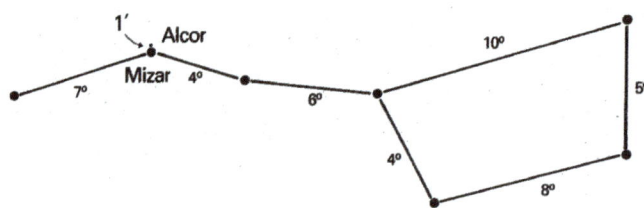

Figure 8.14 Celestial acuity—Alcor and Mizar

Very close to Mizar, the middle star in the handle, sits a faint, tiny star named Alcor. The distance between these two stars is one minute of arc. In the ancient world, resolution of these two stars was equivalent to normal vision. This became part of the Roman "physical examination" for soldiers. If only one star was seen, vision was subnormal. It is not known whether ancients used other naturally occurring visual parameters to quantify lesser visual acuities.

It might appear at first glance that one minute of arc is the best that the eye is capable of, but this is not so. *In fact, for many of us, 20/20 visual acuity is not normal at all.* If tested carefully, most of us are capable of resolving less than one minute of arc. We can read the 20/15 or even the 20/13 lines on the eye chart.

For the moment, let us consider one minute of arc as a benchmark against which to compare our visual abilities in various nautical situations. In certain circumstances we don't do quite that well, whereas in others, we do a bit better.

As a mariner approaches a prominent landmark or buoy from a distance, there are three phases of visual appreciation. The first is when the object is *detected* as distinct from its surroundings (detection range). The object on the horizon is just beyond the resolving power of the eye in minutes of arc. In other words, there is something that could be a buoy—or it might turn out to be a fishing boat! Upon closer approach, it can be *recognized* as an aid to navigation, possessing a certain shape and color (recognition range). At the recognition range, the eye can resolve the dark buoy—analogous to the bar of the E—against the lighter gaps of the sky. There is enough information in minutes of arc to indicate that the object is indeed a buoy. Later in the recognition phase, the color of the buoy becomes apparent. Finally, the buoy can be *identified* when the mariner is close enough to read the numbers or letters (identification range). All three ranges—detection, recognition, and identification—depend on the resolving power of the eye, and each presents a different amount of information to the sailor.

Binoculars and Other Nautical Instruments

When visual discrimination is limited due to the eye's inability to resolve fine detail, binoculars are of value. Binoculars can do only one thing—increase the apparent visual angle of the object and, hence, the size of the image on the retina. This increases the range of perception of an object, such as a buoy, by a factor equal to the magnifying power of the binoculars (seven times with seven by thirty-five or seven by fifty binoculars). For example, a buoy that is barely detected with the naked eye may now be recognized with binoculars because the size of the image on the retina is now large enough (usually about one minute of arc) for the eye to resolve. Likewise, a buoy within the recognition range may now be identified. It is important to realize that in each of these cases, the contrast between the object and the background needs to be sufficient—binoculars work only in conditions where it is merely the size of the object that limits visual resolution. Binoculars are of little or no assistance in situations where the contrast is low, such as in penetratingly, dense haze or fog.

Binoculars are not capable of increasing the contrast between the object and its background (in this example the buoy and the horizon). In fact, because all optical instruments introduce a slight amount of light scatter from the surfaces of the lenses, they tend to decrease rather than increase contrast. *Therefore, if visibility conditions set the limit for visual resolution, binoculars are of no use.*

Color

One question that arose early in the investigation of color was: if the human eye can distinguish among 150 different colors, how many types of cones are present in the eye? If each hue were analyzed by a separate cone, the job of packaging 150 different cones would be enormous. If each point on the retina were represented by each of these cones, the "grain" of the color image would be extremely coarse.

Instead, nature subcontracted the work of color discrimination to various portions of the eye and brain. Three types of cones perform the "blue-collar" job of receiving the different wavelengths of light; each type receives a different portion of the light spectrum. The red cone is maximally sensitive to wavelengths around 570 nanometers, the green cone to wavelengths at 535 nanometers, and the blue cone to the shorter wavelengths, which center around 445 nanometers (Figure 8.15 and endnote 1). Note that there is a great deal of overlap in the territory that each of the cones serves, so any single wavelength usually stimulates two and sometimes three types of cones. The amount of stimulation of each of the cones determines the color that a person perceives. Other cells in the retina perform the "white-collar" job of sorting out all of this, whereas the "executive-level" decisions regarding color are reserved for the brain.

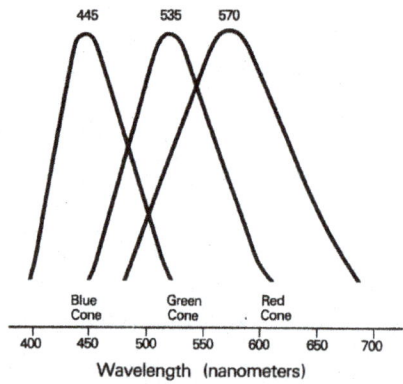

Figure 8.15 The three types of cones: red, green, and blue

All the other hues are produced from the stimulation of two or three cones in different proportions. Mixtures of blue and green wavelengths produce various shades of blue-green, whereas green and red wavelengths produce yellow and orange. Violet results from mixing wavelengths from both ends of the spectrum—blue and red. Note that these rules of color mixing hold only when the colors are *additive*, as are pure spectral bands of light (e.g., the kind of light navigational lights produce at night). If you could superimpose a red and a green navigational light, the resulting light would appear yellow. In a sense, the appearance of the sun during the day is due to such a superimposition since it is missing the scattered blue.[10]

If the eye has a range of approximately 300 nanometers (from 400 to 700 nanometers) and if within that range more than 150 colors can be distinguished, it follows that the eye must be exquisitely sensitive to very small differences in wavelength. Figure 8.16 demonstrates that the eye is not equally sensitive to all portions of the spectrum. Roughly speaking, it is most sensitive to the portions of the spectrum between the three cone curves (i.e., in the blue-green zone and in the yellow zone, between green and red).

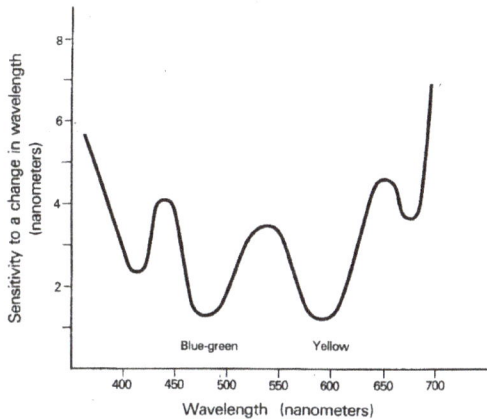

Figure 8.16 Sensitivity to color by wavelength

In these regions, the eye is capable of discriminating colors at 1-nanometer increments! This sensitivity to minute color variations allows us to use changes in the color of the water as natural aids to navigation when sailing in certain regions—often referred to as eyeball navigation. *The Yachtsman's Guide to the Greater Antilles* provides an example of this kind of visual piloting:

> It is almost impossible to describe in words what only experience can really teach, but let us take a stab at it. All of what we say here is assuming there is good light—high and behind the observer—and relatively calm water.
>
> In depths of over 60 feet, the water has a deep "inky" blue-black color. Over sand this color takes on a lighter but still deep blue color—if the bottom is rocky the color is more of a dark green. On coming into water of about 25 to 30 feet a sandy bottom will show as a light green—if it is a rocky bottom it will be more of a mottled brown color. In going into shallower water, the sandy bottom reflects a very pale green at about 10 feet. Over rock or coral at this depth, the water will take on a yellow-brown, mottled tinge and you should be able to distinguish very clearly the outlines of the rocks.[11]

Eyeball navigation is superior to traditional depth sounding in several respects. Not only is the eye capable of sampling data over a much greater area, but the sailor can also judge the depth and composition of the bottom before it is—ugh—beneath the keel.

Anyone who wishes to practice eyeball navigation should keep the following points in mind: a good pair of polarized lenses is essential, preferably in neutral gray: a hat or visor contributes to diminishing the glare; visibility is usually good over coral bottoms, except after heavy rain when the water may be muddy. Human activities such as dumping, dredging, or blasting may also impair clarity. *Anticipating the time of passage through the reef is absolutely crucial.* Plan to cross the reef only when the sun is high and behind, shining over your shoulder.[12] This means that in the morning, you can expect good visibility through water in a westerly direction and in the afternoon in an easterly direction. The higher the sun gets, the wider the "arc" of visibility; the lower the sun, the narrower the arc. Also, if the sun's noontime passage lies to the north of your position, visibility will be somewhat better to the south, and vice versa. If the water is calm and "glassy," it may be difficult to see below the surface. Fortunately, it is rare for the water to be perfectly calm, and even the slightest ripple on the surface enhances vision. Finally, beware of cloud shadows that may resemble coral heads.

There is one other role that color plays with which the sailor should be familiar—the appreciation of distance. During normal atmospheric conditions, all distant objects such as hills or mountains are lightly veiled in a blue haze due to the preferential scattering of blue light. Through experience we have come to associate this indistinct blue quality with distance (as did Leonardo da Vinci, who first emphasized it as an important technique in creating depth perception in a painting). When the atmosphere is unusually dry and clear, however, the blue haze is absent and distant objects stand out starkly against the horizon. This starkness creates the illusion of nearness, so distant objects may be interpreted as being much closer than they really are.

Twilight

During twilight, the eye is in the unfortunate position of being "between systems."[13] It is still too bright for the nighttime rod system and too dark for the optimal performance of the daytime cone system. Nevertheless, it is a critical period for the mariner. It may be the only time of day when the navigator has the opportunity to obtain a fix from simultaneous celestial observations.[14] In addition, if the boat overstands the estimated time of travel, twilight can be an anxious transition period during which everyone worries as to whether there will be enough light to identify the various aids to navigation.

Both the navigator and the helmsman should be aware that the rate of change in illumination is not constant. The brightness of twilight changes relatively slowly until the sun is about 4 degrees below the horizon. From that point on, the decrease in illumination proceeds at an accelerated pace, and visual piloting rapidly becomes a losing battle. Importantly, both of the major cone functions needed for piloting—visual acuity and color vision—degrade together so that the nautical environment becomes increasingly indistinct and gray.

Figure 8.17 illustrates the relationship between visual acuity and illumination. Note that at about a half hour after sunset, visual acuity is reduced to about 20/100, a visual angle of five minutes. This means that a daymark that was previously identified at 0.1 nautical mile (185 meters) now has an identification range of 0.03 mile or 190 feet (57 meters).

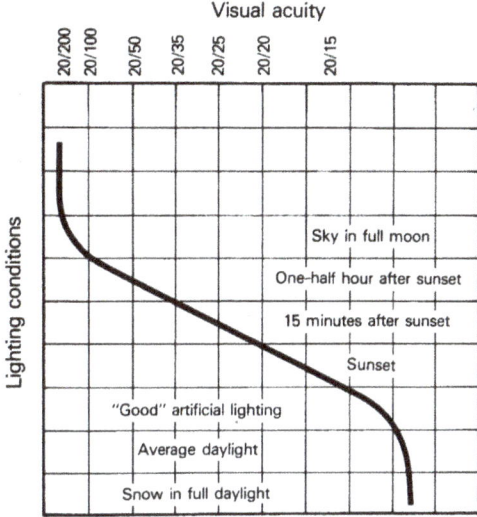

Figure 8.17 Loss of visual acuity with diminished illumination

Nighttime Sailing

The versatility of the eye is truly astonishing if we consider that it is capable of responding to light as dim as 10^{-8} foot-candles and as bright as 10⁷ foot-candles. This remarkable adaptability represents a range of 10 to 15 (1,000,000,000,000,000) log units of intensity!

The cone system, which has a higher threshold (i.e., is less sensitive), functions between 10^{-2} foot-candles (medium moonlight) and 10^7 foot-candles (intolerably bright light). The rod system, which operates between 10^{-8} and 10^{-2} foot-candles, provides the eye with nighttime sensitivity.[15] In exchange, we surrender both high visual acuity and all perception of color. With rod vision, the world appears in various shades of black and white. Since there are no rods in the exact center of the retina—in conditions of dim illumination—there is a blind spot of about 5 degrees in the center of our visual field (Figure 8.18). No matter where we move our eyes, this blind spot remains. *Because of this, navigators and pilots are trained to look about 5 degrees to one side of (or above or below) the object for which they are searching for in the dark.*

The changeover from one system to the other does not occur instantaneously. For example, when passing from the bright sunlight into a darkened movie theater, it is difficult at first to see anything at all. But, after a few minutes, we can see the surroundings fairly well, meaning that we have adapted to the dark (dark adaptation). Conversely, on leaving the theater, we are initially dazzled by the bright sunlight and must readapt to the light (light adaptation). Light adaptation is rarely a problem—it occurs in seconds. Dark adaptation, however, requires a longer period of time.

The rod system requires more than thirty minutes to adapt to dark—up to an hour for complete adaptation—but during this time, it increases sensitivity by one million

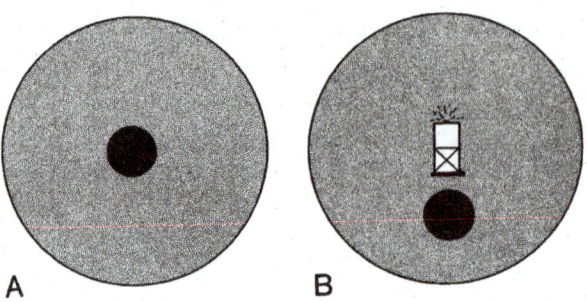

Figure 8.18 The "blind spot"

times! Unfortunately, a few *seconds* of exposure to bright light can undo an entire hour of dark adaptation. For this reason, any sailor who wishes to remain dark-adapted must avoid all white light, even cabin light. *Whenever there is a change of watch at night, the relieving watch should allow thirty minutes for their eyes to become fully dark adapted prior to assuming duty.*

There is a way to use the high visual acuity system and still retain the rods in a dark-adapted, high-readiness state. This requires the use of monochromatic red light, and hinges on the fact that the rods are insensitive to the long, red wavelengths of light.

For this reason, the compass light is red, and the prepared mariner has a flashlight with a red filter. In the eventuality that a brief chart consultation is required, the mariner can utilize the filtered light source, and resume duty immediately. An alternative is to use red goggles that filter the light at the eye instead of at the source. Without red light or goggles, another little-known trick may be used (which supports the fact that we really do have four eyes and not two!) Dark adaptation is entirely a property of the retina, and each eye dark-adapts independently. Thus, if the navigator is fully dark-adapted and must go below to consult a chart, the navigator can simply close one eye. The covered eye remains dark-adapted. When the navigator returns on deck, he or she can switch eyes or leave both eyes open. (This trick is also useful when a midnight trip to the head is necessary either on land or at sea.)

One concept needs to be explored further: the relationship between the two systems. It is wrong to conceptualize the cone system at work only by day and the rod system only on a lonely watch at night. During the daytime, the cone system is dominant, but the rods are not entirely quiescent. They function primarily as movement detectors in the peripheral visual field. At night, the rod system is dominant, but the cone system is poised for action, awaiting an appropriately intense stimulus. Even in starlight the cone system must be working; otherwise, we could never distinguish Alcor from Mizar nor could we appreciate the blueness of Venus or the redness of Mars, both properties of the cone system. The key is that the stimulus must be sufficiently intense. Individual stars do not provide much background illumination, but since they are point sources of light, they *intensely* stimulate a small area of the retina, often just one or two cones.

To appreciate the relationship between the night and day vision systems, imagine that you are searching on a clear night for a flashing green light with a *nominal range* (the maximal distance at which a light can be seen at night when the visibility is clear) of 3 miles (4.9 kilometers). At some distance beyond the nominal range, perhaps at 4 miles (6.4 kilometers), the rod system may detect the light. At this stage, the approximate direction of the light is apparent, but a precise bearing is not possible. All the same, this information may prove useful. At perhaps 3.5 miles (5.6 kilometers), the light will be intense enough to stimulate the cones (allowing a bearing), *but the light will appear white*. The period after a light is visible as white but before its color is appreciated is known as the *photochromatic interval*. It is characteristic of all colored lights at night. At the nominal range of the light, in this case 3 miles (4.9 kilometers), all its characteristics including color will be apparent.

The scenario is similar for a red light, with one exception. If the lights were of the same intensity, the red light would be invisible at 4 miles (6.4 kilometers) because the rod system is insensitive to red light. At about 3.5 miles (5.6 kilometers), it would be visible to the cone system as a white light, and after the photochromatic interval it would appear red.

In many respects, finding a navigational light at night is an easier proposition than finding that same aid to navigation by day because there are fewer variables. By day, the variables include the size, shape, color, and reflectivity of the object; the background against which it is seen; the elevation and angular relationship of the sun and object; the general level of illumination, including cloud cover and glare; visibility conditions; and the height of the observer's eye.

In contrast, at night there are only three variables: the *power of the light*, the *visibility*, and *the position of the observer's eye* relative to the light.

It is axiomatic that a powerful light will be seen at a greater distance than will a weak one, but why? The explanation is that even during conditions of normal visibility, the atmosphere impedes the progress of light waves. After all, the only reason we can see the stars is that they spend 99.999 . . . percent of their journey traveling through interstellar space, which is so rarefied that there are few molecules with which the light can collide. This is certainly not the case on earth. Therefore, one limiting factor (or variable) is the strength of the light, or its nominal range.

If the visibility is normal, only one factor can prevent the light from reaching the observer: the relationship between the height of the light and the height of the observer's eye. This relationship, known as the *geographic range*, is purely geometric and has nothing to do with the power of the light. Since the earth is curved and since light *usually* travels in a straight line, there is a distance beyond which the light is below the horizon of the observer. The formula for calculating distance to the horizon (for both eye and light) is

$$D \text{ (miles)} = 1.22 \times \sqrt{h} \text{ (feet)}$$
$$D \text{ (kilometers)} = 3.57 \times \sqrt{h} \text{ (meters)}$$

where D is the distance in nautical miles and h is the height of the observer's eye. *On a clear night, one of these two factors determines when a light is visible to the sailor.*

For example, for an observer who stands 5'7" tall (1.70 meters) above the water, the distance to the horizon is approximately 3.1 miles (5 kilometers). If that same observer could look from a tower 98 feet (30 meters) above sea level, the distance to the horizon is now 12.2 miles (19.6 kilometers).

What if visibility is reduced? Lowered visibility has no effect on the geographic range, but it does have an impact on the strength of the light, since the "thicker" the atmosphere, the more difficult it is for the light rays to penetrate. The strength of the light, corrected for prevailing visibility conditions, is known as the luminous range and can be determined from a luminous range diagram such as the one provided in any volume of the *United States Light List*.[16]

With this in mind, estimating the expected appearance of a light at night becomes straightforward. In clear visibility, the limiting factor will be either (1) the power of the light (nominal range) or (2) the geographic range. With reduced visibility, the limiting factor will be either (1) the reduced power of the light (luminous range) or (2) the geographic range.

Notes

1. As sailors, we utilize a substantial portion of the electromagnetic spectrum for a variety of purposes (see figure below). The velocity of all electromagnetic radiation is the same, 3×10^8 meters per second (186,000 miles per second). The only difference between, say, light, ultraviolet radiation, and radio waves is their wavelength. Radio beacons and VHF radio equipment produce energy of progressively shorter wavelengths. Each of these systems is designed to transmit or receive energy only in a limited band. To a VHF radio, medium-frequency and high-frequency radiation simply does not exist. So, it is with the human eye as well. It is sensitive to a mere octave in the grand electromagnetic scale. Looked at in this fashion, we are nearly blind.

2. Courtesy of Annie Liao at https://annieliao.com/.

3. Courtesy of Annie Liao at https://annieliao.com/.

4. You can perform a simple test to see whether the sunglasses are actually polarized. Find a good reflecting surface (like the horizontal commercial display surface) and hold the glasses in front of your face. Look through one of the lenses while you rotate it 90 degrees. If there is not a perceptible change in the reflective glare, then the lens is probably not polarized.

5. Here's more information for science types—others may safely skip. If light is reflected, the angle of the reflected ray is equal to the angle of the incident ray such that angle i (incident ray) equals angle r (reflected ray). It should be kept in mind that with both reflection and refraction, all angles are measured from the perpendicular (normal) to the surface and not from the surface up. The degree of refraction depends on the angle of incidence as well as the index of refraction of the two media, in this case air (1.000) and water (1.333). (This is known as Snell's law, the

mathematical expression of which is *n sin I = n' sin I'*, where *n* and *n'* are the indices of refraction of the two media and *sin I* and *sin I'* are the sines of the angles of incidence and refraction, respectively.)

     6. https://upload.wikimedia.org/wikipedia/commons/thumb/0/0d/Clare314.jpg/300px-Clare-314.jpg.

     7. https://medical-dictionary.thefreedictionary.com/pinguecula.

     8. https://upload.wikimedia.org/wikipedia/commons/6/6a/Pterygium%28from_Michigan_Uni_site%2C_CC-BY%29.jpg.

     9. The visual acuity fraction we commonly use is simply a numerical expression of the resolving power of the eye: visual acuity equals the distance at which the test is made (usually 20 feet) divided by the distance at which the minimum detail of the smallest recognized letter is one minute of arc.

The detail in the E in Figure 8.13C subtends one minute of arc at 20 feet and, if recognized, visual acuity is 20/20. The big E at the top of most eye charts has visual detail that subtends one minute of arc at 200 feet, and if it is the smallest letter that can be recognized, then visual acuity is 20/200, very poor indeed.

     10. The primary colors of wavelengths of light are blue, green, and red. Yellow is composed of a mixture of green and red light. If this seems odd, that is because many of us have been raised to conceptualize color only in terms of pigment mixture, a somewhat different system. Color is discussed more fully later in the chapter.

     11. H. Kline, ed., *Yachtsman's Guide to the Greater Antilles* (Coral Gables, FL: Tropic Isle, 1979), 135-136.

     12. With the sun behind you, there is significantly less glare with which to contend. Unless the sun is relatively high, there are too few light rays reflected off the coral toward the observer, and those that are reflected stand a good chance of undergoing total internal reflection (see Figure 8.4).

     13. Twilight is so important that various groups have defined it according to their own interests and needs; thus, we have three different twilight periods: civil, nautical, and astronomic. The duration of civil twilight, a time in which there is still sufficient light for most terrestrial outdoor activities, is defined as that interval between the time when the upper edge of the sun is on and the true position of its center is 6 degrees below the horizon. Nautical twilight is longer, since there is a longer period of light at sea than on land due to the lack of obstructions such as mountains and the reflectivity of the water. Nautical twilight lasts from sunset until the sun is 12 degrees below the horizon. Astronomic twilight is still longer, since astronomers are interested in knowing when the sky will be dark enough for star observation. The darker limit of astronomic twilight occurs when the sun is 18 degrees beneath the horizon.

     14. For those of you still practicing your celestial navigation!

     15. When nature set about to build a high-sensitivity system, she not only succeeded, but in the end created the most sensitive system possible. In order to appreciate the sensitivity of the rod system, we must ultimately reexamine the nature of light itself and redress an egregious error of omission. Earlier, light was considered exclusively as a wave phenomenon. But to stop there belies the dual nature of light and glosses over one of the classic controversies in the history of science. For more than three hundred years, there were two rival theories of the nature of light. On one side was the imposing figure of Isaac Newton (1642-1727), who argued that light must be composed of a train of particles. His adversary and contemporary was Christian Huygens (1629-1695), who

maintained that light behaved primarily as a series of waves. The battle raged on, and for a time it looked as though Newton's theory of particles was wrong. However, at the beginning of the twentieth century, it was shown conclusively that the wave theory could not explain all of the characteristics of light. It is now clear that light is both particle and wave. Sometimes the behavior of light is best described by its wave motions, while under other conditions it is best considered to be composed of particles or photons. A photon is the smallest possible parceling of light energy. Amazingly, the rod is capable of responding, under ideal conditions, to a single photon of light! The system is so sensitive that it can be stimulated by the smallest quantity of light possible in our universe. To be fair, a single photon doesn't produce a visual sensation. This requires the activation of at least two, perhaps as many as five, rods at the same time.

16. https://www.navcen.uscg.gov/?pageName=lightLists

Chapter 9

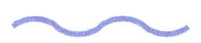

Sailing Nutrition

> "Let food be thy medicine,
> And medicine be thy food."
> —Attributed to Hippocrates, 460-370 BCE

> "Serve God daily, love one another,
> and preserve your victuals [provisions]."
> —Sir John Hawkins, 1562 (advice to his crew prior to embarkation)

Nowadays it seems that people are interested mostly in the gastronomic aspects of food (at least that's the impression from viewing all the photos of food on social media). If you ask the current youth whether they "eat to live" or "live to eat" (in the words of an older generation), they would most likely throw you a quizzical look and ask, "What's your point?" Although there is nothing wrong with epicurism (except perhaps when it borders on total decadence), the nautical community's general neglect of nutrition is a pity. Boaters of every stripe need to know at least something about the food they eat. This includes power boaters, commercial sailors, cruising sailors, and racing sailor athletes. It is especially relevant today, when the food industry continually barrages us with unproven claims concerning such-and-such a diet, vitamin, or nutritional supplement. Americans spend more than $30 billion a year on dietary supplements including vitamins and mineral and herbal products—most of which are of dubious or no value whatsoever. Some of them can actually make you sick.

Nutrition is also part of our nautical heritage. In the past, food and drink were of vital concern in the planning of ocean voyages. Inadequate storage, food spoilage, and vitamin deficiencies (either unrecognized or ignored) were ever-present problems. The early explorers of the New World, for example, were limited by the amount of food they could carry. A voyage to the West Indies was just about the longest and farthest possible, and several times food gave out on unduly prolonged return voyages. No mariner prior to Sir Francis Drake managed to feed his crew properly on any voyage into the Southern Hemisphere, especially those that reached the Pacific Ocean. As Captain Morison points out:

> There simply was not room enough, or storage tight enough, to preserve basic foodstuffs, such as wine, hard bread, flour, and salt meat, for so long a time. Hence the resort to penguin meat, seal, and other loathsome substitutes; and occasionally to the desperate eating of rats and chewing leather chafing-gear. Drake's men made out comparatively well, only because he stripped every prize ship of all desirable food stores, gear, and weapons. There is not one of these southern voyages on which the modern blue-water yachtsman, used to refrigeration and canned goods, would have been happy.[1]

As longer voyages became routine during the seventeenth and eighteenth centuries, the problem of storage was replaced by that of food spoilage and infestation. The food allowance for each man in the Royal Navy during this period was:

Biscuit	1 pound daily
Salt beef	1 pound twice weekly
Salt pork	1 pound twice weekly
Dried fish	2 ounces thrice weekly
Oatmeal	1/2 pint thrice weekly
Butter	2 ounces thrice weekly
Cheese	4 ounces thrice weekly
Peas	8 ounces four times weekly
Beer	1 gallon daily

The caloric value of this ration (if we include the beer at about 130 calories per pint) is roughly 3,800 calories. The quantity of food was not at fault; the amount was "greater than to satisfy an ordinary eater." Rather, the principal objection lay in its quality. This ration contained no fresh foodstuffs and, apart from traces in the beer, was totally lacking in vitamin C. As Captain Roddis remarked, "The pickling process destroyed much of the flavor and palatability of the beef and pork and unfavorably affected their nutrient value. Many stories are told of the beef. It was said that when old and allowed to dry, it could be carved into small boxes or figures which, if shellacked, had much the appearance and the consistency of mahogany."[2]

Sailing Nutrition

The staple of the sailor's diet at the time was his sea bread, or biscuit…what we know today as hard bread, or hardtack. "It was often as hard as flint and all too frequently infested with weevils. Knocking the bread against the edge of the mess table in order to remove the weevils was a regular practice and the noise made by the procedure was as regular a sound at mealtime as the rattle of mess gear."[3] The amount of beer may seem surprising, but it compensated in part for the lack of fresh water aboard the ship. The quality of the beer was poor, however, and eventually rum, generally known as *grog*, was issued instead.[4]

So, where should we turn for help? The U.S. Department of Agriculture (USDA) first published nutritional guidelines in 1894. In 1943 during World War II, the USDA introduced a new set of guidelines promoting the "Basic 7" food groups to help maintain nutritional standards during the war:

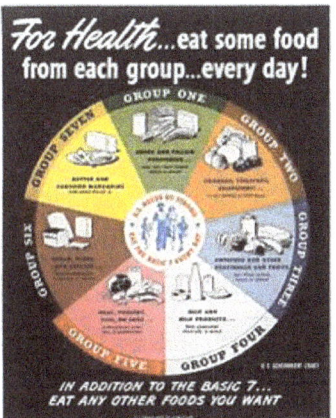

The "Basic 7" was in effect from 1943-1956 and included:

1. Green and yellow vegetables
2. Oranges and tomatoes
3. Potatoes and other vegetables
4. Milk and milk products
5. Meat, poultry, fish, or eggs
6. Bread, flour, and cereals
7. Butter and fortified margarine

Figure 9.1: The "Basic 7"

Then, in 1956, the USDA recommended the "Basic 4" food groups:

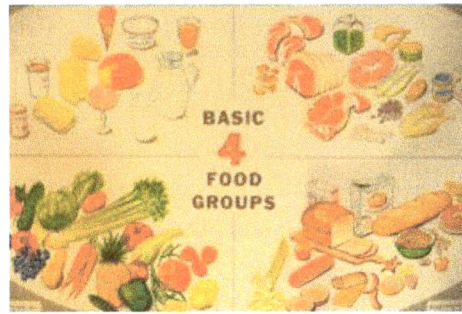

1. Vegetables and fruits
2. Milk
3. Meat
4. Cereals and breads

Figure 9.2: The "Basic 4"

In an attempt to address serving size, the USDA proposed a food pyramid in 1992. But this chart was not the first chart suggested by the nutritional experts. The original chart featured fruits and vegetables as the biggest group, not breads. This was later *overturned* by the special interests of the grain, meat, and dairy industries.

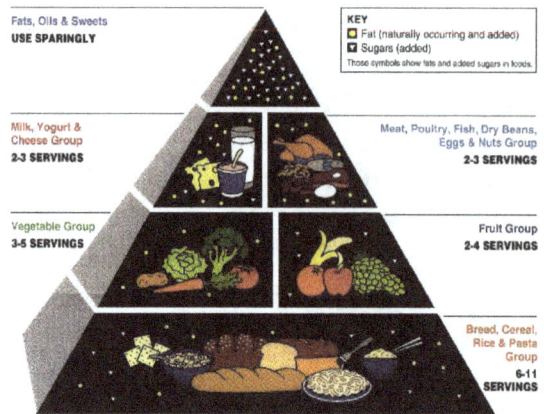

Figure 9.3 This is the pyramid that was released after all the special interest groups had their say. It remained operative until 2005

In 2005, the pyramid was redrawn to slightly change the share of the different food groups and to emphasize the need for exercise.

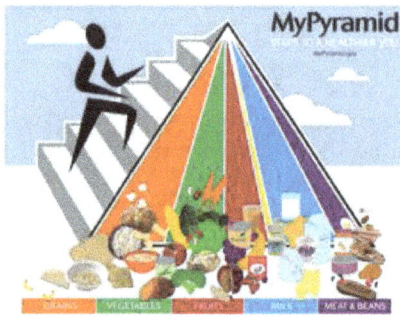
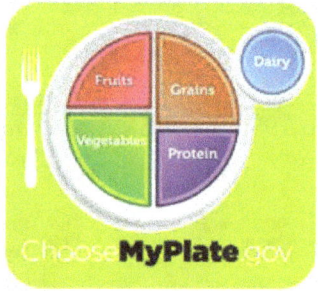

Figure 9.4 "MyPyramid" Figure 9.5. "MyPlate"

MyPlate is the current nutritional guide logo; it replaced the MyPyramid diagram in 2011. So, we are almost back full circle to the "Basic 4" that I grew up with from the 1950s through the 1980s. Instead of berating the USDA's recommendations for some of the political compromises that it likely made with industry groups (and I would maintain that the MyPlate logo is not that helpful—see the DASH Diet and Mediterranean

Diet pyramids later in the chapter), I would refer the reader to the ChooseMyPlate.gov website and the PDF *Dietary Guidelines for Americans 2015-2020*, 8th edition. Both the website and the extensive PDF are chock-full of useful information, and the PDF can be downloaded and consulted offline.

One last thing before we get to the meat of the matter. In nutritional terms, the word *diet* refers to the sum of food consumed as opposed to a program for losing weight (although that may be one expectation). For the purposes of this book, nutritional discussions will focus on heathy eating, but be aware of the fact that the USDA uses the term *healthy eating patterns* synonymously with *diet*. Although "healthy eating pattern" is probably a better term, I am going to stick with the simpler term "diet" throughout this chapter.

The Basics

Protein

There is nothing magical about protein. It is composed of various combinations of twenty amino acid "building blocks." The way in which the different amino acids are put together determines the *structure* and *function* of the particular protein. The adult body cannot synthesize nine of the amino acids, which *therefore must be provided in the diet*. These are referred to as the *essential* amino acids. The amount and the proportion of amino acids in a protein determines its nutritional value. *Complete protein* contains all of the essential amino acids in approximately the correct ratio for use by the human body. All of the building blocks are supplied at the same time, and are available for the construction of any protein the body needs. *Incomplete protein* either lacks one or more of the essential amino acids, or contains them in an unusual ratio. However, combining a variety of incomplete sources of protein, such as fruits, vegetables, and grains, accomplishes virtually the same result as consuming a complete protein would. The strengths and weaknesses of one protein complement those of the other, a concept known as *protein complementarity*. In this way, a vegetarian diet need not be inferior in protein quality to a diet that contains animal products. For example, rice is low in the amino acid lysine while high in the amino acid methionine; beans are low in methionine and high in lysine. The combination of rice and beans turns out to be a complete source of protcin, on par with beef.

By and large, animal protein is more complete than plant protein. The most complete sources are eggs, fish, beef, poultry, milk, and cheese. The following have a high amino acid content although they are incomplete: nuts, seeds (such as sunflower or sesame), lentils, peanut butter, beans, and peas.

Since protein is the major constituent of muscle, there must be protein in the diet to retain and increase muscle mass. The average daily requirement is 20 to 30 grams, preferably spread out through the day. But, consuming huge amounts of protein does not augment muscle mass. *Only muscle work increases muscle mass*. Since the typical Western diet contains more than twice the amount of protein necessary, and since active boaters frequently consume considerable quantities of food, their diet invariably contains two to three times the amount of protein needed to increase muscle mass. All additional protein in the diet is simply broken down and used as fuel, or stored as fat. We will address the protein requirements and the effect of protein supplementation for sailing athletes below.

Carbohydrates

The main function of carbohydrates is to provide energy. Carbohydrates that the body does not use immediately are stored in the liver and muscle as glycogen, which consists of hundreds and thousands of glucose sugar molecules that are linked together. Once the capacity for glycogen storage is reached, the remainder is stored as fat.

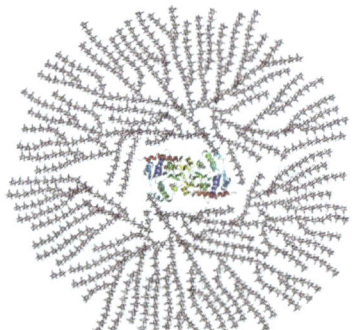

Figure 9.6 Glycogen core surrounded by thousands of linked glucose molecules[5]

During exercise, glycogen, especially that stored in the particular muscles being exercised, breaks down, supplying fuel for the muscles. (The rest of the energy is supplied by the breakdown of fat into fatty acids, which are then burned as fuel.) Fatigue occurs if the glycogen in these muscles becomes depleted.[6]

Carbohydrates come in two basic types, *simple* and *complex*. The simple carbohydrates include all of the sugars, such as glucose, fructose, sucrose, and lactose. There are two kinds of complex carbohydrates:

- *Starch* (where 300 to 1,000 glucose units join together)
- *Cellulose* (where some 1,500 glucose rings chain together)

It really doesn't matter how the racing sailor gets his or her carbohydrates, although the starches are generally more nutritious than the simple sugars. Everyone is familiar with the starches, but few people appreciate the importance of cellulose, especially for the cruising sailor.

Cellulose is found in the fibrous part of plants and is present in the leaves, stems, seeds, roots, and the covering of fruit. It gives trees and plants their rigidity. Cellulose is insoluble in water, and because cellulose is resistant to human digestive enzymes, it provides the food residue with *bulk* or *fiber*, which aids in bowel movement. Cellulose is one form of fiber—*insoluble fiber*. Other insoluble fibers include wheat bran, vegetables, and whole grains. Cellulose is especially important for individuals who routinely become constipated at sea. One explanation for sea constipation is that in a nautical environment we become mildly dehydrated. Fluid intake is often less than on land and, if the weather is warm, a significant amount of water may be lost via sweating (see Chapter 4). In order to preserve total body water, extra water is reabsorbed from the food residue, and this in turn produces constipation. This, by the way, is the main job of the colon—to regulate water in our waste material. Cellulose fiber, since it is hydrophilic (attracts water), tends to counteract this action, retaining the water and promoting a more normal bowel movement. The other type of fiber is *soluble fiber*, which attracts water and turns into a gel that slows digestion. It is found in oat bran, barley, nuts, seeds, beans, peas, lentils, and certain fruits and vegetables. Psyllium seed is a common soluble fiber supplement (e.g., Metamucil). If the sailor tends toward constipation, use either dietary or supplementary fiber or both.

One final topic is the concept of *glycemic index* (GI). Not all carbohydrates are equal in how rapidly they are absorbed from the gut. The GI is a relative ranking of carbohydrates based upon the rapidity of absorption (and what the insulin "spike" is like). As you may recall, insulin is secreted by the pancreas in order to send glucose into the cells of the body.

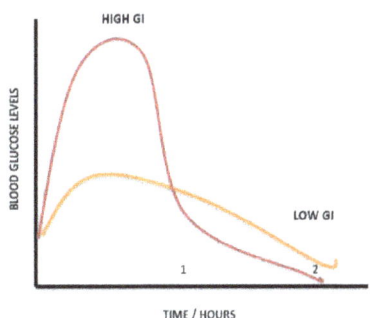

Figure 9.7 GI curves: high GI versus low GI

High-glycemic foods induce a spike in insulin and produce a rapid and high rise in blood sugar. In general, this is not desirable as it can lead to obesity, heart disease, and diabetes. However, there is one situation when it is advantageous to have high glycemic index carbohydrates: during prolonged periods of intense exercise or between repeated bouts of exercise such as would occur with two races in the same day. In that situation, when you need to replenish your glucose as rapidly as possible to aid exercise performance, you need carbs to be absorbed and metabolized rapidly. In this situation, high-caloric sports drinks or sugar-intense foods such as candy like jellybeans are a good choice.

The values are obtained by taking blood samples from subjects after they have eaten a specific food to see how their blood sugar rises. If there is a sharp spike, then it has a high GI; a slower rise is typical of a lower-glycemic food. (see Figure 9.8). Unfortunately, there is a great deal of variability in food absorption, which is why dieticians and nutritionists have not found the GI very helpful—especially in managing diabetics. But although the values are not absolute, they are still useful for our purposes. Sailors, especially racing sailors, need to be aware of foods that have a high GI so they can rapidly replenish their glucose. For everyone else, lower GI foods are definitely preferable.

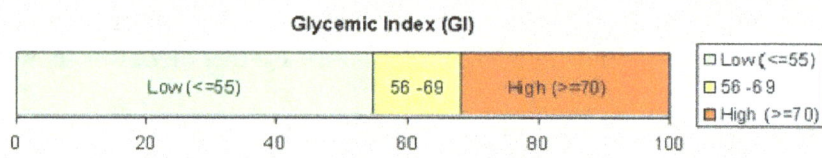

Figure 9.8 GI scale

Fats

Fats are an essential part of our diet although some types of fat are healthier than others.

Saturated fats are the ones most highly linked to an increased risk of cardiovascular disease. You can recognize saturated fats because they are usually *solid at room temperature*. Products include dairy foods such as butter, cream, and cheese as well as fatty cuts of beef, pork, and lamb and processed meats like salami. Packaged goods high in saturated fats include pastries and pies, croissants, cakes, high-fat muffins, deep-fried foods, and fatty snacking foods such as potato chips.

Unsaturated fats are an important part of a healthy diet. They help reduce the risk of cardiovascular disease and help lower cholesterol levels when they replace saturated fats in the diet. They come in two varieties:

- *Monounsaturated fats* are found in olive oil, canola oil, avocados, cashews, and almonds
- *Polyunsaturated fats* are found in fish (omega-3 fats), safflower and soybean oils (omega-6 fats), and some nuts, such as Brazil nuts

Trans fats are unsaturated fats that have been processed and behave like saturated fats. These fats increase LDL cholesterol ("bad cholesterol") and decrease HDL cholesterol ("good cholesterol"). They are found in many packaged foods and should be avoided if possible.

Cholesterol is a type of fat that has many, many important functions in the body although high levels of LDL cholesterol are associated with cardiovascular disease. It has been recognized for some time that the majority of cholesterol in the human body is actually manufactured in the body, rather than derived from the diet.

Vitamins

Vitamins are the most misunderstood of all of the food substances. They neither supply energy to the body nor contribute to its mass. What they actually do is play a crucial role as catalysts in many of the body's metabolic reactions. As catalysts, vitamin stores are used up very slowly, so their daily requirements are small.

There are thirteen vitamins: vitamin A (retinols and carotenoids), vitamin B1 (thiamine), vitamin B2 (riboflavin), vitamin B3 (niacin), vitamin B5 (pantothenic acid), vitamin B6 (pyridoxine), vitamin B7 (biotin), vitamin B9 (folic acid or folate), vitamin B12 (cobalamins), vitamin C (ascorbic acid), vitamin D (calciferols), vitamin E (tocopherols and tocotrienols), and vitamin K (quinones). Nine of the vitamins are water soluble (all the B vitamins and vitamin C), while four of the vitamins are fat soluble (A, D, E, and K). Since the fat-soluble vitamins are stored in the fatty tissues of the body, they do not need to be taken every day. In fact, it takes years for symptoms of a fat-soluble-vitamin deficiency to occur. Excessive intake, however, has risks, especially true of vitamins A and D. Although a true "overdose" of vitamins E and K is unusual, intake above recommended levels offers no particular benefit. The water-soluble vitamins—the B-complex and C—are not stored as extensively. Unlike the fat-soluble vitamins, excessive intake does not produce continued accumulation. Once the body's stores are replete, whatever is left over is excreted in the urine.

Athletes, because they have a higher total calorie intake, have a slightly higher requirement for three of the B-complex vitamins—thiamine (B1), riboflavin (B2), and niacin. Nevertheless, vitamin supplementation is not necessary since a varied diet contains an abundance of B-complex vitamins.

Experiments have demonstrated that on a diet that contains no vitamin C whatsoever, it takes four to six months to deplete the body's stores. For this reason, scurvy (a vitamin-C deficiency) did not become a nautical health problem until the age of exploration, when extended voyages were attempted. The saddest part of the scurvy story is that it didn't need to occur at all!

As early as 1593, during a voyage to the South Pacific, Sir Richard Hawkins recommended the following treatment for scurvy: "That which I have seen most fruitfull for this sicknesse, is sower [sour] oranges and lemmons."[7] Better yet, only seven years later,

Captain James Lancaster unintentionally performed a controlled study of lemon juice as a preventive for scurvy. His fleet of four ships departed on April 2, 1601, and scurvy began to appear in three of the ships by August 1 (four months after sailing). By the time of arrival, September 9, the three ships were so devastated by scurvy that the men of Lancaster's ship had to assist the rest of the fleet into the harbor. "And the reason why the General's [Lancaster's] men stood better in health than the men of other ships was this:—he brought to sea with him certaine bottles of the juice of limons, which he gave to each one as long as it would last, three spoonfuls every morning, fasting, not suffering them to eat anything after it till noone."[8]

Incredibly, the naval authorities ignored these discoveries, and scurvy continued to decimate the ranks of seamen. The account of Admiral George A. Anson's round-the-world voyage in the *Centurion* is gruesome testimony. In 1740 he embarked with six ships and 1,955 men in all. Four years later the flagship alone returned; 1,051 sailors died, mostly of scurvy.

Losses of this magnitude encouraged the Scottish naval surgeon James Lind to seek a cure. Aware of the earlier work, he performed his now classic experiment in 1747 aboard the *Salisbury*, studying the effects of several types of treatment, including one composed of "two oranges and one lemon given every day" on sailors with the typical signs of scurvy—"putrid gums, the spots and lassitude, with weakness of their knees." The curative power of these citrus fruits was clear, although with typical bureaucratic inertia, it was another forty-eight years before the Admiralty prescribed lemon juice for all British sailors. What finally persuaded the Admiralty was the experience of Captain James Cook. Less than thirty years after Anson's voyage, Cook made his first voyage of a little more than three years, losing but one man from disease, probably tuberculosis. On board, Cook pursued a slightly different tack. He relied heavily on malt and sauerkraut as preventives. For actual cases of scurvy, he used orange and lemon juice, the limited supply of which the surgeon kept. Cook also sent men ashore at every opportunity to procure local fresh vegetables. In order to persuade his men to eat these exotic foods, he insisted that his officers eat them with tremendous gusto in front of the men. This ingenious strategy was so effective that rationing was sometimes necessary. Cook was the first commander to demonstrate conclusively that long ocean voyages did not necessarily result in scurvy or other health problems, an achievement in which he took pride.

Undoubtedly, the scurvy story should end there, but there is one additional twist. For years, the victualing commissioners obtained their lemon juice from Sicily. However, in the nineteenth century, it seemed feasible to replace the lemon with the lime, which was in plentiful supply in the West Indies. Since the juice of the lime was supposedly as good as that of the lemon, it was made the official antiscurvy treatment for the Royal Navy in 1860 (hence the term limey). Unfortunately, no one realized that *preserved* lime juice, unlike preserved lemon juice, contains little vitamin C. Outbreaks of scurvy reappeared until 1918, when it was proven conclusively (using guinea pigs) that preserved lime juice had little to no antiscorbutic effect! The British Navy estimates that during the worst years of the scurvy, between 1600 and 1800, nearly five thousand lives were lost each year. That means that nearly one million men died of an easily preventable disease—largely due to official indifference.

Now, it is relatively easy to obtain a sufficient amount of vitamin C in the diet. Good sources include oranges, orange juice, grapefruits, grapefruit juice, cantaloupe, strawberries, broccoli, brussels sprouts, and green and sweet red peppers. Fair sources include tangerines, tomatoes, honeydew melon, watermelon, asparagus, cauliflower, cabbage, spinach, and potatoes cooked in their skins.

For the cruising sailor with adequate food supplies—including citrus fruits, vegetables, and tubers—there is no need to take any vitamin supplementation. If food supplies are marginal, one multivitamin tablet per day provides a wide margin of safety. The racing sailor must realize that because vitamins are used over and over again in metabolic reactions, the vitamin needs of an athlete are virtually the same as the requirements of more sedentary people. (The slightly higher requirement for B-complex vitamins is provided by any balanced, varied diet.)

Minerals

About 4 percent of the body is composed of a group of elements known as minerals. The minerals can be divided into the major minerals, such as calcium, phosphorus, iron, iodine, magnesium, sodium, potassium, and chloride (the last three known collectively as electrolytes), and the trace minerals, which, as the name implies, are present in minute amounts.

As with vitamins, mineral supplementation is generally unnecessary, because most minerals are readily available in a varied diet. The only exceptions are the electrolytes and iron. Electrolyte replacement and water balance are covered in depth in Chapter 4. About 15 percent of women in the childbearing years have poor iron stores or iron depletion. Iron depletion does not mean that the person has or will develop anemia, although it may predispose to the condition. It does mean that the amount of iron stored in the body is less than normal. Iron-depleted women may have a lower exercise tolerance than normal women. It is certainly true that iron-deficiency anemia does impair performance. In most instances, iron stores can be augmented with a diet rich in iron, such as dried uncooked fruits, beans, peas, green leafy vegetables, egg yolk, liver, and kidneys. If it is documented (usually during a medical examination) that there is either iron depletion (and the woman is an athlete) or has frank iron-deficiency anemia, then iron supplementation is usually required.

Calories and Exercise

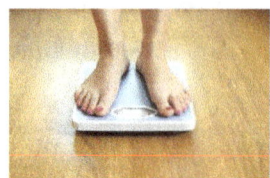

A *calorie* is a measure of energy expenditure and stored energy. Calories referred to in the diets discussed below represent calories eaten in the diet as well as calories burned during exercise. Actually, these are *kilocalories*. Often when you encounter the word calories what someone is really talking about are kilocalories so that:

calories (common usage in the United States) = kilocalories

(Scientifically, one kilocalorie is equal to the amount of heat that will raise the temperature of 1 kilogram of water by 1 degree Celsius at sea level.)

Different nutrients, as discussed above, have more or fewer calories packed into the same weight. Nutrition labels use these conversions:

- 1 gram of carbohydrates (sugars and starches) = 4 calories (kilocalories)
- 1 gram of protein = 4 calories (kilocalories)
- 1 gram of fat = 9 calories (kilocalories)
- 1 gram of fiber (a poorly digested carbohydrate), approximately = 1.5 calories (kilocalories)
- 1 gram of alcohol = 7 calories (kilocalories)

Each pound (0.45 kilogram) of body fat stores approximately 3,500 calories (kilocalories). Therefore, if you wish to lose 1 pound (0.45 kilogram) of body fat in a week you would need to eat approximately 500 fewer calories per day (7 days x 500 = 3,500). There are really three aspects of calorie burning that we need to consider:

(1) *Basal metabolic rate* (BMR). These are the calories that are spent keeping our body running, including breathing, pumping blood, temperature regulation, and so forth—basically, all the functions of our autonomic nervous system. This area represents 60 to 70 percent of our daily caloric expenditure.

(2) *Thermic effect of food* (TEF). About 10 to 15 percent of our calorie expenditure is actually spent digesting our food—it takes work to digest a meal.

(3) *Exercise and activity* (EAT & NEAT). We are all familiar with burning calories during exercise—technically known as *exercise activity thermogenesis or* EAT. There are numerous charts to quantify caloric burn during different exercises. It is worth noting that walking on a level surface only burns about 100 calories per mile. So, in order to

burn 1 pound or 3,500 calories, you would need to walk 35 miles! If you walk 3 miles, burn 300 calories, and then return home and eat a large chocolate chip cookie you have totally negated your exercise.

There is, however, one more concept that is generally ignored, and that is *non-exercise activity thermogenesis*, or NEAT. This is the energy that is expended for everything that we do during the day that is not sleeping, eating, or sports exercise. It includes energy expended fidgeting, pacing, doing housework, and so forth. We are familiar with people who seem to be in constant motion; this definitely does burn calories and needs to be taken into consideration. EAT and NEAT can represent up to 30 percent of total body calorie expenditure per day in very active people.

Calories in includes everything you eat or drink, and calories out is represented by the formula:

Total Daily Energy Expenditure (TDEE) = BMR + TEF + NEAT + EAT[9]

Simply stated, body weight depends on only two parameters: the number of calories taken in and the number of calories expended, or TDEE. Altering one or the other (or both) results in a change in body weight. In other words,

Stable weight: calories in = calories out
Increase in weight: calories in > calories out
Decrease in weight: calories in < calories out

That's it, pure and simple. It doesn't matter how the calories are provided nor when in the day they are taken in (for the most part). All that matters are the total daily calories in and the total daily calories out!

The active adult man consumes and expends about 2,700 to 3,000 calories per day; the average active woman 2,000 to 2,100. These figures assume that a healthy, active person spends about eight hours sleeping, six hours sitting, six hours standing, two hours walking, and about two hours in light recreational activities per day. Certainly, active sailors and sailing athletes expend more than that, but even athletes at the peak of training rarely consume and expend more than 4,500 to 5,000 calories per day.

A sailor who wishes to lose weight as part of a physical fitness program has three options: (1) decrease caloric intake, (2) increase activity, or (3) do both. It turns out that the third option is the most preferable since it results in the greatest loss of fat and the least loss of lean body mass (i.e., the muscles and connective tissue).

Is there a way to calculate your TDDE? Yes. In order to figure out how much energy we are currently using, we need to first calculate our BMR (see above for definition). There are a number of equations to calculate BMR, but the most widely used is the Mifflin St. Jeor equation.

System	M/W	BMR Formula
Metric	Men	BMR= (10 x weight in kg) ÷ (6.25 x height in cm) − (5 x age in years) +5
Metric	Women	BMR= (10 x weight in kg) ÷ (6.25 x height in cm) − (5 x age in years) -161
US	Men	BMR= (4.54 x weight in lbs.) ÷ (15.88 x height in in.) − (5 x age in years) +5
US	Women	BMR= (4.54 x weight in lbs.) ÷ (15.88 x height in in.) − (5 x age in years) -161

Table 9.1 Mifflin St. Jeor Equation for BMR

For example, let's assume boater John is 30 years old, weighs 200 pounds, and is 6 feet tall (i.e., 72 inches). His daily caloric requirement *while at rest* would be: (4.54 x 200) + (15.88 x 72) − (5 x 30) +5 = 1,906.36 cal (kcal). But John is no couch potato. He needs to calculate his energy needs while active. How active? If John actually is engaged in moderate exercise, then to maintain his weight he would have to consume 2,955 calories per day (1,906.36 x 1.55 = 2,955).

Little to no exercise	Daily cal (kcal) needed = BMR x 1.2
Light exercise (1-3 days per week)	Daily cal (kcal) needed = BMR x 1.375
Moderate exercise (3-5 days per week)	Daily cal (kcal) needed = BMR x 1.55
Heavy exercise (6-7 days per week)	Daily cal (kcal) needed = BMR x 1.725
Very Heavy exercise (twice per day, extra heavy)	Daily cal (kcal) needed = BMR x 1.9

Table 9.2 Exercise intensity

If you don't fit exactly into one of these categories, then extrapolate (e.g., heavy exercise three days a week might lead you to an activity factor of around 1.65 [between 1.55 and 1.725]).

Designing a weight-reduction program is simple. All you need to recall is the conversion factor for calories and pounds of fat, which is approximately 3,500 to 1. [For the rest of the world, there are 7,700 calories per kilogram] The most prudent rate of weight loss is about 1 pound per week. This requires a net deficit of 3,500 calories per week or 500 calories per day. One way to achieve this deficit is to limit intake by 500 calories per day. However, half an hour of moderate exercise (about 350 calories) performed three times a week produces a 1,050-calorie deficit; consequently, the weekly caloric intake could be reduced by only 2,400 calories instead of 3,500 in order to lose 1 pound a week. If the number of exercise days is increased to five, causing a 1,750-calorie deficit, the food intake needs to be reduced by only 250 calories per day. If these five-day-per-week workouts are prolonged to a full hour, then no reduction in food intake is required, because the 3,500-calorie deficit is created entirely through exercise.[10]

Healthy Diets

There are innumerable diet programs available, but I would like to explore the three most popular because I believe that a recurring theme is present in these, as well as many other diets. The two top diets every year are Dietary Approaches to Stop Hypertension (DASH) (Figure 9.9) and the Mediterranean (Figure 9.10). The DASH diet encourages reducing dietary sodium, as well as eating a variety of foods rich in nutrients that help to lower blood pressure, including potassium, calcium, and magnesium. The DASH diet emphasizes fruits, vegetables, and low-fat dairy foods, as well as moderate amounts of whole grains, fish, poultry, and nuts. In the standard DASH diet, you consume up to 2,300 milligrams of sodium per day, and in the lower sodium DASH diet, you can consume up to 1,500 milligrams of sodium per day. Both versions reduce the sodium compared to a typical American diet, which can contain up to 3,500 milligrams of sodium each day.

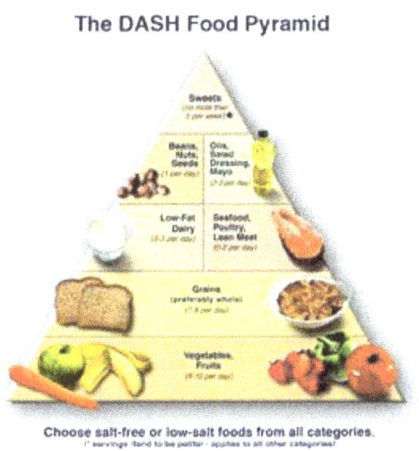

Grains: six to eight servings per day
Vegetables: four to five servings per day
Fruits: four to five servings per day
Dairy: two to three servings per day
Lean meat, poultry, and fish: six servings or fewer a week
Nuts, seeds and legumes: four to five servings a week
Fats and oils: two to three servings a day
Sweets: five servings or fewer per week

Figure 9.9 DASH food pyramid[11]

Research has shown that both the DASH and Mediterranean diet reduce the risk of heart disease. The Mediterranean diet has been shown to lower the level of LDL cholesterol—the "bad" cholesterol—and was associated with a reduced risk of not only cardiovascular mortality but also overall mortality. The focus is on making wise choices especially in terms of the types of fat, favoring monounsaturated and polyunsaturated fat (see above). It also encourages wine (in moderation but not if there is a personal history of alcohol abuse).

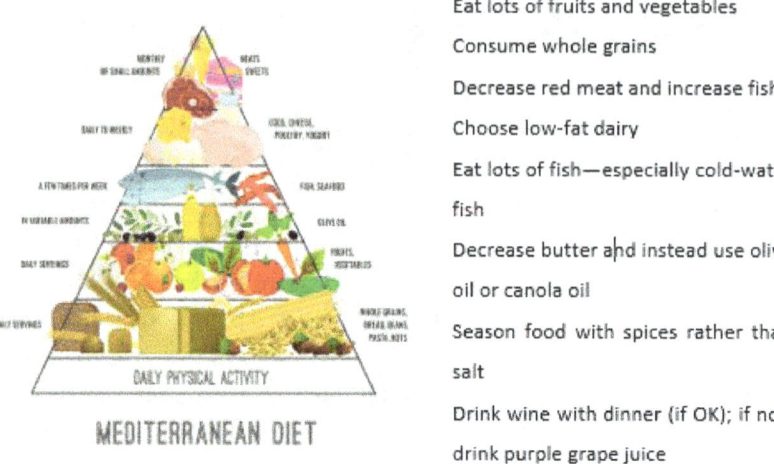

Figure 9.10 Mediterranean diet pyramid[12]

The third diet I'd like to mention is the Mediterranean-DASH Intervention for Neurodegenerative Delay (MIND) diet developed by Martha Clare Morris, ScD, and her colleagues at Rush University Medical Center in Chicago. MIND is a hybrid of the first two diets. The diet specifically addresses the effect of food nutrients on brain health and cognition. It appears that adhering to the diet may slow cognitive decline among aging adults (even if the person is not at risk for Alzheimer's) and actually reduces the risk of developing Alzheimer's—at least in the initial study at Rush it appeared to reduce the risk of Alzheimer's substantially. According to Laurel Cherian, MD, one of the study authors and vascular neurologist at Rush, the people who were most adherent to the MIND diet cognitively functioned as if they were 7.5 years younger!

The common themes in these three diets should be self-evident. Time will tell if one turns out to be more superior than the other. Obviously choose the one that best fits your lifestyle. For example, if you come from a Mediterranean background (possibly Italian or Greek), then that might be the easiest to follow.[14]

Nutrition and the Sailing Athlete

For the power boater or cruising sailor, the above diets (and others not discussed here) should be a good starting point. If you follow one of those heart- and brain-healthy diets, watch your overall caloric intake, and exercise, you should be good to go. It is still wise to have a regular check-up with your primary care physician, monitor your blood pressure, and have routine laboratory studies. Evidence has become clear that early treatment of chronic diseases such as hypertension, diabetes, and hypercholesterolemia will prevent or ameliorate problems down the road. And if you follow those diets listed above, you will probably have no need for any nutritional supplementation whatsoever.

Sailing Nutrition

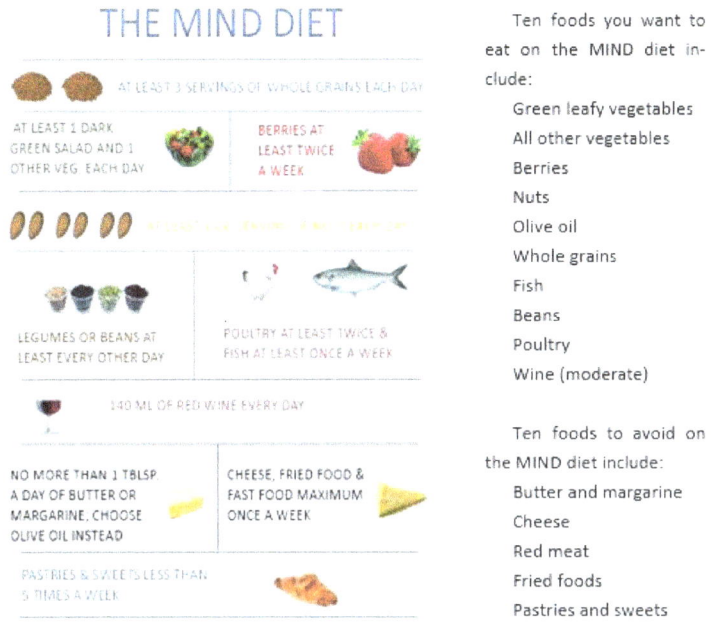

Ten foods you want to eat on the MIND diet include:
  Green leafy vegetables
  All other vegetables
  Berries
  Nuts
  Olive oil
  Whole grains
  Fish
  Beans
  Poultry
  Wine (moderate)

Ten foods to avoid on the MIND diet include:
  Butter and margarine
  Cheese
  Red meat
  Fried foods
  Pastries and sweets

Figure 9.11 The MIND diet[13]

The nutritional demands for the sailing athlete, however, get a lot more complicated very quickly. And the nutritional demands are quite different for a long-distance ocean voyager (think Volvo Ocean Race), an America's Cup crew member, an Olympic Laser sailor, or even a sailboarder. And if you are one of the crew on an America's Cup boat, you could be a grinder, sail trimmer, or a helmsman, all with very different nutritional needs.

How Do Our Energy Systems Work?

The proper care and feeding of our energy system (our body) is the bottom line. The outlines are very simple. We take in nutrients (foodstuffs), our body metabolizes those nutrients during this process, and the body creates *adenosine triphosphate* (ATP). ATP is the main "energy currency" that powers the ship. That's it. Well, that's not exactly it. The chemical reactions that occur behind the scenes are extremely complicated and would curl your hair. We don't need to know all of that, but we do need to understand ATP.

Energy in the body is produced by splitting a chemical bond on the ATP molecule (Figure 9.12). In the figure, the bond between the last phosphate to the left and the next to the last is a *high energy bond*. When ATP is metabolized into adenosine diphosphate (ADP), energy is released to carry out work by the muscles (although up to 75 percent is given off as heat, which is why your muscles feel warm).

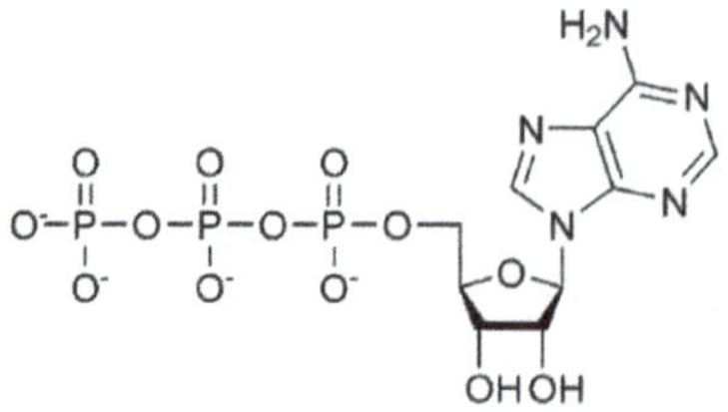

Figure 9.12 ATP

Once the ATP is converted into ADP and the energy is released, then the ADP is converted back to ATP and the process is ready to begin all over again.

$$ATP \leftrightarrow ADP + P + Energy$$

All of the stored energy in our body comes from one of three sources (Figure 9.13): carbohydrates (4 kilocalories/gram), fats (9 kilocalories/gram), or protein (4 kilocalories/gram). Ultimately, all of the energy stored in these nutrients is harvested in order to synthesize ATP, which, as we saw, is the "energy currency" of the human body.

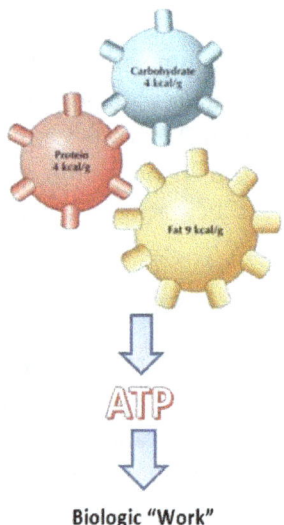

Figure 9.13 Energy sources

Let's look more carefully at storage (Table 9.3). The first thing to notice is that there is astonishingly little ATP stored in the body. For everyday tasks, it is constantly being used and replenished but very little is sitting around waiting. This is so-called "just-in-time" manufacturing.

Energy Source	Storage Site	Energy (kcal)
ATP/Creatine Phosphate	Tissues	5
Carbohydrate	Blood glucose	80
	Muscle Glycogen	410
	Liver Glycogen	1,500
Fat	Serum Fat (free fatty acids)	8
	Serum Triglycerides	75
	Muscle Triglycerides	2,500
	Adipose Tissue (fat)	80,000 or more
Protein	Muscle Protein	32,000

Table 9.3: Energy storage in the "normal" human

Carbohydrate storage is composed of blood glucose—the blood sugar that is in your blood for ready use—as well as stored carbohydrate in the liver and muscle in the form of *glycogen*. Glycogen is a multibranched polysaccharide of glucose. Figure 9.6 earlier in the chapter demonstrates a glycogen molecule with the core surrounded by up to thirty thousand branches of glucose units. The total body store of glycogen is about 500 grams (400 in the muscles and 100 in the liver). This is only about 2,000 calories. Increasing muscle mass will increase your glycogen storage, which, as we will see shortly, is something you can modify *depending on your exercising needs*. Each of the glucose units are cleaved off and thrown into the stew to make more ATP.

Fat storage is much more "robust." The average person stores about 10 to 15 kilograms of fat as adipose tissue, mostly beneath the skin and around internal organs. Fat reserves contain a huge amount of stored energy (Table 9.3). It is the major fuel for long-term, low intensity exercise. Also, as it is integral to all cell membranes everywhere in your body, including your brain and nerves, some fat is essential. It also cushions the internal organs. Fat provides those fat-soluble vitamins A, D, and E, which is why athletes should consume some fat, or risk developing deficiencies of those vitamins and essential fatty acids. Figure 9.14 is an illustration of a triglyceride molecule (which is how most fat is stored), with the glycerol backbone and the three rows of fatty acids (hence *tri*glyceride).

As with glycogen, the triglycerides are broken apart and thrown into the stew to produce more ATP.

The human body also requires protein—it is needed for building and repairing muscle and other organs. But unlike carbohydrate and fat, excess protein is not able to be stored and therefore is not a major source of energy. The protein in Table 9.3 is stored in the muscle, but as muscle protein, it is not a ready storage source for energy/activity. However, proteins can be broken down for energy in two situations. First, if you eat

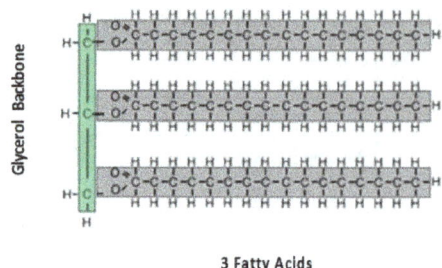

Figure 9.14 Glycerol/fatty acid structure

more protein than is needed for repair of damaged tissues, then it will be turned into ATP and used as fuel. Second, as we will see shortly, in very strenuous and prolonged events—mainly in long endurance events when glycogen has been depleted—protein will be liberated from the muscle and used as fuel.

The Energy Systems

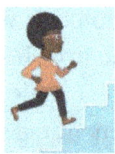

Now that we've discussed how the body banks all of this energy, it's time to look at how it's used. Perhaps the banking metaphor is a good one. If we need money quickly, we could go to an ATM. But there is a limit to what we can withdraw. If we need more, we must go into the bank. (This takes time, and you are bound to get behind some old person who wants to cash a check and can't find their ID.) If you need to borrow even more, you could establish a line of credit…you get the idea. You might think, for example, that a fair amount of ATP would be stored in the muscles, but as we have seen, that is not the case. (It would be equivalent to walking around with thousands of dollars in your pocket.) Only a small amount of ATP is present in the muscles for immediate use—just enough to last for very short bursts of activity, such as the *initial few steps* of sprinting or running up the stairs, for example, but for no more than a few seconds.

Once past the first few seconds of any activity, ATP must be regenerated from one of the three main energy systems:

(1) ATP-PC (phosphocreatine), aka phosphagen system
(2) Anaerobic (without oxygen) glycolysis system
(3) Aerobic (oxidative) glycolysis (carbohydrate) or lipolytic (fats) system

ATP-PC (Phosphocreatine/Phosphagen)—Short Burst of Power

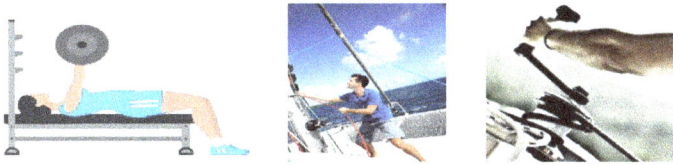

During short bursts of power, the body rapidly produces additional ATP by adding phosphocreatine to the ADP and reconstituting ATP for use by the muscle. A typical example might be when completing a bench press, a sail raise, or a grinder on a short tack. This provides enough energy for five to ten seconds of maximum effort and is depleted within twenty to thirty seconds (see Figure 9.15, phosphagen line). Energy is restored quickly with perhaps 50 percent available thirty seconds later and up to 100 percent within two to three minutes, thus allowing many short bursts of activity lasting five to ten seconds each without a person becoming exhausted. (Phosphocreatine is produced when the phosphate molecule binds with a creatine molecule. This is precisely the reason that *creatine supplementation* is commonly used—see below.) So far, we have been talking about energy as ATP stored in the muscle (very little) and ATP in the muscle that can be rapidly synthesized by adding phosphocreatine to ADP (the phosphagen system: fast but limited in duration).

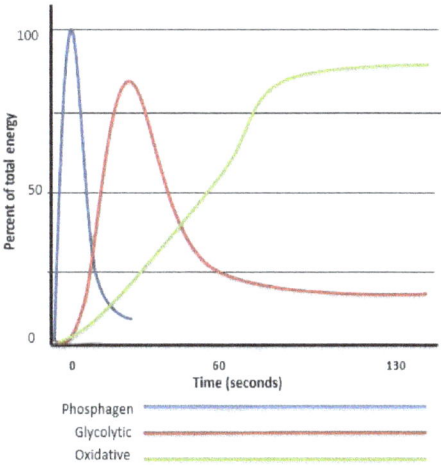

Figure 9.15: The energy response of three systems: phosphagen, glycolytic, and aerobic (oxidative)

Anaerobic Glycolysis—Short-Term, High-Intensity Activity

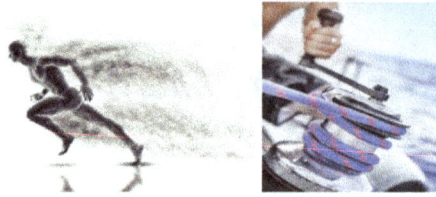

Carbohydrates (mainly glucose) are the major fuel for short-term, high-intensity exercise. An example might be a 200-meter sprint, a 50-meter swim, or anything high intensity on a boat lasting thirty seconds to two minutes. This kind of activity is primarily anaerobic (without oxygen). That is, the chemical reaction does not require oxygen to proceed, although that doesn't mean you are not breathing hard! It just takes time for the oxygen to get into the lungs, hook a ride on the hemoglobin in your red blood cells, get to your muscles, and unload the oxygen. The oxygen hasn't arrived in sufficient amount to help out right away. What supplies the energy in this high-intensity activity? Carbohydrates; i.e. glucose stored in the muscles as glycogen. However, the chemical reactions only produce a limited amount of ATP; it is just not a very efficient system (although it is pretty fast). This is the glycolytic curve shown in Figure 9.15. It is over in two minutes. (If I wasn't prepared to discuss seaweed sex in Chapter 2, I'm certainly not going to add any sexual innuendos at this point!) In addition to producing ATP, the glucose is metabolized into pyruvate and then lactate. As the lactate accumulates in the muscle, it decreases the pH of the muscle and causes muscle fatigue (lactic acidosis). (Some of the lactate is released into the blood stream and taken up by the liver and resynthesized into glucose—no one said this was easy.)

Aerobic (With Oxygen) Glycolysis—Prolonged Lower-Intensity Activity

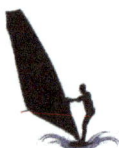

Although the aerobic system does not kick in as rapidly, it can produce larger amounts of ATP. So, to recapitulate when you start to exercise, you use the *ATP–phosphocreatine (phosphagen) system*, then transition to the *anaerobic glycolysis system*, and, after a few minutes of continuous activity, your body transitions to the *aerobic (oxidative) system*.

Most of the glucose that fuels aerobic glycolysis comes from glycogen stored in the muscle. In events lasting less than thirty minutes, the muscles rely primarily on the glycogen that is stored in that muscle. After about one hour, when the muscle glycogen begins to dwindle, glucose from the bloodstream becomes more important, and by two hours, almost all of the muscle glycogen is depleted. Once glycogen stores are exhausted, the athlete can continue, but at perhaps 50 percent of maximal capacity. This is commonly known as "hitting the wall." If possible, before all of the glycogen is depleted, taking some rapidly dissolved glucose (high GI) will allow the body to "save the muscle glycogen" for a sudden burst or a second workout later in the day. Once the glycogen is depleted, you are totally dependent on glucose in the bloodstream (ultimately from the liver and any carbs you eat or drink during the activity). In general, with most aerobic activity, the demand for energy is slower and smaller and there is more than enough time for oxygen to be transported from the lungs to the muscles and then to react with glucose to manufacture ATP. *Aerobic energy production is up to twenty times more efficient than anaerobic, but it is also much slower.*

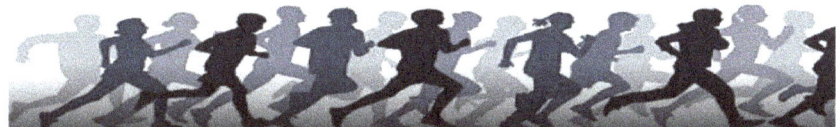

During prolonged exercise, fat becomes the predominant fuel source for muscle. During very long events, such as long-distance running, marathons, ultramarathons or Ironman events, fat may supply up to 50 to 90 percent of the energy; the better trained the muscle is, the better it can utilize fat and spare the glycogen. On the other hand, the more unfit the muscle, the more it will rely on carbohydrate rather than fat. Training actually increases the level of fatty acid oxidative enzymes, allowing athletes to use fat more readily as a fuel. Think of it this way: during long events, the energy demands are lower, production is slower, but "Jumpin' Jehoshaphat"—that fat's got staying power. One fatty acid molecule can produce two to five times as much ATP as glycogen.

Glucose or Fat?

So how does your body decide whether to use glucose or fat during aerobic activity? There are a number of factors including:

- Intensity of exercise
- Duration of exercise
- Fitness level
- Preexercise diet

Intensity. The higher the intensity, the greater the reliance on glycogen in the muscle. As we saw during anaerobic exercise, energy is produced by the ATP-PC (phosphocreatine) and anaerobic glycolysis systems. During aerobic activity, the body uses a mixture of glycogen and fat. Exercising at low intensity mainly relies on fat. As the intensity of the exercise increases—running faster and faster—the proportion shifts from fat to glycogen. At moderate levels, the mixture may be fifty-fifty. When the exercise becomes very intense, glycogen supplies provide 70 to 75 percent of energy needs (Figure 9.16).

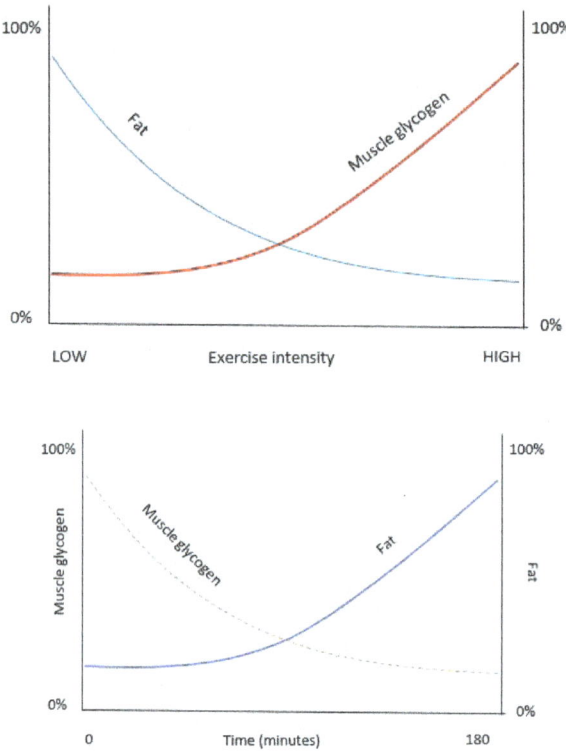

Figure 9.16 Fat versus glycogen in exercise intensity and duration

Duration. The stores of muscle glycogen are limited, as we have seen. They can become exhausted as you continue to exercise. As muscle glycogen falls, fat plays a greater role in energy production.

Fitness level. Aerobic training creates a number of adaptations in the fat-oxidizing enzymes, which makes your body more efficient in converting fat into fatty acids. In fact, the mitochondria (energy area of the cell) actually increases in size, which means that each cell now has a greater capacity to burn the fat that both improves aerobic fitness and spares glycogen.

Preexercise diet. A low-carb diet will result in less glycogen storage, and this can create a serious impairment in the body's ability to sustain exercise. When muscle glycogen is low, the body relies on fat and protein for energy.

Sailing Nutrition

Activity Level	Daily Carbohydrate Intake
Very Light training (low intensity or skill based)	3-5 g/kg body weight daily
Moderate intensity training (approx. 1 hr/day)	5-7 g/kg body weight daily
Moderate-high intensity training (1 -3 hr/day)	6-10 g/kg body weight daily
Very high intensity training (> 4 hr/day)	8-12 g/kg body weight daily

Table 9.4 Guidelines for daily carbohydrate intake[15]

Table 9.4 provides some guidelines for daily carbohydrate requirement, based on training intensity.

There is one other school of thought that is somewhat controversial: *training low*. That is a *low* carbohydrate diet that apparently, for some athletes, increases the efficiency of fat metabolism. This type of training may have some appeal to long distance/endurance types who depend on fat burning for a good deal of their activity; however, *for virtually all boating and sailing activities, a low carbohydrate diet would appear to be counterproductive.*

Protein consumption facilitates muscle repair and synthesis. Athletes need to consume approximately double the protein amount when compared with sedentary individuals. Generally, the upper limit is about 40 grams of protein in any one meal. Multiple meals throughout the day, each with 20 grams, is the best way to stimulate muscle protein synthesis.

Vegetarian athletes usually meet or exceed protein requirements; however, since the quality of plant protein has slightly less bioavailability, they should increase their protein needs by 10 to 15 percent. One other disadvantage is the low level of creatine in their diet (creatine is most abundant in muscle and more readily available to those of us carnivores). Creatine supplementation—especially for resistance exercises, predominant among the sailing athlete—has been demonstrated to be beneficial. There is also some concern regarding sufficient levels of iron, zinc, Vitamin B12, and calcium in the vegetarian diet. Vegetarian athletes may need additional nutritional guidance from a certified nutritionist who has experience in advising athletes.

Activity Level	Daily Carbohydrate Intake
Very Light training (low intensity or skill based)	3-5 g/kg body weight daily
Moderate intensity training (approx. 1 hr/day)	5-7 g/kg body weight daily
Moderate-high intensity training (1 -3 hr/day)	6-10 g/kg body weight daily
Very high intensity training (> 4 hr/day)	8-12 g/kg body weight daily

Table 9.5 Protein recommendations for athletes[16]

Notes

1. As cited in S. E. Morison, *The European Discovery of America: The Southern Voyages* (New York: Oxford University Press, 1974), 174.

2. L. H. Roddis, *A Short History of Nautical Medicine* (New York: Hoeber, 1941), 127.

3. Roddis, *A Short History of Nautical Medicine*, 129.

4. Rum had been issued in the British Navy since the early eighteenth century, initially at 1/2 pint per day. It was issued straight until 1740, when Admiral Edward Vernon ordered that it be diluted with water. The term *grog* has come to mean the mixture of spirits (usually rum) with water. Grog is said to allude to the fact that Vernon was known as "Old Grog" to his men, from the word grogram, a type of cloth from which his coat was made.

5. M. Häggström, "Medical Gallery of Mikael Häggström 2014," *WikiJournal of Medicine* 1, no. 2 (2014), DOI:10.15347/wjm/2014.008. ISSN 2002-4436. Public Domain.

6. Athletes who are involved in endurance events (runners or bicyclists, for example) have discovered that by modifying their carbohydrate intake prior to an athletic event, they can increase the amount of glycogen in their muscles and improve their performance. This has been confirmed experimentally. Subjects were divided into three groups and given three different diets. The first group had a normal caloric intake, but most of the calories were in the form of fat. The second group was provided with the recommended percentages of fat, carbohydrate, and protein. The third group was given over 80 percent of their calories in the form of carbohydrate. The glycogen concentration in the leg muscles of these subjects averaged 0.6, 1.75, and 3.75 grams per 100 grams of muscle, respectively. Those in the high carbohydrate group had significantly more glycogen in their muscles, and their endurance capacity was also markedly improved. The technique of *carbohydrate loading*, or *glycogen supercompensation*, consists of two phases. In the initial phase, exhaustive exercise and a low carbohydrate intake for three to four days deplete the muscles of glycogen. Phase two consists of reduced activity and high carbohydrate intake for the three to four days right before competition. This regimen can increase glycogen stores in those muscles that are exercised by well over 100 percent. For most competitive sailors who perform primarily brief, nonendurance tasks, carbohydrate loading is usually not necessary. For endurance events, a modified loading is more practical than the two-phase technique. Instead of restricting carbohydrates early in the week and restricting activity later in the week, the athlete continues intense training for the entire week prior to competition, increasing carbohydrate intake by 1,000 to 1,500 calories (above normal caloric intake) for 3 to 4 days before the event. This increase will produce a glycogen concentration in the exercised muscles about 75 percent as high as the full carbohydrate-loading regimen. Remember, carbohydrate loading is to be used only prior to selected events. It is not intended as a routine diet.

7. As cited in R. S. Allison, *Sea Diseases* (London: John Bale, 1943), 26.

8. As cited in Allison, *Sea Diseases*, 28.

9. E. T. Trexler, A. E. Smith-Ryan and L. E. Norton, "Metabolic Adaptation to Weight Loss: Implications for the Athlete," *Journal of the International Society of Sports Nutrition* 11, no. 7 (2014).

10. U.S. Department of Health and Human Services, Physical Activity Guidelines for Americans, 2nd ed. (Washington, DC: U.S. Department of Health and Human Services, 2018), https://health.gov/paguidelines/second-edition/pdf/Physical _Activity_Guidelines _2nd_ edition.pdf.

11. The DASH diet was developed in the early 1990s under the auspices of the National Institutes of Health. It has been endorsed by the Mayo Clinic and other leading institutions. See https://www.nhlbi.nih.gov/health-topics/dash-eating-plan.

12. In 1993 Oldways, a health-conscious non-profit in coordination with Harvard School of Public Health created the Mediterranean Diet Pyramid in part as a healthier alternative to the original food pyramid of the USDA (see Figure 9.3 above). This original USDA pyramid was the food pyramid that was "adulterated" by special interest groups.

13. K. Pearson, "The MIND Diet: A Detailed Guide for Beginners," *Healthline*, accessed March 17, 2019, https://www.healthline.com/nutrition/mind-diet.

14. There are two additional diets that have become popular lately. The first is the ketogenic diet (keto diet) and the second is intermittent fasting (IF). The ketogenic diet remains controversial since it is a high-fat, low-carbohydrate diet. There are a number of variations, but at this time, there is insufficient evidence that it is either healthy or sustainable. The second is IF. IF does appear to be healthy but requires the individual to fast for sixteen hours per day—eating is restricted to a contiguous eight-hour period during the daytime from say 10 a.m. to 6 p.m. or 7 a.m. to 3 p.m. It's just not easy for boaters or cruising sailors to stay on that schedule, and that is even more true for sailing athletes.

15. J. R. Berning, *Sports Nutrition in Netter's Sports Medicine*, 2nd ed. (Philadelphia: Elsevier, 2018), 28-33.

16. Berning, Sports Nutrition in Netter's Sports Medicine, 28-33.

Chapter 10

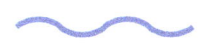

Exercise at Sea

"Seafaring people are that class of mankind who are supposed to be in perfect health when they enroll themselves for any particular voyage or cruise; notwithstanding their hardiness, they are liable to many and numerous excruciating maladies.... Sailors are very apt to become careless of their health, especially while in port, and expose themselves to every intemperance that can possibly produce the occasional causes of disease."

—Samuel H. P. Lee, medical doctor and apothecary, 1795

All boaters and sailors have reasons to stay in good physical shape. Small-boat-racing sailors recognize that sailing is like any other sport that requires a high degree of training and physical conditioning. They are interested in developing an exercise program that improves endurance and flexibility while also strengthening those muscle groups crucial to the small-boat racer. Crew members of larger boats, by contrast, may wish to design an exercise program that focuses on upper-body strength. Grinding or tailing a winch requires short, repetitive bursts of power. Their exercise needs differ in many fundamental respects from those of the small-boat racer. The cruising boater or sailor may not have any interest in training for competition; nevertheless, there are other reasons for keeping in shape. For one thing, exercise improves the overall efficiency of human machinery, making it less vulnerable to injury or accident. Additionally, most people simply feel better when they are engaged in a regular exercise program.

It is important for the mariner to adopt an exercise program that reflects both his or her specific goals as well as being tailored to his or her individual constraints of time and space. An exercise program, after all, is time consuming, and most of us have to choose from myriad exercises that will further our identified goals. Exercises chosen willy-nilly take up valuable time, with little demonstrable effect. Space may also be a consideration. Many of the exercises discussed here require heavy equipment. Since there is no place for such equipment aboard a boat, the cruising sailor is forced to plan ahead and seek imaginative alternatives. When designing a program, the sailor should identify specific goals: strength, flexibility, balance, speed, or endurance. Individual programs emphasize one or more of these goals. The importance of identifying one's primary and secondary goals in advance cannot be overemphasized.

What precautions should be taken prior to commencing an exercise program? Children and adolescents participating in sports of any kind should have a pre-participation physical examination. The primary objectives are: (1) to screen for any disorder or condition that could be disabling or life-threatening and (2) to screen for any disorder or condition that could predispose to injury. The specific details are still a matter of some debate. At the collegiate level, virtually every school requires a pre-participation physical. As an adult, you are on your own. Everyone over the age of thirty who is either beginning an exercise program, or increasing exercise to an appreciable extent should be evaluated. If you are engaging in sports (or if you are engaging in "life" for that matter), you should be aware of those risk factors that are modifiable and those that are not—and then do something about those that are! If you are smart enough to be reading this text but are not dealing with the modifiable risk factors listed in Table 10.1, then put down the text and address those risks first. You are presumably reading this text because you wish to stay healthy on the water, and yet you are not treating your cholesterol or your blood pressure? (I'm sorry…I promise that this scolding won't happen again!)

Nonmodifiable Factors
- Male gender
- Increasing age
- Family history of cardiovascular disease

Modifiable Factors
- Cigarette smoking
- High blood pressure
- Hyperlipidemia
- Prolonged physical inactivity
- Obesity
- Diabetes mellitus

Table 10.1 Risk factors (American Heart Association)

The organization of this chapter will be as follows:

- Training theory (basic exercise physiology)
- Components of a training program

- Cruising and conditioning
- The sailing athlete (big boat and Olympic classes)

There are a few basic exercise concepts that the sailor should consider when designing an individualized exercise program.

One way to think about your overall exercise program is to consider frequency, intensity, time, and type, otherwise known as the FITT principle. *Frequency* refers to how often you undertake the exercise (i.e., how many times per week you perform, or plan to perform the exercise). That is relatively easy to understand. *Intensity* is more difficult. We will discuss below a number of different approaches—some of the most accurate are expensive and not very practical—but the simplest is a basic heart rate monitor or even a wristwatch. If you place your hand over your heart or feel the pulse in your neck or wrist for fifteen seconds and multiply by four, that is your heart rate in beats per minute. The *time* you spend exercising is obviously an important component of the FITT principle, although it depends a great deal on the specific exercise. For example, for cardiovascular fitness, you may need thirty minutes or so of nonstop cardio to see any improvement, whereas when dealing with strength training, the time is less important than "sets" and "reps," which sometimes require you to slow down and do fewer. *Type* may be the most important component and raises the question of what we mean by "fitness". *The American Heritage Dictionary of the English Language* (online edition) lists three definitions for "fitness":

1. The state or condition of being fit; suitability or appropriateness

2. Good health, especially good physical condition resulting from exercise and proper nutrition

3. Biology: The extent to which an organism is able to produce offspring in a particular environment.

We can dismiss number 3 (as I have mentioned many times, I am keeping sex out of this book) and instead concentrate on some combination of numbers 1 and 2. As per the specificity principle (see below), we want our exercises to closely approximate the sailing tasks at hand. For example, if we need to hike out, then some of our exercise training should strengthen the hiking-out muscles—that is the "suitability or appropriateness" definition (number 1). On the other hand, those of us who are not racing need to exercise in a way that more generally deals with overall cardiovascular and musculoskeletal good health. Even athletes who have very specific musculoskeletal sailing requirements still need to improve their overall cardiovascular fitness.

Finally, every good FITT program needs to have a goal, which I discuss in more detail in Chapter 14.

Let's look more closely at the five exercise principles that underlie every exercise program (beyond the concept of "No pain, no gain.")

(1) *Overload.* In order to gain fitness, you must overload the system. That is, you must exceed or overload whatever your body is used to. In order to improve muscular strength—for example biceps strength using arm curls—there must be enough weight to overload the biceps. Multiple repetitions with too light a weight results in little or no improvement. We will return to this concept below when discussing resistance (weight) training.

(2) *Recovery.* Rest and recovery are an *essential* part of any workout. Your recovery routine has a big impact on your overall fitness gains and your performance. Every workout—including resistance training and aerobic training—leads to tissue damage, and the muscles need anywhere from twenty-four to forty-eight hours or more to repair and rebuild (hopefully slightly stronger than before). Recovery is one of the overlooked issues in training. There is a related principle referred to as *periodization*, which deals with organization and planning in preparation for a specific goal or competition. There are annual cycles peaking toward a specific competition, perhaps a year ahead, referred to as *macrocycles*. The sailor plans, for example, a yearlong campaign, building in periods of rest as well as varying the workouts—all with a specific goal in mind. Within the larger macrocycles, there are smaller cycles with a training duration of two to six weeks referred to as *mesocycles* and shorter weeklong plans known as *microcycles*. A well-developed plan will emphasize and de-emphasize certain muscle groups. And it will emphasize and de-emphasize aerobic training versus resistance training, for example. This allows the sailor to build in rest and recovery periods as well. If the plan is followed, the athlete should be able to approach the goal or competition in top physical shape while avoiding stress and overtraining.

(3) *Specificity.* The specificity principle is the most misunderstood of the training concepts. This is unfortunate, since it has resulted in much wasted time and unrealistic expectations. Simply stated, specific exercises produce specific changes in the body that result in specific improvements in performance. Since the improvements in performance are specific for the type of exercise performed, the sailor should try to formulate an exercise program that mimics the kinds of activities he or she will need to perform. If you are an America's Cup grinder, then you want to concentrate in the weight room on those exercises that mimic what you will need to do in competition on the water—since there is a limited amount of time on the water. Although specificity is most definitely important in designing your overall program, aerobic activities such as running, swimming, or bicycling are still important. Whether you are a beer-bellied sea captain (no offense intended), an Olympic Laser sailor, or an

ocean racing crew member, improving your aerobic fitness will contribute to your overall health and your performance on the water (more on this below). So, there are exceptions to the specificity principle, and aerobic fitness is one of them.

(4) *Reversibility*. The fourth principle is the reversibility principle. After only two weeks of "detraining," significant reductions in exercise performance are observed. Almost all of the training improvement is lost within several months. Thus, the beneficial effects of exercise are both transient and reversible. For this reason, the program must be realistic. Only then is there the likelihood that it will be incorporated into a hectic schedule.

(5) *Individuality*. Individuality is also a factor in the training program. Clearly, if exercise must overload the system, the absolute exercise level varies from individual to individual according to his or her relative fitness at the start of the training. The amount of aerobic exercise needed to overload the cardiorespiratory system is markedly different for a marathon runner, a sedentary adult, and a cardiac patient! The benefits of any training program are optimized when the program is planned to meet individual needs and capabilities.

This would be an opportune time to think about yourself as an individual—or at least yourself as a collection of muscles. What kind of muscles do you have to work with? If we examine our chicken dinner before consuming it, we know that there are at least two types of meat—white meat that comes from the breast and wing and darker meat that comes from the drumstick and thigh. The different colors reflect different functions. Chicken legs (dark meat) are equivalent to the muscles of our endurance athletes—these chickens need to walk around, all day long, every day until they "die." The dark meat is dark because the muscle fibers utilize more blood. In Table 10.2, the dark meat characteristics are in the first column (Type I). These muscles (also referred to as "slow twitch") have more capillaries, more mitochondria, and are high in oxidative capacity. Contraction speed is slow, but resistance to fatigue is high. Similarly in humans, the dark muscles are our *endurance* muscles. There is plentiful oxygen that can be used by the mitochondria, allowing us to exercise longer. They are highly fatigue resistant, which is why your gastrocnemius (calf) muscle contains more Type I slow twitch fibers allowing you (and the chicken) to keep running, or even just walk around all day. Recall from the chapter on nutrition that these fibers rely on fat to provide an abundance of adenosine triphosphate (ATP). While these slow twitch fibers are excellent for prolonged exercise, they won't be as effective for short bursts of energy—like those commonly needed while operating a boat.

The lighter breast and wing meat of the chicken reflect the function of these muscles (e.g., a chicken's short burst of energy when flapping the wings). For sailors, these muscles would be used in short bursts, such as when sprinting or raising a main sail. As you can see in Table 10.2, there are two varieties of Type II fibers, A and B. They are the "fast twitch" fibers. Type IIA can produce energy through both glycolytic and oxidative pathways (they are intermediate in color and in the number of capillaries), and so they are more fatigue resistant than type IIB. Type IIB muscle fibers do not use oxygen. They rely on glycogen for fuel and fatigue more quickly, but they are suited for short-term intensely powerful movements. (See Figure 10.1 and see also Chapter 9 "Sailing Nutrition.")

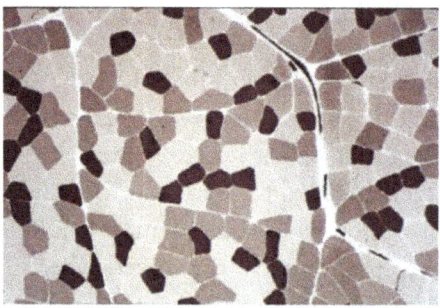

Figure 10.1 Type I (dark), type IIA (intermediate), and type IIB (white)

Characteristic	Type I	Type IIA	Type IIB
Contraction Speed	Slow	Fast	Fast
Resistance to Fatigue	High	Intermediate	Low
Force Production	Low	High	High
No. Of Mitochondria	High	Medium	Low
No. of Capillaries	High	Medium	Low
Oxidative Capacity	High	Intermediate	Low
Glycolytic Capacity	Low	High	High

Table 10.2 Type I (slow twitch), type IIA (fast twitch), type IIB (fast twitch)

Does our individuality play a role? Yes. Our genetics determine the distribution of Type I and Type II fibers that we have—not the total distribution, but perhaps up to 40 percent is genetic endowment; the rest is training. This is still being worked out, as is the question of whether fast twitch fibers can be transformed through exercise into slow twitch fibers, and vice versa.[1] What's most important to boaters and sailors is that Type IIA can, through appropriate exercise, be transformed into Type IIB and vice versa. It is also clear that if you desire to increase the size and efficiency of Type IIB fibers, then you need to do exercises that incorporate both high speed and high strength.

Strength Training

What is strength? It is the ability to apply force against a resistance. Everything we do on the water requires strength, from hauling a line, to hiking out, to steering a sailboard. The only way to become stronger is through resistance training (RT), aka weight training. The type of training is less important—barbells, dumbbells, machine weight…it doesn't matter. Ultimately, you have got to move weight through space. RT, however, has a number of variables that are determined by what you want to accomplish. These variables include:

- The amount of weight that can be lifted (measured in kilograms or pounds)
- The speed with which the strength must be applied (power equals work divided by time)
- The repetitions (i.e., endurance)

The first step for each exercise is to determine the maximum amount of weight that can be lifted on a one-time basis. (If using free weights, make certain that you have assistance for this). This maximum weight is referred to as a one-repetition maximum, or 1RM, and is not employed in training since excessive weight contributes little to the development of strength and greatly increases the likelihood of muscle and joint injury. Rather, 70 to 85 percent of the 1RM should be used. If a 1RM bench press, for example, is 100 pounds (45 kilograms), then only 70 to 75 pounds (32 to 34 kilograms) should be used initially for that exercise. This weight is still too heavy if the person cannot perform ten to twelve repetitions. However, if the repetitions feel too easy, a heavier weight should be selected. Determining the initial weight is a process of trial and error. How many sets, how many reps? There is no easy answer. Unless otherwise instructed by a trainer, you could consider beginning with two to three sets of eight to fifteen reps. After one to two weeks of training, when the muscles have adapted and the correct movements are second nature, the target number of repetitions can be decreased to eight to ten. The weight will then have to be adjusted periodically as the muscles become stronger. Increments of 5 pounds (2.25 kilograms) for the arms and 10 pounds (4.5 kilograms) for the legs can be considered. The program can be performed with individual weights or on a machine. Here are some other considerations:

- Training for power is accomplished with fewer reps and more sets, which optimizes the power output of each set (because of rest between sets, there is less muscular fatigue).
- The length of rest between sets is important, as it determines how much time the phosphagen system has to recover energy (see Chapter 9 "Sailing Nutrition").

- Many bodybuilders use the pyramid system or a variation of it. In the traditional pyramid system, the resistance is low to start (warm-up) with a number of reps. Then the number of reps decreases as the weight increases.

Set 1	135	15 reps
Set 2	185	12 reps
Set 3	205	10 reps
Set 4	225	8 reps
Set 5	245	6 reps
Set 6	265	4 reps

Table 10.3 Sample bench press pyramid

- The reverse pyramid is exactly the opposite. You start with your heaviest weights for a few reps, decrease the weight, and do more reps in the sets that follow. The reverse pyramid is problematic for beginners and intermediates, as you are approaching your maximum (1RM) without a warm-up (cold muscles don't lift well and are more easily injured).
- However, you are not a bodybuilder; you are perhaps a grinder. Yes, you need to be strong, but in addition you need to be explosive (i.e., power), and remember the equation above, power equals work divided by time, and you may have to continue for a while (that is endurance).

    For more strength, do fewer reps per set (perhaps four sets of only four to eight reps)

    For more endurance, do more reps per set (perhaps two sets of twenty to thirty-plus reps)

    For power, mix it up

    In general, you need to build strength first and then add endurance so you can "endure" with enhanced strength
- Over the past twenty-five years, the concept of *variation in training* has taken hold, and is used in different ways. The overarching concept is that each individual adapts differently to physical training, and that after a period of time, as the body adapts, the exercise program needs to be varied in some way. Sometimes the variation occurs in cycles, which can be weeks or months (see "periodization" above) – anything so that the muscles are exposed to differing routines. It could be changing the sets and reps, or it could be changing the workout program (e.g., arms greater than legs greater than abdominals greater than arms; *changed to* legs greater than arms greater than back greater than abdominals greater than legs).

Most resistance training is a form of *isotonic* strength training. Isotonic contraction involves either a shortening or a lengthening of the muscle against a fixed resistance.

Two other forms of strength training are available: isometric and isokinetic exercise. *Isometric* strength training differs from isotonic in that the length of the muscle (isometric) and the angle of the joint do not change when contraction takes place. If the sailor attempts to push or lift an object that he or she cannot move, his or her muscles would be in a state of isometric contraction. In general, isometric exercises are not that valuable. First, they are time consuming. A contraction must be held at each and every angle of the joint through its entire range, because the strength developed is specific to the joint angle at which contraction takes place. In addition, isometrics are not effective for developing speed of contraction. The kind of strength that is developed with isometrics is best suited for isometric tasks (the specificity principle). They are not, for the most part, the kinds of tasks the sailor must perform. The one major exception, which will be discussed below, is hiking, especially in the dinghy class such as the Laser. In this particular case, the isometric contraction of specific groups of muscles of the legs, hips, and core are *critical* to performance.

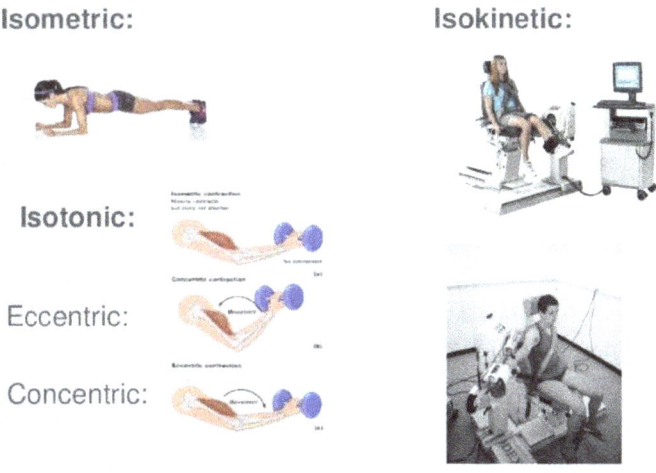

Figure 10.2 Isometric, isotonic, isokinetic muscle contractions[2]

Isokinetic strength training (also known as accommodating resistance exercises) has become familiar through the Nautilus isokinetic program. With this method, the machine varies the resistance throughout the entire range of the exercise (i.e., every effort encounters an equal and opposing force). This is not true of isotonics, where the greatest force is generated in the initial part of the movement when inertia is overcome. Fewer repetitions are needed with isokinetics—three sets of five to six repetitions would be adequate for each exercise.

Which is superior, isotonics or isokinetics? The question is useful only if we add the question "For what purpose?" For weightlifting tasks, isotonics is superior to isokinetics since it more nearly imitates the task (the specificity principle, again). However, many of the sailor's tasks (such as grinding a winch, tailing, sweating a halyard, or weighing an anchor) produce continuous resistance throughout the entire range of motion. Isokinetics does closely imitate this kind of resistance, suggesting that isokinetics may be equal to or even superior to isotonics for many boat-related tasks. The advantage, however, is probably slight, if at all. If machines are readily available, by all means use them. However, probably the most important use for isokinetics is for rehabilitation. An isokinetic contraction is a dynamic contraction (it uses a dynamometer to measure and control the contraction) and the speed of the entire movement is controlled by the machine. This prevents injury and so is especially useful in rehab situations.

Circuit Training

Circuit training consists of alternating between several exercises (usually five to ten) that target different muscle groups. For example, you might move from an upper body exercise, to a lower body exercise, to a core exercise, then back to an upper body exercise, and then do a sprint. That would be one circuit. Then you repeat the entire circuit. Each exercise might take one minute, and if you did six circuits with each circuit consisting of five exercises, that would add up to thirty minutes. The key is that there is a minimum (or no) rest between exercises. But because you are alternating body parts, you are resting one muscle group while the other is working. For example, your arms get to rest during squats while your legs get to rest during pull-ups. Not only does it build strength, but there clearly is a major cardio component that is an additional benefit of circuit training. The reason is that you are moving from exercise to exercise with very little rest and so circuit training produces a significant cardiorespiratory improvement. Assuming you use enough weight during the exercise, you will also be improving muscular strength.

But circuit training does not build maximum strength. The only way to build maximum strength is with "reps and sets." It takes much more time because you need to rest between the sets to allow for recovery. So, for one muscle doing eight reps per set and three to four sets with rest of two to five minutes between sets, you are looking at a lot of time. Reps and sets are also much better than circuit training for building skills since you are spending more time concentrating on the exercise as opposed to rushing through.

High-Intensity Circuit Training

High-intensity circuit training (HICT) is a hybrid. It involves combining cardio (aerobic) and resistance training (anaerobic) exercises in the same workout. Popularized by Brett Klika and Chris Jordan,[3] the concept packs into a single workout resistance training of various muscle groups with little or preferably no rest between exercises, allowing time-conscious adults to get the best of both worlds. Traditionally, the American College of Sports Medicine recommends eight to twelve reps at an intensity of 40 to 80 percent of 1RM with two to three minutes of rest between sets. This is for each muscle or group.

Additionally, the group recommends 150 minutes of moderate intensity cardio per week. The idea here is that, using primarily bodyweight resistance, a circuit can be done in seven minutes, and even two to three circuits is only fourteen to twenty-one minutes. And it can be done anywhere. The American College of Sports Medicine provides a sample program to address all of the major muscle groups:

Jumping jacks	Total body
Wall sit	Lower body
Push-up	Upper body
Abdominal crunch	Core
Step-up onto a chair	Total body
Squat	Lower body
Triceps dip on chair	Upper body
Plank	Core
Running in place—high knees	Total body
Lunge	Lower body
Push-up and rotation	Upper body
Side plank	Core

Table 10.4 HICT

Aerobic Training

Aerobic training is at the core (no pun intended) of every boater's physical performance. Without a decent level of aerobic fitness, your ability to respond to emergencies at sea or compete in a sailing race will be compromised. You should consider your aerobic fitness to be the engine that underpins everything you do. Although weight training (RT) produces improvement in muscle strength, it has no significant influence on the cardiorespiratory system. This is because all of the activities discussed so far are of the anaerobic type. Anaerobic activities—such as winch grinding, swim sprints, and power weight lifts—are typically of short duration, lasting less than two minutes. These activities require the immediate release of stored energy sources, such as high-energy compounds like ATP and creatine phosphate (review the ATP section in Chapter 9), and the partial breakdown of glucose into the "waste product" lactic acid (Type IIB). If the activity lasts longer than two to four minutes, aerobic reactions become a source of energy (Type IIA); for pure endurance activities like marathon running or distance swimming, aerobic reactions are virtually the sole supplier (Type I).

So, if the vast majority of sailing tasks are anaerobic, why is aerobic fitness so important that it is at the "heart" of every fitness program for sailors? Because a stronger heart will pump out more oxygen and glucose *not only to your muscles, but also to the rest of your body, including your brain*. And it will pump it out with less effort. Your pulmonary (lung) function also improves, allowing not only more oxygen in, but more efficient elimination of CO_2. As your overall aerobic fitness improves, not only does your physical conditioning improve, but with less fatigue comes a concomitant improvement in attention, concentration, and decision- making.

Where to start? Aerobic training includes any activity such as running, swimming, rowing, or bicycling for extended periods of time under conditions that stress the cardiorespiratory system. This level of stress is reached if the exercise is intense enough to increase the heart rate toward its maximum. Maximum heart rate (MHR) is conveniently determined by the rule-of-thumb: 220 minus the person's age. So, a forty-year-old would have an MHR of 180 (220 - 40). That is the maximum, but the goal is to increase your heart rate into the training sensitive zone which is 70 to 85 percent of MHR. Thus, if Bob is a forty-year-old man who wished to train at moderate intensity, he could select 70% of his maximum predicted heart rate (i.e., 126 beats per minute: 220 - 40 = 180 x .70 = 126). Then, by trial and error, he would arrive at the running or cycling intensity that produced the desired heart rate. If he wished to train at 85 percent maximum, his exercise heart rate would have to increase to 153 beats per minute (220 - 40 = 180 x .85 = 153). Super intense training at heart rates above 85 percent MHR, in general, should be discouraged unless under the direction of a trainer or exercise physiologist. For women, it has been suggested that the numbers are slightly different. The Gulati formula to calculate the MHR for women is 206 minus age times 88 percent. So, Susan, who is forty years old, would have an MHR of 171 (i.e., 206 - .88 x 40 equals 171). If she started out aiming for 70 percent of MHR, it would be 119. Not wildly different than 126 but enough to make a possible difference in training.

If swimming is chosen for aerobic training—and endurance swimming has potential utility for the boater—an adjustment is needed in order to estimate maximum heart rate. In swimming, the maximum heart rate is about thirteen beats per minute slower than in running, an effect that may be due to the horizontal position of the body and/or the cooling effect of the water. Consequently, if Bob wished to swim at 70 percent maximum, he would select a swimming speed that increased his heart rate to 117 (220 - 40 = 180 - 13 = 167 x .70 = 117).

The sailor can determine his or her heart rate by taking his or her pulse every four to six minutes during exercise. The easiest place to take the pulse is over the carotid artery, located on either side of the neck. The radial artery on the wrist is another option. Simply count the number of beats in a ten-second period and multiply by six (or in a fifteen-second period and multiply by four) to obtain the heart rate.

It is advisable to flank the aerobic session with ten- to-fifteen-minute warmup and cool-down phases. The duration of each aerobic session should be at least twenty to thirty minutes, and three to five workouts per week are needed to produce cardiorespiratory improvement. Sailors who wish to do both anaerobic and aerobic training may alternate the two.

Another method to gauge how intensely you are exercising is to use the Borg Scale of Perceived Exertion.[4] It considers your fitness level by matching how much effort you feel that you are exerting, on a relative scale of six to twenty (see Appendix D). Borg devised the scale so that the average adult could multiply that number (correlated to perceived exertion) by a factor of ten to estimate heart rate. A strenuous workout, for example, might rate a fifteen on Borg's scale, which when multiplied by 10, would very roughly correlate with a heart rate of 150.

Finally, the "talk test" is a rough-and-ready way to measure exercise intensity.[5] The person exercising is simply required to speak in order to make a rough assessment. If the person exercising can carry on a brief conversation or sing three to five words with each breath—while exercising—then the pulmonary threshold has not been reached and the intensity of exercise is "moderate" or less. If the person exercising is not able to speak two or three words without pausing to breathe, then the person is engaged in "high" intensity exercise. When you do not have enough air to speak and can only grunt, then the amount of exercise constitutes an effective workload. This is true, independent of the individual's fitness level.

If you desire to take your training to a higher level, then there are two measurements you need to be aware of. The first (and one of the gold standards of fitness endurance) is VO2 max, or maximum oxygen uptake. It is simply the amount of oxygen your body can deliver to the working muscles per minute. It is an excellent measure of fitness since it provides a measure of cardiovascular efficiency. The heart is the body's pump sending oxygen-rich and nutrient-rich blood out to the tissues via arteries and bringing back CO_2 and metabolic waste products via the veins. It is calculated in a fitness laboratory by measuring the volume (V) of oxygen (O_2) you consume while running on a treadmill while attached to a breathing mask (see Figure 10.3). The treadmill speed is gradually increased and eventually you max out—and at that point the physiologist calculates the oxygen and the carbon dioxide in the inhaled and exhaled air and comes up with a number: your VO2 max. The higher the value, the better. For most people, the VO2 max reading falls between 30 to 60 and is measured in milliliters of oxygen per minute per kilogram of body weight (ml/min/kg).

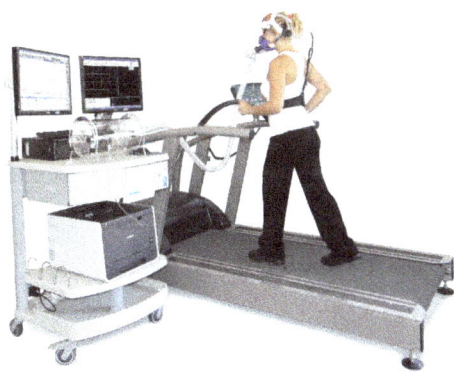

Figure 10.3 Ergospirometry[6]

All things being equal a higher VO2 max is a good thing as it means that your body can take in more oxygen and deliver it quickly to your muscles and other organs, enabling better aerobic performance. Aerobic exercise improves VO2 max significantly. It is a great measure of physical fitness, but it is not the only predictor of cardiovascular fitness nor is it always a dependable predictor of athletic performance.

That is where lactate threshold (LT) enters the picture. LT is defined as the intensity of exercise at which lactate begins to accumulate in the blood faster than it can be removed. You will recall that anaerobic glycolysis is the energy system used when we perform rapid high intensity tasks—think grinding, or short bursts of any activity. As lactate is added in increasing quantities to the blood, the blood becomes acidic and this causes nausea and vomiting. Lactate was previously thought to be merely a "waste product," but that is not so. (Interestingly, much of the lactate is taken back up by the liver and converted into glucose that can then be burned as fuel.) However, if the muscles are producing lactate at a faster rate than the liver can process it, the lactate level rises. The advantage of having a high LT is that you can work at a higher intensity for a longer time period before the lactate begins to build up. The lactate is measured in the blood by taking a finger stick or an earlobe stick and collecting a small amount of blood while the person is exercising on a treadmill or bicycle. The blood lactate is plotted against the VO2 max, and the LT is identified where the curve has an inflection point upward (Figure 10.4). Let's say that your LT occurs when you are at 80 percent VO2 max. Then, if you perform your aerobic training at say 80 to 85 percent—or even slightly above that—at 90 percent VO2 max, you can improve your LT, and hopefully your overall performance.

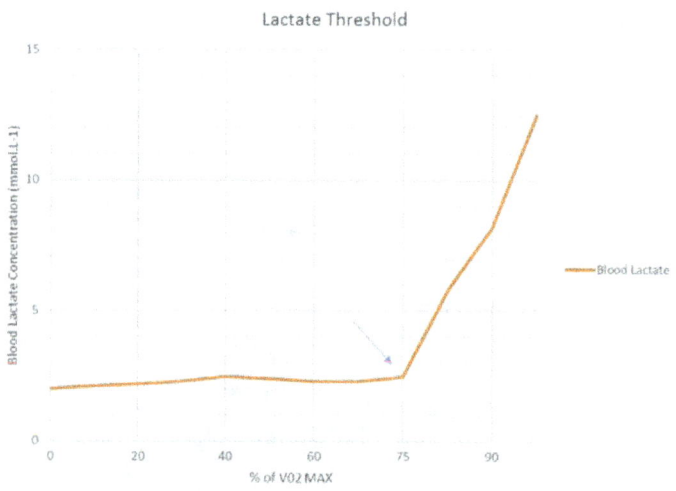

Figure 10.4 LT measurement

High-Intensity Interval Training

Interval training (IT) is a type of training (running, cycling, rowing, etc.) that involves higher intensity exercise periods interspersed with recovery periods of lower intensity. High-intensity interval training (HIIT) describes any workout that alternates between *intense* bursts of physical activity and fixed periods of *lesser-intense* activity. HIIT is like IT "on steroids" (not literally). One example would be running as fast as possible for one minute and then walking for two minutes. Repeating that three-minute interval five times will produce a fifteen-minute HIIT workout. The intense HIIT bursts accomplished in only fifteen minutes, three times a week, will actually burn more calories than jogging on the treadmill for an hour. In one study, two weeks of HIIT intervals improved aerobic capacity as much as six to eight weeks of endurance training. So, this training method takes little time (is very efficient) and is effective in fat burning. Whereas steady-state cardio may produce some muscle loss with the fat loss, HIIT workouts (and resistance training) spare the muscle. The reason it is so efficient is that the effects of an intense HIIT session continue throughout the day, long after training is complete. Moreover, HIIT has been shown to be very heart healthy. Another plus: you do not need any specific equipment—running, biking, rowing, or jumping rope all work well for HIIT. But don't assume it's easy…This training method is intense and extremely challenging if done appropriately.

Cross Training

Cross training is an exercise regimen that uses several different exercises to develop overall fitness. So, an ocean racing team workout might include some time boxing or swimming, which has nothing to do with the sport or the expected demands of the sport. You can change it up within a workout, or alternate on different days of the week. In fact, it flies in the face of one of our most important principles—the specificity principle. But like circuit training, it does have certain benefits:

- *Reduced injury risk*—spending as much time as possible training on the water may produce cumulative stress at muscles and joints, and cause overuse and other injuries. By spreading out the stress to different muscle groups within a balanced schedule, you lessen the likelihood of overloading one particular joint or muscle group.
- *Improved total fitness*—cross training is similar to circuit training, especially HICT (see above).
- *Enhanced exercise adherence*—with circuit training, there is less chance of getting bored with the training regimen, and an increased likelihood that you'll comply long term.

Flexibility Training

Improved flexibility is an important part of any conditioning program, and numerous studies have shown that improved flexibility decreases injury and improves performance. For the small-boat sailor who must contort his or her body into a number of unnatural postures, the value of flexibility is obvious. But even the sailor whose main interest is strength training has need for flexibility.

The problem is that stretching, the major method to increase flexibility, has become thoroughly controversial. Even the basic terminology is confusing. Let's look at some of the different types of stretching:

(1) *Static stretching.* Static stretching simply means taking a muscle (or a group of muscles) to its farthest point—its fully lengthened position—and then maintaining that position for up to ten to thirty seconds. It has been the mainstay of "warm-ups" for decades—and that is the problem. It makes no physiologic sense to stretch a cold muscle. On the other hand, it is an excellent stretching technique *once the muscles have been warmed up.* At the end point of each stretch, there should be a mild feeling of "tension," but extreme pain must be avoided. The body is relaxed and then stretched again, perhaps two to three times. During the stretching, breathing should be slow, deep, and rhythmic. This helps loosen tight muscles. Static stretching should be used as part of your cool-down routine—that's where it belongs.

(2) *Active versus passive static stretching.* In active-static stretching, you assume a position without assistance other than the use of your *antagonist* muscles (the opposing muscle to the *agonist* muscle, which is the one you are trying to stretch). This is the form of stretching used in yoga and many martial arts. In passive-static, you assume the position and hold it with another body part (usually your hand) or with the aid of a partner. Imagine a standing quadriceps stretch in which you bend your leg behind you and hold the foot, pulling the heel in close to your buttock, stretching the quadriceps (thigh) muscle.

(3) *Isometric stretching.* Isometric stretching is a type of static stretching that involves the resistance of muscle groups through the tensing of stretched muscles. The most common way to provide the needed resistance for an isometric stretch is to apply resistance manually to one's own limbs, or to have a partner apply the resistance, or to use a fixed object such as a wall or the floor. Once the position is assumed (pushing against the wall, for example), the tension in the stretched muscle is maintained for five to fifteen seconds while resisting against the immovable object. Then, one relaxes for fifteen to twenty seconds and repeats the motion.

(4) *Ballistic stretching.* Ballistic stretching uses momentum of a moving body part, such as a limb, to force the limb beyond its normal range of motion. There is often a bouncing motion. This type of stretching is not considered useful for many athletes, and may lead to injury. The American College of Sports Medicine states that it can increase flexibility when performed properly, but is best reserved for those participating in activities that are by nature ballistic, such as basketball.

(5) *Dynamic stretching.* If ballistic stretching is out, dynamic stretching is in—especially for warm-ups. Dynamic stretching is stretching with movement. It consists of controlled arm and leg movements that take the arm or leg through its normal range of motion, starting slowly and only increasing the range of motion after the movements have been happening after some repetitions. Then and only then are the movements taken toward the full range of motion. Basically, the athlete performs those stretches (e.g., torso twists, walking lunges, leg swings, etc.) that replicate the kinds of things he or she will have to do in competition. This kind of stretching prepares the muscles for upcoming competition, so you can see why these would be good for warm-up situations. Dynamic stretching is often performed in group exercise classes.

(6) *Proprioceptive neuromuscular facilitation (PNF) stretching.* PNF is often referred to as partner stretching. Two people are needed to perform the movements, so it is usually used in a fitness setting and for rehabilitation. There are a number of variations, but most involve an isometric hold of a position followed by a static stretch of the same muscle group.

Balance Training

Balance training has been the stepchild of the fitness world. The concept of training or even just improving your balance has been relegated to the realms of rehabilitation, and fall prevention in the elderly. That is unfortunate because on the water our balance system is constantly being tested, since our center of gravity is constantly shifting beneath us. "Toto, I've a feeling we're not on terra firma anymore."

For balance on or off the water, we depend on the interaction of three systems to keep us upright and prevent us from falling: vision, vestibular (inner ear balance mechanism), and proprioception (position information coming from our muscles and tendons about our position in space). If this seems familiar, it should, as it was discussed in depth in Chapter 1, "Seasickness."

There are two types of balance—static and dynamic—and they are both important on the water.

Static balance is the ability to maintain fixed postural stability and orientation over the base of support with the body at rest. (In neurology, we evaluate static balance by doing the Romberg test, which tests the ability to stand erect for one minute after closing the eyes.) To test static balance, just have the person stand on one leg (flamingo stand). What this does is reduce the proprioceptive input by 50 percent. If that is stable with either leg, then you can have the person move the free leg through space pointing ahead, behind, and to the side. Some of the yoga poses represent static balance as well. To further test and train the balance system, the person can perform the same static exercises on an *exercise balance foam pad*, which makes the static task more difficult because the surface is irregular and varying. There are many other strategies to test and train the static system, including mini squatting, tandem stance, and half-tandem stance. More difficult still is the *rocker board* or the *wobble board*. The rocker board is less challenging since it only offers one degree of movement (i.e., banking left to right). The wobble board (my favorite, and given my age, I was surprised I could improve) is a little more difficult as it can rotate as well as going from side to side. More difficult still and more dangerous are the rocker-roller boards (sometimes referred to as Bongo Boards, which look like surfboards with a cylinder beneath them). (If you are in the United States and over the age of 30, do not even think about attempting the Bongo Board without good insurance coverage!)

Dynamic balance is more difficult to define. Basically, it is the ability to maintain postural stability and orientation while the body is in motion. Examples would include forward or backward stepping with a brief stop to maintain alternate leg balance, side-to-side stepping also with a stop to maintain alternate leg balance, the grapevine walk, lunges, many of the Tai Chi moves, and basically any disco move (for those of you of a certain age).[7] Now, speaking to those of a certain age: if you can't perform even the basic static and dynamic balance exercises then I would favor cruise ships for your nautical experience (Harsh advice, I know, but with your best interest in mind).

It has been said that balance training is not necessary because at sea the perturbations of a moving boat cannot be replicated by any balance training (specificity principle). Theoretically, that is true, but I can vouch from personal experience that the type of side-to-side and fore and aft movements that we experience at sea are fairly close to what I experience on my wobble board, and as I have stated, I have definitely improved my balance over time. There are a number of tools used by therapists to assess balance, especially in the elderly, including the Tinetti Assessment Tool for Balance.[8]

The Cruising Sailor

The cruising boater or sailor must be creative in order to continue with an exercise regimen at sea. Machines and free weights that are the mainstay of resistance training are usually not available (unless on a ship), and aerobic training is also difficult if not near a town or fitness center. Flexibility and balance exercises should not be a problem, so let's concentrate on resistance training and aerobics (cardio). Resistance training can be accomplished in basically one of two ways—assuming weights are not available—by using resistance bands or trying bodyweight training, which is roughly the modern incarnation of twentieth-century calisthenics.

Resistance bands (e.g., those made by DynaPro) are basically composed of hard rubber tubing connected to an anchoring mechanism and secured to an immovable object, such as a door at home or a fixed point on the boat. You perform exercises with the bands providing the resistance rather than traditional weights. The bands come in varying "thicknesses," which provide a range of resistance (e.g., 5 to 10 pounds up to 35 to 50 pounds). These can be used to replicate virtually any exercise that can be performed in the gym, although of course, you are limited in the absolute amount of resistance. Many trainers use these for clients on land, and if you have been using them already, then the decision is easy. They are inexpensive, lightweight, and easily stored on your boat. The limiting factor is the maximal resistance of the bands.

Calisthenics—alternatively, you could use your body weight for the resistance in place of the resistance provided by the bands. This is often referred to as bodyweight fitness. Most examples of bodyweight fitness are similar to older calisthenics. Calisthenics are physical exercises depending primarily on your own body to strengthen muscles and keep them in good condition.[9] It is usually performed with little or no equipment, and at least in the United States, has been the mainstay of physical education in most school systems: running, jumping jacks, push-ups, sit-ups, and so forth. Originally, the only equipment included perhaps a chin-up bar, but not much else. Calisthenics are still included in the training of the U.S. military (I trust that's not classified information) and others around the world. Since calisthenics is training with your own body weight, you are already doing a form of calisthenics every day in one sense, since you are walking, sitting, and standing—all of which require the strength of various muscles. Calisthenic programs can be easily adapted for use on a boat with limited space. If you wish to purchase one piece of equipment, it would be resistance straps rather than bands. The straps do not provide any resistance, but rather allow you to use your body weight to perform the calisthenic-type exercises.

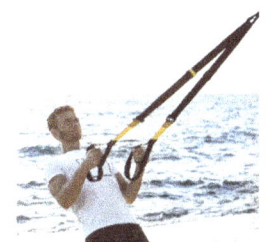
Figure 10.5 Resistance straps

Aerobic/cardio—bodyweight fitness with calisthenics if performed rapidly can also provide a moderate cardio workout as well. And that is fortunate, as cardio on a boat is very problematic. Swimming is certainly possible in some locations, as is kayaking. A newer option is stand-up paddling (SUP), which is becoming popular as well (Figure 10.6). The boards are either a hard board (similar to a surfboard) or inflatable—a so-called iSUP. The inflatable would be preferable for the cruising sailor as it can be compressed down to a small form.

Healthy Boating & Sailing

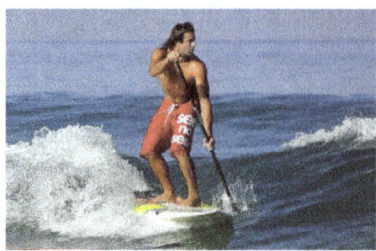

Figure 10.6 Stand-up paddleboard[10]

The cruising boater can consider either HIIT or HICT. Both of these can be performed on a boat. For HIIT, the sailor can consider jumping rope, since running or bicycling is not an option. Jumping rope performed in the HIIT regimen would certainly be an option. Since the HICT program depends on body weight, it too would be something that the cruising sailor could consider.

Yoga is another approach that can be accomplished easily on a boat. All you need is a yoga mat and a few square feet on deck. There are many different programs, but most yoga enthusiasts (at least in the West) practice Hatha yoga. A number of sailing yogis have listed their yoga routines online.[11] Some poses are pictured in Figure 10.7

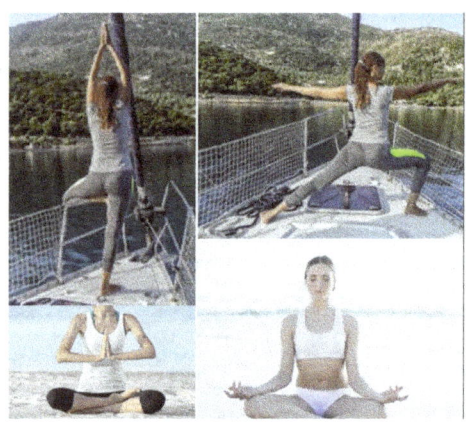

Figure 10.7 Yoga poses on a boat[12]

Yoga doesn't fit neatly into cardio or resistance training; it is more akin to flexibility and balance exercise. However, practitioners have related that with difficult programs and difficult progressions, your heart rate is definitely elevated. And although there is no way to "build" muscle with most yoga programs, toning muscles is definitely something to expect. The same would also be true of Tai Chi and Pilates. Katherine Knight's "Sailing Fitness Toolbox" is an excellent source for fitness information and sailing workouts, including multiple yoga poses. Her sequences of poses, known as *asanas*, include a hiking series, a trapeze series, and a series chosen for keelboats. There is even a series of Pilates exercises.[13]

Big Boat Racing

Big boat racing is one of the most grueling sports in the world. Whether the sailors are involved in match racing, like the America's Cup or long-distance open water racing like the Volvo Ocean Race, the level of physical training required is unparalleled. The obvious physiologic advantage of match racing is that at the end of the day, you get to go home and try to recover for the next race (assuming there is not a second race later in the day!). The 2015 Volvo was the first around-the-world race with strictly one-design boats, so the pressure was on the sailing athletes to a greater degree than ever. The six-month pre-race workouts were rigorous. However, one of the most important goals was injury prevention, because with a very limited crew, losing a set of hands would be a major problem, not only for the boat as a whole, but also for all of the remaining crew. Pete Cunningham, the sports science manager on the winning vessel *Team Abu Dhabi*, related that

> the lower body will deteriorate a bit when you spend three or four weeks at a time at sea, but squats and lunges can combat that problem on board (although mostly, precious free time goes to sleeping). It's critical, though, to maintain upper body mass and strength. "You start the race quite healthy and fit, in the best shape," says bowman/helmsman Luke Parkinson, 25. "And over nine months of intense racing, you slowly decline in fitness level and health. Just having a cough can slowly wear you down."[14]

Here was the crew's typical prerace training plan:

Cardio (four times per week—minimum of eight hours total): Prolonged steady state aerobic exercise: ninety- to one hundred and twenty-minute gym sessions on a bike, rower, or treadmill. Can be mixed up on different machines. Outside cycling requires a minimum of two hours.

Weights (three sessions per week, weights vary): Chest and shoulders—push-ups (two sets, twenty reps), bench press (four sets, eight to ten reps), incline bench press (three sets, ten reps), push press (three sets, eight reps), shot put (three sets, eight reps), rear delt row (three sets, ten reps), curls (three sets, eight reps), pushdowns (three sets, eight reps). Legs and back—deadlifts (four sets, eight to ten reps), cable squat to row (four sets, eight reps), one-arm dumbbell snatch (4 sets, 8 reps), bent over row (three sets, eight reps), lateral pull-downs (three sets, eight reps), seated row (three sets, eight reps), uni-rotational row (three sets, eight reps).

Abs and core (three sessions per week, directly after weights): twenty reps each of crunches, bicycle crunches, oblique crunches, sit-ups, flat back leg lifts, flat back toe touches, jack knifes, bridge crunches, and hollow holds. Thirty reps each of planks, one-leg planks, side planks, side planks and abduction.

Circuit training (substitute for an aerobic session once per week): sixty-minute circuit: two sets of twenty reps for each of the following: squat, uni-rotational row, push-up, bent-over row, rower machine, overhead press, rear delt row, flat fly, seated row, cable pushdown, sit-up, spin bike, curl, lying leg raise, hi-lo chop, lower body twist, chop, treadmill jog 500 meters.

Both the ocean racing teams and the Olympic teams have a staff of exercise physiologists, trainers, and nutritionists. The physical and nutritional demands are well beyond what you can accomplish yourself. But if you have a large boat and wish to race, outlining this type of training will give you some ideas on building your own program. Alternatively, just be as healthy and fit as possible when you take to the water.

Small Boat and Olympic Class Sailing

If you race smaller craft, you may be aware that the format for the next Olympics is yet to be determined. But one thing is for certain: over the years, the contribution of overall fitness to success, and the importance of strength, endurance, and aerobic capacity has been continuously advanced. The physical demands have increased the level of competition to a fierce level. Table 10.5 outlines the sailing classes to be represented in the 2020 Tokyo games. There are a couple of themes: there will be no side-hiking— hiking is down from 65 percent of the events in 1968 to 33 percent in the 2002 games—and the number of trapeze events has increased and now will represent 53 percent of all sailors. Not only has the event format changed, but the racing format has as well, with more races of briefer duration and more maneuvering at higher intensity. Bojsen-Moller reviewed the physical requirements in Olympic sailing and noted the following points:[15]

> (1) With respect to hiking performance, moderate to strong correlations were observed between knee extensor strength and hiking performance. Hiking places a tremendous amount of strain on the knee joint and the muscles needed to support it, as well as on the trunk flexors needed to keep the body up. (Michael Blackburn was one of the first to measure the unique stressors required of hikers, in both "laboratory" and on-the-water studies.) The problem with hiking is that it places a unique, quasi-isometric strain on the knee stabilizers (mainly isometric with dynamic actions as well). It also restricts blood supply to the legs, as well as blood returning from the foot and leg. With training, however, hikers were able to improve their hiking endurance by 100 percent compared with highly trained non-sailors.

(2) Aerobic and anaerobic capacity has been evaluated and the best aerobic values (VO2 max) went to the board sailors, the next best to the hikers, and the trapeze sailors were slightly behind. Earlier studies were quite different; in the past, elite sailors were able to perform at a high level despite having VO2 max well below that of other sports. This highlights the increasing fitness requirements of current sailboat racing. Not many studies of anaerobic capacity of elite sailors exist. Those that do exist suggest that sailors compare well anaerobically with swimmers and middle-distance runners. Anaerobic capacity is highly relevant in modern sailing, including hoisting sails.

(3) On-the-water assessments are by nature difficult. One thing is certain—boardsailing requires tremendous aerobic and anaerobic capacity, with VO2 max at or above 80 percent and heart rate maximum (HR max) above 90 percent.

(4) Fatigue was evident in two studies. One demonstrated a 35 percent reduction of hiking strap forces after only ten minutes of sailing. A second (simulated in the laboratory) looked at repeated spinnaker pulls (three at five-minute races separated by five-minute pauses) and found that in elite 49er crewmen, the average peak power was reduced by 26 percent by the end of the repeated trials.

Class	Type	Event	Sailors	Trapeze	First OG	Olympics so far
RS:X	Sailboard	women	1	-	2008	4
RS:X	Sailboard	men	1	-	2008	4
Laser Radial	Dinghy	women	1	-	2008	4
Laser	Dinghy	men	1	-	1996	7
Finn	Dinghy	men	1	-	1952	18
470	Dinghy	women	2	1	1988	9
470	Dinghy	men	2	1	1976	12
49er	Skiff	men	2	2	2000	6
49erFX	Skiff	women	2	2	2016	2
Nacra 17	Multihull	mixed	2	2	2016	2

Table 10.5 Sailing classes 2020 Summer Olympics[16]

Where do you turn for fitness advice? Your sail coach/trainer would be your obvious first choice. In terms of training for small boats, the most authoritative author is Dr. Michael Blackburn. His *Sailing Fitness and Training* is now in its 3rd edition (Kindle).[17] He was a world champion sailor and coach and performed some of the earliest scientific sailing physiology studies. His text has something for every small boat sailor or racer, with an emphasis on the physical techniques of hiking, trapezing, and sailboarding. There are chapters on training sessions, yearly training, and injury avoidance. Here are some of his top tips for sailing fitness:

- Develop your back strength. As we will see, it is the most frequently injured area.
- Work on shoulder stabilization. This is a frequently injured area.
- Work on hiking and also on strengthening abdominal muscles and hip flexors.
- Use ice and cold-water recovery practices after a strenuous practice or race.
- Have a plan and stick to it: although, if you are on the water and there are few options for exercising onboard, go to the gym and compensate.
- Keep a record of your fitness and goals.

Another excellent choice would be the previously mentioned Katherine Knight's "Sailing Fitness Toolbox." Some of the fitness tests they recommend are located in my Appendix D, along with a series from Texas A&M. And there are other excellent sources of information on training fitness. Many are listed on *The Final Beat* website, which also includes some helpful videos.[18]

Notes

1. J. M. Wilson et al. "The Effects of Endurance, Strength, and Power Training on Muscle Fiber Type Shifting. *Journal of Strength and Conditioning Research* 26, no. 6 (2012): 1724–1729.

2. S. Landrum, Student Physical Therapist, AMEDD Officer, Clerical Staff: Tri-County Therapy, February 1, 2015.

3. B. Klika and C. Jordan, "High-Intensity Circuit Training Using Body Weight: Maximum Results with Minimal Investment," *American College of Sports Medicine Health and Fitness Journal* 17, no. 3 (May/June 2013): 8-13.

4. G. A. Borg, "Psychophysical Bases of Perceived Exertion," *Medicine and Science in Sports and Exercise* 14 (1982): 377–381.

5. B. A. Roy, "Monitoring Your Exercise Intensity," *ACSM's Fitness & Health Journal* 19 (2015): 4.

6. https://commons.wikimedia.org/wiki/File:Ergospirometry_laboratory.jpg.

7. R. Lomas-Vega, et al., "Tai Chi for Risk of Falls: A Meta-Analysis," *Journal of the American Geriatrics Society* 65, no. 9 (2017): 2037–2043.

8. You can find the Tinetti Assessment Tool for Balance online. It is easy to administer and score. I recommend it mainly for the protection of skippers with older in-laws who wish to come boating. If they can't pass the Tinetti, then you have an objective rationale for disinviting them; even your spouse can't argue with that!

9. The word *calisthenics* is derived from the Greek words *kallos*, which means beautiful, and *sthenos*, meaning strength. It was practiced by the ancient Greeks, including both the armies of Alexander and the Spartans at the Battle of Thermopylae.

10. https://en.wikipedia.org/wiki/Standup_paddleboarding#/media/File:J%C3%A9r%C3%A9my-Massi%C3%A8re_stand-up-paddle_biscarrosse-2.JPG.

11. "Yoga for Sailors," *Sail*, August 2, 2015, https://www.sailmagazine.com/cruising/yoga-for-sailors.

12. These poses are only a few of the many yoga poses which have been developed. Most can be adapted for nautical use.

13. Katherine Knight, "Sailing Fitness Toolbox, Techniques of Champions That Will Make You Faster," *Sports Fitness Tools*, 2012.

14. Julie Dugdale, "How to Sail Like a Sailor," *Outside Magazine*, June 30, 2015, https://www.outsideonline.com/1994626/.

15. L. Bojsen-Moller, A. Agaard. Physical requirements in Olympic sailing. European Journal of Sport Science, vol.15, No. 3, 220-227, 2015.

16. "Sailing at the 2020 Summer Olympics," *Wikipedia*, accessed April 14, 2019.

17. Michael Blackburn, *Sailing Fitness & Training*, 3rd ed. (2010). Kindle.

18. *The Final Beat*: http://thefinalbeat.com/categories/fitness.

Chapter 11

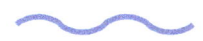

Accidents and Injuries

"A ship in harbor is safe, but that is not what ships are built for."
—*John A. Shedd* (often misattributed to Einstein)

"The art of the sailor is to leave nothing to chance."
—*Annie Van de Wiele*

As we begin this chapter, let's review a few recent U.S. boating and sailing accidents:

- June 17, 2017—the *USS Fitzgerald* of the 7th Fleet collided with a giant cargo ship off the coast of Japan. Seven sailors drowned in their sleeping quarters.
- August 21, 2017—just two months later, the *USS John S. McCain*, also of the 7th Fleet, turned right in front of a thirty thousand-ton oil tanker, and in the collision ten sailors died.
- April 27-28, 2012—during the Newport to Ensenada race, a 37-foot Hunter, *Aegean*, ran aground at night (good visibility) and was wrecked, with the loss of all four sailors.
- July 16, 2011—during the Chicago to Mackinac race, the boat *Wingnuts* capsized with the loss of two sailors.
- July 19, 2018—a "duck boat" capsized in severe weather on Table Rock Lake with the loss of seventeen lives.
- June 23, 2011—a Club 420 capsized with the tragic loss of a fourteen-year-old when her harness became entangled and she drowned.
- September 30, 2018—a man drowned after being thrown from a fishing boat by a large wave in Rockport, Massachusetts.

Can all of the above equally be termed accidents? Are some more "accidental" than others?

Accidents represent the third leading cause of death in the United States after heart disease and cancer—up from fourth place in 1983. For those younger than forty-four, accidents are the leading cause of death (unchanged). No group is likely more sensitized to the problem of accidents than the boating community. The ultimate goal, of course, is accident prevention. However, we remain hampered in achieving this goal by the concept of the accident. Traditionally, the definition of an accident has implied that something undesirable occurred that was unanticipated and thus probably uncontrollable—in other words an unpredictable encounter between a human and the environment. At times, this concept is useful: a tourist struck and killed by a cable that snapped while he was walking across the Brooklyn Bridge was certainly the victim of an accident. The victim had no way to anticipate it and, hence, protect himself. It was a freak occurrence.

But many incidents that we label as accidents probably could have been anticipated. For example, if you are involved in boating under the influence (a BUI) and crash into a pier, should that be referred to as a "boating accident?" Such an incident was clearly avoidable. When I addressed this issue in the first edition of this book thirty-five years ago, I wrote that "to label it an accident, however, would be in a very real sense to abdicate responsibility."[1]

> If we label all of life's unpleasant surprises as accidents, then we come to perceive ourselves as the playthings of fate and we cultivate a philosophy of carelessness and irresponsibility. On the other hand, if we look for causes and hold ourselves accountable for the mishaps in our lives, we become people of resource and confidence, increasingly able to control the direction of events. If these conclusions are as true as I think they are, it matters very much how we define the word accident.[2]

Times have changed. Look at a 1993 editorial in the *British Medical Journal*: "Evans explained why 'motor vehicle crash' is an appropriate expression but 'motor vehicle accident' is not: 'The word crash indicates in a simple factual way what is observed, while accident seems to suggest in addition a general explanation of why it occurred without any evidence to support such an explanation.'"[3] In 2001 the *British Medical Journal* banned the word *accident* from its publication.

Purging the term has not been easy. The U.S. Centers for Disease Control and Prevention no longer refers to accidents as the third-leading cause of death in the United States; rather, it refers to "unintentional injury." However, most of the rest of the world (at least the English-speaking world) seems to have missed the memo. The word *accident*, and unfortunately much of the intellectual baggage associated with it, seems to be here to stay. Of course, in the nautical field we have an excuse—our oft-cited "nautical tradition".

Accidents and Injuries

Let's look at the 2017 Coast Guard Recreational Boating Statistics "Executive Summary" (Figure 11.1).[4]

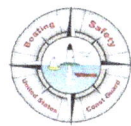

2017 EXECUTIVE SUMMARY

- In 2017, the Coast Guard counted 4,291 accidents that involved 658 deaths, 2,629 injuries and approximately $46 million dollars of damage to property as a result of recreational boating accidents.
    - The fatality rate was 5.5 deaths per 100,000 registered recreational vessels. This rate represents a 6.8% decrease from the 2016 fatality rate of 5.9 deaths per 100,000 registered recreational vessels.
    - Compared to 2016, the number of accidents decreased 3.9%, the number of deaths decreased 6.1%, and the number of injuries decreased 9.4%.
- Where cause of death was known, 76% of fatal boating accident victims drowned. Of those drowning victims with reported life jacket usage, 84.5% were not wearing a life jacket.
- Where length was known, eight out of every ten boaters who drowned were using vessels less than 21 feet in length.
- Alcohol use is the leading known contributing factor in fatal boating accidents; where the primary cause was known, it was listed as the leading factor in 19% of deaths.
- Where instruction was known, 81% of deaths occurred on boats where the operator did not receive boating safety instruction. Only 14% percent of deaths occurred on vessels where the operator had received a nationally-approved boating safety education certificate.
- There were 172 accidents in which at least one person was struck by a propeller. Collectively, these accidents resulted in 31 deaths and 162 injuries.
- Operator inattention, improper lookout, operator inexperience, machinery failure, and alcohol use rank as the top five primary contributing factors in accidents.
- Where data was known, the most common vessel types involved in reported accidents were open motorboats (46%), personal watercraft (18%), and cabin motorboats (16%).
- Where data was known, the vessel types with the highest percentage of deaths were open motorboats (47%), kayaks (15%), and personal watercraft (7%).
- The 11,961,568 recreational vessels registered by the states in 2017 represent a 0.84% increase from last year when 11,861,811 recreational vessels were registered.

Figure 11.1 2017 Coast Guard Recreational Boating Statistics "Executive Summary"

A couple of points stand out:

(1) People are not wearing their personal flotation devices (PFDs)
(2) Alcohol remains a leading factor in accidents
(3) The majority of the incidents were in open motorboats

(4) Operator inattention, improper lookout, inexperience, machine failure, and alcohol were the top five contributing factors of accidents

(5) 81 percent of deaths occurred in boats where the operator had not received any prior boating instruction

Let's examine the theories of accident causation and see which of those tragedies at the top of this chapter are really "accidents."

Theories of accident causation go back to the pioneering work of Herbert Heinrich. He was an official with the Travelers Insurance Company who, in the 1920s after studying seventy-five thousand industrial accidents, proposed the domino theory of accident causation. Following his lead, the field of industrial safety has grown and expanded on theories about accidents,[5] which now include:

- *Domino theory*—like successive dominos toppling, one factor leads to another
- *Human factors theory*—see below
- *Accident/incident theory*—an extension of the human factors theory
- *Epidemiologic theory*—study of the causal relationship between the environment and accidents or diseases
- *Systems theory*—see below
- *Combination theory*—sometimes more than one theory is necessary

For nautical use, the *human factors theory* and the *systems theory* are the most constructive.

The *human factors theory* (Figure 11.2) attributes the accident to a chain of events ultimately caused by *human error*. It encompasses three factors that contribute to human error: overload, inappropriate response, and inappropriate activities.

The *overload* factor is just what it sounds like: an imbalance between the responsibilities expected of the boater and the capacity at any given time to deliver on those expectations based on the individual's training, state of mind, stress, and even physical abilities. The load stressors can be environmental (e.g., unexpected severe weather, mechanical failure), they may come from internal stress (e.g., personal problems), and they may even arise from situational factors (e.g., unclear instructions).

All of these stressors were present at the time of the USS *Fitzgerald* and the USS *John McCain* accidents. Unfortunately, evidence in the records of the incidents also shows that there were inappropriate activities and inappropriate responses as well.

Inappropriate activities include taking on a task for which the boater is untrained or undertrained or misjudging (often because of lack of experience) the degree of risk inherent in the task. In the two large-scale naval accidents described above, evidence was presented that the training of naval personnel was curtailed or abbreviated because of a personnel shortage, and there was a simultaneous shortage of more senior officers to provide the training.

Finally, there may be *inappropriate responses*—for example, disregarding established protocol or disregarding a safety procedure. Another example of an inappropriate response is to note a specific hazard and then to respond inappropriately or not at all. Sleep deprivation is one such hazard. The profound effect of chronic sleep deprivation in naval personnel—which was system wide—is ironic in the face of the extensive recent scientific research on sleep by the Naval Postgraduate School.

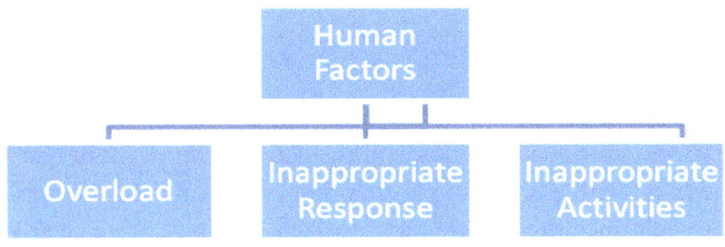

Figure 11.2 Human factor theory

So, one way or the other, we are dealing with primarily a human failure—human error.

An alternative theory that is sometimes a better fit to understanding an accident is the *system theory* (Figure 11.3). In this theory, three components: the person (sailor), the machine (boat), and the environment (weather) are interrelated in the system of carrying out a task. The likelihood of an accident occurring depends on the interaction of all three components.

A failure in the case of the sailor alone (as occurred in the Newport-Ensenada race when the crew of the *Aegean* apparently did not have an adequate lookout) could probably best be described by the human factor theory. On the other hand, the *Wingnuts* incident is clearly more complicated. Weather was certainly a major factor, with gusts powerful enough to knock over a great many of the boats in the race. But in this case, the boat was simply not appropriate for the conditions. It had a wide beam, and once it was knocked over, it remained inverted ("turtled") since it was more stable when inverted. It appears after the fact that its stability (the least of all the boats invited to the race) was technically overrated—especially once the beam width was taken into consideration. The boat was simply not designed nor appropriate for that weather, despite the fact that it had withstood many knockdowns in the past. So, in this case, the system came up short, not because of any deficiency in the sailors (they were experienced sailors who had participated in this race before) but because the boat's design and the severe weather made the overall system unstable.

What about the duck boat incident? This is also best described as a systems problem. The duck boat is not especially stable. These boats were developed and used as a landing craft in World War II so that soldiers could not only be brought ashore quickly, but

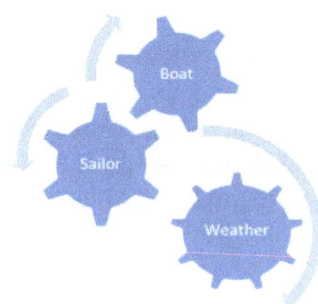

Figure 11.3 System theory

could also be driven up the beach, closer to the action. The vessel in question had been extensively modified with a roof and plastic siding, which altered the stability and made escape very difficult once the vehicle had capsized. So, there were clearly design flaws. Weather was also a factor, as severe weather was forecast, and it is debatable whether the boat should have left the dock. Ultimately, it was up to someone to cancel the cruise, but that never happened, and seventeen people lost their lives.

What about the last two incidents? These two are best described as true "accidents"—*undesirable*, *unanticipated*, and *uncontrollable*: that is, they were *unpredictable*.

In the case of systems problems, a detailed analysis of the entire system is necessary to sort out which aspects of the system need repair. That is precisely what has been done with the naval accidents (although in those cases, implementation of changes, unfortunately, is still a work in progress). It has also been performed in many of the cases cited above.[6] This often requires a team approach in order to bring to bear expertise in nautical design, engineering, meteorology, psychology, and so forth.

What about human factors? To some degree, it boils down to simply doing the right thing:

- Wear your PFD. With newer models, there is simply no excuse.
- Limit alcohol.
- Pay attention and always have a lookout.
- Don't take to the water without at least basic boating instruction.
- Get enough sleep.

These are obvious. But let's get back to the problem of prediction. It is important to remember that the human brain is really a prediction machine. We are constantly making predictions concerning our environment and modifying those predictions based on updated input from our surroundings. That is the final step in staying safe on the water: making predictions as to what can happen—worst-case scenarios—sometimes moment by moment, sometimes as needed, sometimes simply as a verbal thought experiment, and sometimes using mental imagery. We will discuss mental imagery in the psychology chapters—it is used by every champion athlete, and that certainly includes sailing athletes. It can be used prior to the event or during the event. It should be utilized while boating in order to imagine *in advance* what you would do if . . . The old salt can draw upon extensive familiarity: you may have to imagine some of the possible scenarios that the old salt has already experienced.

Injuries

One takeaway message from the preceding section is that many of the incidents that we refer to as accidents are predictable and avoidable with an element of forethought. But despite the best laid plans of mice and men, stuff happens. Backs become strained, boaters fall, rotator cuffs tear—the list of possible injuries at sea is long. I believe, however, that we need to take the same approach with injuries as we did with accidents. Knowledge is power. To be forewarned is to be forearmed (especially for you grinders out there!).

Any discussion of injuries on the water is bound to be complicated. Not only are the injuries different when comparing boaters to sailors, but within the sailing community, there are day sailors, long-distance cruisers, Olympic class sailors, America's Cup racers, and long-distance ocean racers. And within the last three categories, the injury frequency will depend heavily upon the position of the crew member. For example, a bowman can be expected to have a different set of injuries from a helmsman.

Before we look at who is liable to get what, we need to discuss the basic types of injuries. What is an injury? In regard to boaters and sailors, one could think of it as a state of damage to the body whereby the sailor can no longer perform optimally due to pain or physical impairment. Injuries may result from *lack of general fitness* (especially aerobic fitness), *trauma, overuse, or overtraining.*

Trauma (macrotrauma)—this is what most people think of when they think of injuries. They are by nature *acute* rather than *chronic*. There is a specific episode of trauma with tissue damage. These are the bruises, contusions, lacerations, fractures, and concussions that we are all familiar with. (As a neurologist, I am embarrassed to admit that I sustained a concussion after being struck by a boom while racing on the Chesapeake in the early 1980s. That may explain why it took thirty-five years to rewrite this book.) Trauma also includes injury to the soft tissues (muscles, tendons, ligaments) and often goes under the name "strain and sprain." To be precise, a *strain* is an injury to a muscle or tendon—tendons attach muscle to bone—or both. Typical signs and symptoms include pain and muscle weakness. There may or may not be visible bruising over the muscle. Generally, the muscle or tendon *overstretches*, causing the injury. There may be a partial or even a complete tear of the muscle or tendon. One example would be a pulled hamstring or hamstring strain (Figure 11.4).

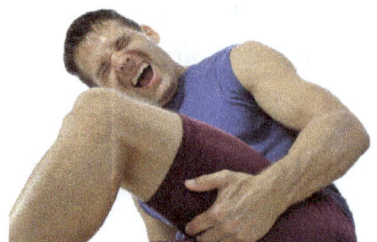

Figure 11.4 Hamstring strain

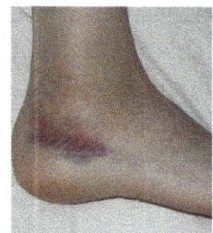

Figure 11.5 Ankle sprain

A *sprain*—also known as an injured or torn ligament—is damage to one or more ligaments in a joint, caused when the joint is taken beyond its normal range. An example would be a sprained ankle (Figure 11.5). Sprains vary from mild, which require a few days' rest, to those that require surgical intervention, like a complete ACL tear. Oftentimes, a neck or low back injury will be referred to as a "strain and sprain" injury. The diagnosis really means "you seem to have injured your back muscles or ligaments, but it doesn't look like a disk out of place and there is no nerve injury like sciatica" (see below).

Overuse (microtrauma)—this occurs when a structure of the body (e.g., muscle or tendon) is exposed to repetitive, cumulative stress. Over time, the reparative efforts of the body are overwhelmed by the ongoing tissue breakdown. This is often referred to as overuse because of the repetitive nature of the injury. Other names for this disorder include *cumulative trauma disorder* and *repetitive strain injury*. Microtrauma can include microtearing of the muscles, connective tissue, tendons, bones (stress fractures), and even the disks of the spine. The overuse syndrome occurs when the body part is overused without sufficient time for healing. This can occur because of overuse during competitions or overuse during training, in which case it is often referred to as *overtraining*. The process is essentially identical. On the one hand, as we saw in the chapter on exercise, muscles and tendons adapt to stress—that is how they become stronger, *but they also need time to rest and rebuild between episodes of stress*. With overuse, the tissue never gets the chance to heal and repair—the process of recovery.

Overtraining should be differentiated from overtraining syndrome, which appears to be a maladaptive response that occurs in some athletes after extended training for a sport. It is manifested by prolonged fatigue and performance decline and associated with

Accidents and Injuries

apathy, sleep disturbance, loss of appetite, feeling of exhaustion, and increased vulnerability to injury. The athlete becomes "stale." This staleness is seen in all sports, including sailing.

"Burnout" may be related to overtraining syndrome, but differs in a number of factors. Athletes (and nonathletes, including an entire generation of physicians!) with burnout have lost all motivation and typically experience chronic fatigue, helplessness, poor sleep, and clinical depression. Both overtraining and burnout are a nightmare for the athlete and coach, since there is no known treatment. For overtraining, a period of withdrawal from the sport or activity may sometimes be sufficient. Recovery from burnout is a more complex process that can take years. The individual should be under the care of a sports psychologist.

Entrapment neuropathy (*compression neuropathy* or *trapped nerve*)—this condition is caused by direct pressure on a nerve. It is another form of overuse or microtrauma, but the microtrauma is directly related to nerves rather than to muscles or ligaments. Nerves can be pinched or compressed when they travel through narrow areas created by muscles, tendons, and bone. Symptoms include pain, tingling, numbness, and weakness. The presence of tingling and numbness tells you that you are probably dealing with a nerve injury. Sciatica is a nerve compression in the low back that causes back pain that may radiate down the leg. It can be caused by a disk herniation or be due to compression by bone spurs where the nerve exits the spinal canal (Figure 11.6B).

Boaters and sailors of all types are liable to have low back pain, usually in the absence of sciatica (Figure 11.6A). In other words, most back pain is a "sprain and strain" injury to the muscles and ligaments in the lower back because of the prolonged sitting interspersed with vigorous pushing, pulling, bending, lifting, and rotating. Or in older boaters, there is often a combination of "sprain and strain" and arthritic pain of the lumbar spine. (In active boaters, arthritic changes may start as early as the thirties). Sciatica pain, on the other hand, implies that the nerve has been injured.

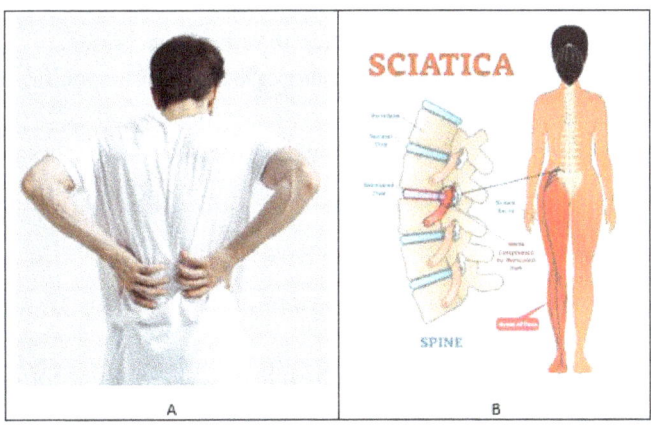

Figure 11.6 Low back pain without (A) and with (B) sciatica

Carpal tunnel syndrome and other entrapment neuropathies are almost always due to overuse/microtrauma and will be discussed below.

Types of Injuries

Since different experiences on the water will be associated with different injuries, it is worth looking at these profiles:

(1) Recreational boating and cruising
(2) Big boat racing (America's Cup and ocean racing)
(3) Olympic-class sailing (including windsurfing)

Recreational Boating and Cruising

In an early study of the injuries in novice dinghy sailors, Schaefer found the injuries were mainly acute in nature, including contusions and bruises (61 percent), followed by cuts and abrasions (32 percent).[7] This is what we would expect of novice dinghy sailors out for a day sail. As Neville and Folland pointed out in their extensive 2009 review, novice and recreational sailors are focusing on skill development rather than elite performance, and so the types of injures would be primarily acute in nature, including abrasions, cuts, bruises, sprains, and fractures as well as injuries to the hands, fingers, and head as a result of impact with and use of the equipment.[8]

An online survey by Nathanson and colleagues looked at responses primarily from dinghies and keelboats.[9] There were 1,188 respondents with a total of 1,715 injuries. The top three injuries for keelboats were leg contusions (11 percent), knee contusions (6 percent), and leg lacerations (6 percent). The most common injuries were from trips and falls, being hit by an object, and getting "caught in lines." The most common contributory factors were tacking, heavy weather, and jibing. Of the seventy severe injuries included in the study—25 percent were fractures, 16 percent were torn tendons or cartilage, 14 percent were concussions, and 8 percent were dislocations.

Figures 11.7 and 11.8 represent the frequency with which specific areas of keelboats and dinghies were associated with injuries.

Nathanson recently reviewed other injury data in addition to the study cited above.[10] He reached the following conclusions about recreational dinghy sailing and keelboat cruising:

1. In dinghy and keelboat sailing, lacerations and contusions are the most common injuries.
2. Many of the injuries are the result of falls due to walking on a wet, angled, or cluttered deck.
3. Impact from the rigging, flogging sails, and collisions with other crew are other causes of injury.

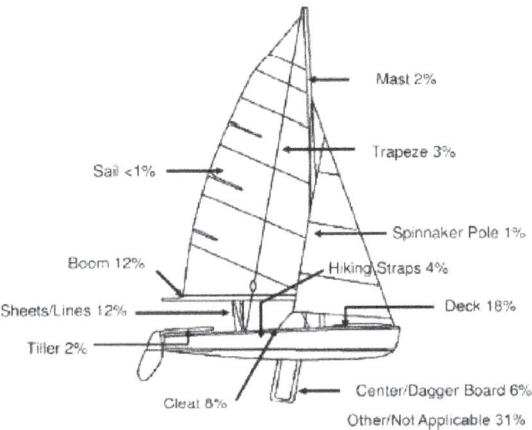

Figure 11.7 Part of keelboat associated with injury, $n = 1226$, from Nathanson et al. (2010)

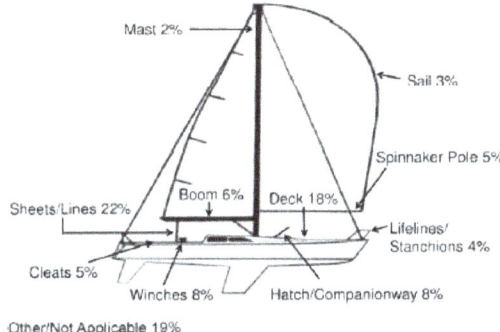

Figure 11.8 Part of dinghy associated with injury, $n = 397$, from Nathanson et al. (2010)

4. Due to the heavier forces, fractures are more common on keelboats.
5. Injuries to the hands and fingers are more likely on larger boats due to the heavier forces involved when handling lines and winches.

Rouvillain and colleagues performed a study of cruising sailboat injuries.[11] They interviewed one hundred consecutive sailboats arriving in Martinique. Inclusion criteria required them to be French-speaking subjects and to live aboard at least half the year. Eighty percent of sailors interviewed had made at least one transoceanic trip. Ninety percent were single-hull sailboats. Since the questionnaire was answered after the events had taken place, the number of injuries was probably underestimated. In all, fifty-six injuries were reported. Head and neck injuries were involved in seven cases (13 percent). One head injury was due to a fall in the companionway, the other when a winch handle kicked back. The boom was responsible for four cranial traumas, three of which were associated with an accidental jibe. There were eight chest traumas (14 percent): six rib cage bruises and two rib fractures. All the above injuries were due to loss of balance associated with a sudden shift of the boat (sailor falling in the companionway or cockpit). There were twenty upper limb injuries (35 percent). Of these, 70 percent involved the hand, including three injuries from a knife while cleaning fish. Two occurred pulling anchor, two pulling rope, and one each due to an accidental closure of the deck cover, rope injury, and bladed weapon attack. There were twenty lower limb injuries, seventeen involving the ankle and foot, thirteen associated with bare feet. There were three cases of sciatica: one case caused by a fall in the cockpit, and the other two cases occurred after raising the anchor. The injuries occurred in the following areas of the boat:

Deck	53 percent
Cockpit	25 percent
Companionway	13 percent
Kitchen	4 percent
Other	5 percent

The study's recommendations included: having adequate technical training, using a windlass to make anchor raising easier, always wearing shoes on deck, making sure crew have three support points when walking on deck or in the cockpit to avoid falls ("One hand for the ship, one hand for yourself"), and using sturdy gloves when using sharp tools. The study also recommended telemedicine.

Although head injuries represent only 10 percent of injuries, they represent 25 percent of severe injuries. Fischer analyzed thirty-four severe sailing head injuries, twenty-four of which were caused by a "flying boom."[12] Of these, more than 50 percent were fatal, the boom being responsible for 80 percent of head injury deaths.

The injuries documented above are basically in line with what we would expect on a recreational keelboat or dinghy, or on a power boat, for that matter. The situation is very different if we turn our attention to the big boat racing classes: the America's Cup, the Golden Globe, the Volvo Ocean Race. For an excellent review of injuries and management of both small boat and big boats, see the review by Allen and De Jong.[13]

Big Boat Racing

Allen and colleagues analyzed injuries sustained by members of the female-majority team during the 1995 America's Cup Challenge, which came close to defending its title.[14] The most common injuries were low back pain and shoulder injuries, felt to be primarily overuse/microtrauma.

A study in 2000 by Allen et al. reported that bowmen and grinders were injured most often. Of the injuries, 76 percent were soft tissue (that basically means "strain and sprain"), and they involved the lumbar spine (16 percent), shoulder (16 percent), knee (10 percent), cervical spine (8 percent), and hand (7 percent).[15] Injury mechanisms

Accidents and Injuries

included grinding (30 percent), lifting (24 percent), and physical impact (16 percent). *However, 18 percent of all injuries occurred during training off the boat.* As the physicality increased with each America's Cup Challenge, the incidence of injury during training increased dramatically. Neville and colleagues were one of the first to catalogue overuse nerve involvement including *posterior interosseous nerve* (PIN) *entrapment* caused by overload of the upper extremity, while pulling sails, grinding, and training on the arm ergometer (for PIN, see below).[16]

Following the 2003 America's Cup, Neville and colleagues documented 220 injuries over seventy-four weeks of training and sailing.[17] The upper limb was affected most commonly (40 percent), followed by the neck and spine (30 percent). Most injuries were overuse type—strains and sprains (47 percent)—similar to the 2000 study by Allen. *The incidence of injury was significantly higher during training than during sailing.*

Table 5 Incidence of injury, illness, and all incidents as a function of crew position

Crew position	Number	Injury			Illness	All incidents
		Sailing	Training	All		
Grinder	12	33 (3.1)	33 (11.2)	101 (7.7)	51 (3.9)	152 (11.5)
Pitman	3	5 (2.0)	9 (12.2)	24 (7.3)	10 (3.0)	34 (10.3)
Utility	4	5 (1.5)	12 (12.2)	28 (6.4)	16 (3.6)	44 (10.0)
Bowman	4	11 (3.2)	1 (1.0)	22 (5.0)	11 (2.5)	33 (7.5)
Navigator	2	1 (0.6)	4 (8.1)	6 (2.7)	8 (3.6)	14 (6.4)
Trimmer	7	10 (1.7)	13 (7.6)	33 (4.3)	19 (2.5)	52 (6.8)
Helmsman	3	1 (0.4)	2 (2.7)	6 (1.8)	4 (1.2)	10 (3.0)
All	35	66 (2.2)	74 (8.6)	220 (5.7)	119 (3.1)	339 (8.8)

Values are number with incidence/1000 hours in parentheses.

Table 11.1 Crew position, from Neville et al. (2006)

Grinders had the highest overall incidence of injury. This should not be surprising, as grinder strength and power requirements mean that training is intense as far as the upper extremity and shoulder are concerned, causing many different types of microtrauma.

Bowmen had the highest incidence of sailing injuries. Their vulnerability to acute traumatic injuries—macrotrauma—given the "sturm und drang" at the bow, should also come as no surprise.

Rotator cuff injuries come with the territory, and virtually every portion of the rotator cuff muscles have been strained and torn by boaters the world over. The rotator cuff is composed of four muscles (supraspinatus, infraspinatus, subscapularis, teres minor), which allow the incredible flexibility of this joint. But with flexibility comes the likelihood of injury. It is a common sailing and boating injury—check out any sailing or boating bulletin board—and is especially common in an America's Cup crew.

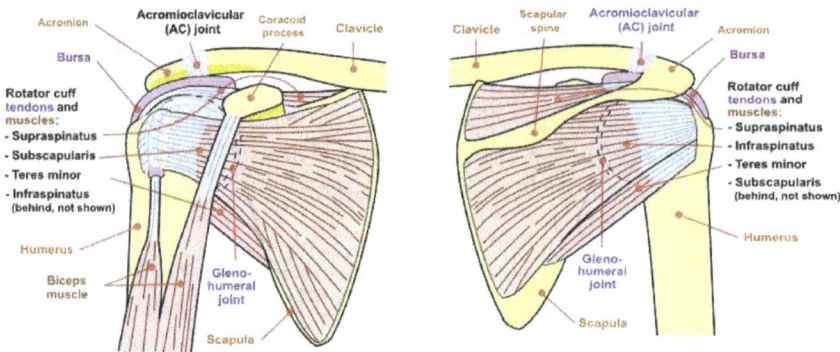

Figure 11.9 The four rotator cuff muscles: front view on left and rear view on right. It is difficult to show the four muscles in one view as the subscapularis is in front of the scapula (wingbone; left illustration), while the other three are behind the scapula (right illustration). This arrangement allows the flexibility and vulnerability of the shoulder.

Another theme for injuries as a result of big boat racing (and training) is the predominance of injuries not only to the shoulder and upper extremity but also the cervical (neck) and lumbar spine (low back). Cervical and lumbar spinal injuries (overuse) are likely due to the forward flexed and rotated position of the spine during the repetitive grinding, trimming, pulling, and lifting. Cervical spine injuries especially in trimmers and helmsmen are undoubtedly secondary to the constant extension of the neck while looking up at the sails.

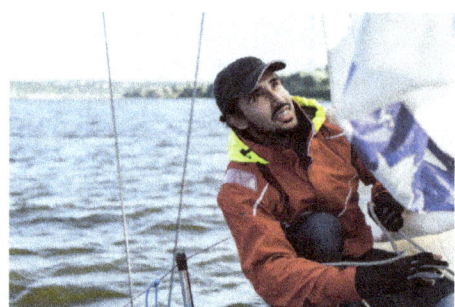

Figure 11.10 Sailor looking up at sails with neck held back in extension

It is likely that the sustained postures contribute to the chronic degeneration of both spinal areas—neck and low back.

Neville and colleagues reported entrapment neuropathy as a fairly frequent occurrence. Posterior Interosseous Nerve (PIN) entrapment was common. It is only one of the *many* entrapment neuropathies that occur in the upper extremity. The nerves of the

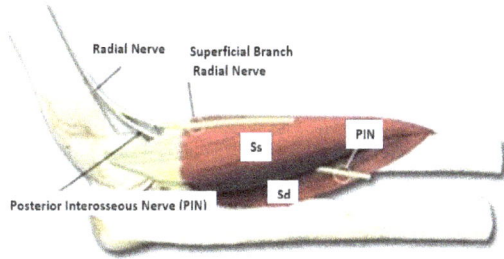

Figure 11.11 PIN: most of the arm muscles have been removed. The radial nerve branches into the superficial branch (sensory) and PIN, the deep motor branch. Notice how the PIN is deep to the supinator muscles; Sd = deep, SS = superficial.

upper extremity have a vulnerable path traveling beneath muscles and tendons that are being strengthened and bulked-up in training and contracted forcibly during training and sailing. Figure 11.11 demonstrates the PIN peeking out beneath powerful muscles.

(If nerves had "feelings," they would probably feel as though they no longer recognize their neighborhood—what with the gym next door filled with body-building bullies.) PIN entrapment appears to have often been reported as "grinder's elbow," described as a "combination of tendonitis, fasciitis, and epicondylitis causing local tenderness near the elbow and forearm." In fact, PIN entrapment is especially difficult to diagnose since the nerve is a pure motor nerve (no sensory fibers); without the numbness and tingling that often accompanies a nerve injury, it may be difficult to differentiate it from a musculoskeletal problem like epicondylitis (inflammation of the elbow). Normally with PIN entrapment, there is pain in the forearm and weakness in extending (holding up) the thumb and fingers.

Another nerve entrapment that is common especially in big boat racing (but also in the boating community in general) is *carpal tunnel syndrome* (CTS). In this condition, the median nerve is compressed at the wrist by bone, tendons, and a transverse ligament.

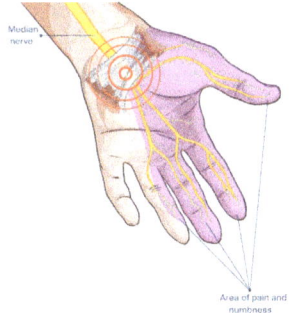

Figure 11.12 Carpal tunnel compression

Figure 11.12 illustrates the compression of the median nerve in the carpal tunnel. CTS is most common in helmsmen who must grip the steering wheel tightly for long periods of time. Often the diameter of the wheel is small, and if the helmsman's hands are large, they must exert a tremendous amount of force to control the often-slippery wheel.

Offshore endurance races such as the Volvo Ocean Race or the Golden Globe Race pose similar challenges to the sailing crew. The injuries are comparable—with low back pain and shoulder pain predominating—but many experience neck pain as well. Overuse injuries such as *epicondylitis* (lateral epicondylitis is also known as tennis elbow and medial epicondylitis as golf elbow) also occur. Again, bowmen are subject to a greater degree of injury based on their job description and unique vulnerability. In these long-distance races, helmsmen are prone to develop upper extremity overuse problems, including CTS.[18]

There are a few points that we can all learn from the big boat experiences:

(1) Acute trauma or macrotrauma are episodes that are less predictable, and closer to what we might consider to be true accidents.
(2) Microtrauma or overuse may be somewhat more predictable (especially if you know your crew position on the boat). But more importantly, there is something you can do about it.
(3) Early recognition is crucial, since the earlier you recognize the diagnosis, the earlier you can change your training program to take that body part out of action for a rest. If you ignore the early signs, it will invariably worsen over time. Discuss any symptoms with your trainer or coach, and do not try to hide the injury or you will be sorry.
(4) Early recognition of nerve entrapment is even more important. The reason is simple. You can rest a muscle or muscle group and substitute another exercise to preserve your fitness and the remainder of your training program., you may be able to simply avoid the offending movement. However, it is much more difficult to rest a nerve. It's not that it can't be done—it's just much more difficult. Recall that the nerve is being compressed by the beefed-up, stronger muscle. The only way that it may improve is if the extremity (the arm, for example) is actually immobilized, rather than just avoiding a specific exercise.

Olympic Class Boats

Olympic class dinghy sailing creates an entirely different set of body stressors. Big boat sailing clearly has a mixture of acute trauma and overuse, whereas dinghy sailing presents much more of a problem in terms of overuse. Although, as we shall see, the newer classes of 49er and Nacra are faster and are associated with more traumatic injuries. The major difference, however, is hiking and to a lesser degree the trapeze. This is how Michael Blackburn, world class sailor and coach, describes hiking—"the most dreaded activity in small boat sailing":

> There is a definite limit to how long small boat sailors can hold an effective hiking position. Feel your legs start to burn even before the end of the first beat? Hiking involves static contractions of the large muscles of the thighs and trunk. Static contractions involve a muscle developing tension without making the joints move [isometric contraction]. These contractions are dominant in small boat sailing—another example is holding the main sheet.
>
> Even at relatively low levels of static muscle tension, the blood vessels can be squeezed shut and the ensuing lack of blood flow and oxygen to the muscles will rapidly cause pain and fatigue. This discomfort must be tolerated in training to develop the muscles so they can better handle demands of competition sailing.
>
> In addition to the continual muscle strain of hiking, there is also the need to carry out active movements of the arms and trunk to trim or pump the sail(s), steer and physically drive the boat through waves. The intensity and nature of the physical activity during sailing and the optimal physical characteristics of the sailors themselves obviously depends on the class of boat sailed.[19]

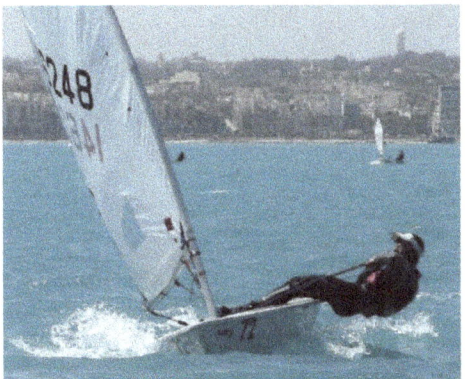

Figure 11.13 Full hiking position[20]

The major muscles that allow the hiking in Figure 11.13 are shaded in Table 11.2. (The reason it is important to understand the musculoskeletal mechanics will become evident shortly, so hang in there.)

Major Muscles	Actions

Knee Extensors (Quadriceps)	Hold the legs straight while hiking or standing
Hip Flexors (Iliopsoas)	Hold the trunk up by stabilizing the hip joint
Trunk Flexors (Abdominals)	Stabilize the spine by linking ribs and pelvis (core)
Back Extensors (Low back muscles)	Support low back and stabilize spine (core)
Foot Flexors (Tibialis Anterior)	Lifts toes while hiking and balance while standing
Elbow Flexors	Critical for arm pulling incl. steering & pumping
Shoulders (Rotator Cuff & Deltoid)	Vital for all arm movements while sailing
Foot Extensors (Calf Muscles)	Up on your toes while sailboarding or trapezing

Table 11.2 Key muscles in small boat sailing and sailboarding

The first muscle is the quadriceps, which consists of four muscles (rectus femoris, right above the quadriceps tendon; vastus lateralis; vastus medialis; and vastus intermedius—not visible beneath the rectus [Figure 11.14]).

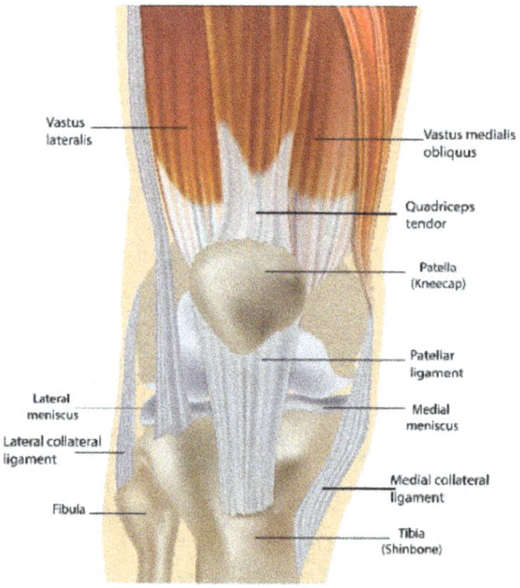

Figure 11.14 Patellar tendon and quadriceps

The quadriceps' main function is to extend (straighten) the knee, keep it straightened at whatever angle is needed, and stabilize the knee joint. Notice the patella right in the middle of the knee. It normally slides in its groove. But with prolonged hiking, the underlying patellar surface may *roughen*, become painful, and may actually be *pulled to one side in the groove*. The vastus lateralis often overpowers the medialis, pulling the patella laterally. Either situation produces the *patellofemoral syndrome*. Patellofemoral syndrome usually causes a dull, aching pain in the front of your knee. This pain can be aggravated when you walk up or down stairs, squat or kneel, or sit with a bent knee for a period of time.

Next is the iliopsoas muscle (Figure 11.15), which allows you to hold your leg up (flexion at the hip joint). It is the main muscle group that controls the amount of flexion at the hip and controls the angle between the sailor's quads and abdominal plane—the hiking angle. See Figure 11.19.

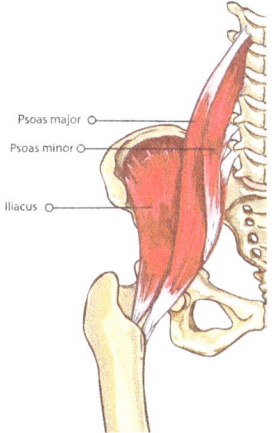

Figure 11.15 Iliopsoas muscle

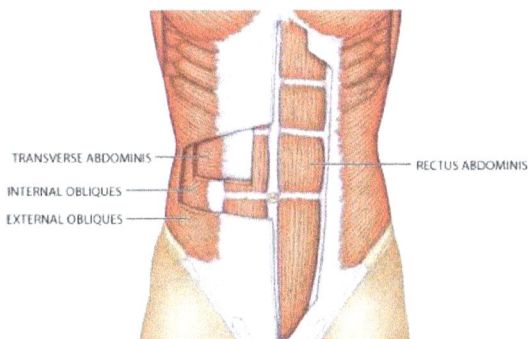

Figure 11.16 Abdominal muscles

The abdominals (and as you can see in Figure 11.16, there are a number of muscle groups oriented in different planes) making up the front and some of the sides of what we call the "core"—rectus abdominis, transverse abdominis, and the internal and external obliques.

Finally, we come to the lower back muscles, which are also an important component of the "core." In addition to the long erector muscles arranged in different directions (Figure 11.17A), there are a series of small muscles (multifidi) that are deep in the back and help to stabilize the entire spine (Figure 11.17B).

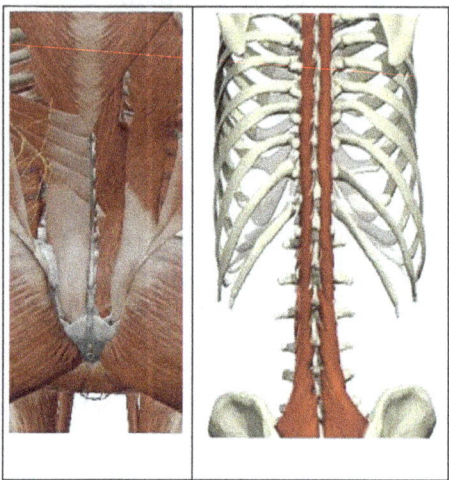

Figure 11.17 Multiple muscles of the low back (A) and the deep multifidi (B)

Those are the four major muscle groups utilized in hiking. The fifth shaded is the foot flexors (the anterior tibialis muscle, Figure 11.18), which brings the foot/ankle back and is critical when hiking, since the foot or sometimes just the toes beneath the hiking strap may be keeping you in the boat. Overuse of this muscle and its tendon is the cause of most cases of ankle pain.

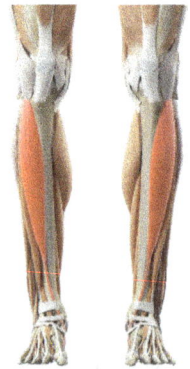

11.18 Tibialis anterior muscle

If we look at Figure 11.19, the illustration demonstrates the angle between the plane of the quadriceps and the chest controlled by iliopsoas and abdominal muscles. But notice there are additional angles between the buttocks and the back, the angle of the knee, and the angle of the foot in the hiking strap (not shown).

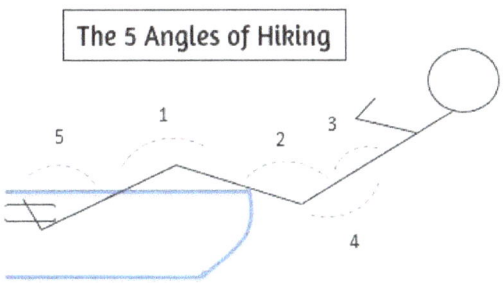

11.19 Hiking angles

The muscle contractions are referred to as quasi-isometric because although the sailor must hold the position for a period of time without moving, as the wind and waves shift there will be periodic movements from a short hiking position to a long hiking position or somewhere in-between. So, dinghy sailing is quasi-isometric and quasi-dynamic.

Leong et al. performed a twelve-month retrospective study of injuries sustained at the forty-third ISAF Youth Sailing World Championship.[21] There were 351 sailors who completed the questionnaire, and 50 sailors reported a total of 69 injuries. The three most injured sites were the lower back (24 percent), knee (18 percent), and ankle (9 percent). In these youth sailors there was no association with age, gender, class, or crew position (Figure 11.20).

Tan et al. surveyed injuries and illness at the Sailing Federation World Championships 2014.[22] The researchers noted that since 2000 when the 49er, 49erFX, and the Nacra 17 were introduced as Olympic classes, there has been a rise in injuries. These newer classes are faster and inherently less stable. The Nacra17 class is now hydrofoiling and will be so in the 2020 Olympics. That can only increase the demands upon the body. The physiologic demands on the sailor are both class specific and position specific. The distribution of injuries, however, was similar: lumbar spine/lower back (29 percent), knee (13 percent), shoulder/clavicle (12 percent), ankle (10 percent). By class, the highest injuries were in the 49erFX (women; 21 percent), 49er (men; 13 percent), laser radial (women; 12 percent), laser (men; 10 percent).

Healthy Boating & Sailing

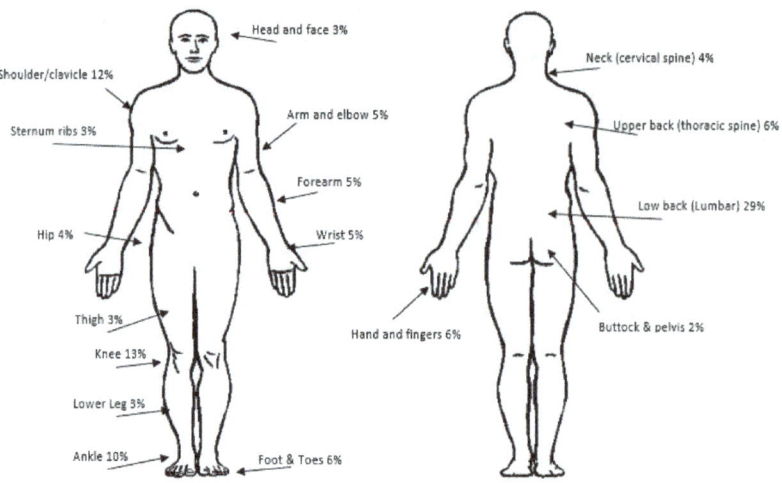

Figure 11.20 Injuries by site; After Tan et al. (2016)

The reason that body mechanics is so important is that these overuse injuries are cumulative, and they begin early. In a study of young Swedish sailors, Skarp questioned Swedish elite sailors, male and female, aged thirteen to twenty-eight. 76 percent had one or more injuries. A knee injury followed by a back injury accounted for more than 50 percent of all injuries. The main injuries were overuse. Males had more injuries than females. The most strenuous activity was "knees while hiking." The majority of sailors with knee injuries responded that it started at twelve to fifteen years of age, and 75 percent still suffered from knee problems. Back pain started before age fifteen in many but there was no evidence for chronic back pain. However, 50 percent missed at least a week of sailing because of back pain. Shoulder disorders were less common. The most important takeaway message is that 80 percent of males and 60 percent of females believed that more knowledge and better training would have helped![23]

The trapeze has not been associated with as frequent overuse injuries, since the position of the body is more neutral. Wearing a harness and standing up on the boat takes a bit of getting used to, but is much less stressful on the knees and low back. Like hiking, however, there are long periods when your muscles will be working isometrically—especially neck, abdominal, and calf muscles—so it is important to move around, periodically relaxing the muscles to allow and enhance blood flow to the isometrically contracted muscles.

Windsurfing (boardsurfing) has been associated with a somewhat different variety of injuries. Rib fractures and head injuries are more common. In the upper extremity, shoulder, elbow, and forearm are the most frequent cited.[25] In the lower extremity, there are foot and ankle injuries (overuse) as well as a variety of more serious injuries to the foot and ankle, often having to do with the foot straps that lock the foot to the board. This gives better control of the board, but it can impart severe leverage and cause

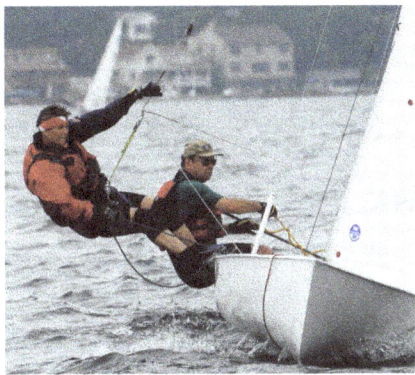
Figure 11.21 Trapeze harness versus hiking[24]

severe ligamentous tears, midfoot sprains, and disruption of the tarsal bones (Lisfranc fractures).

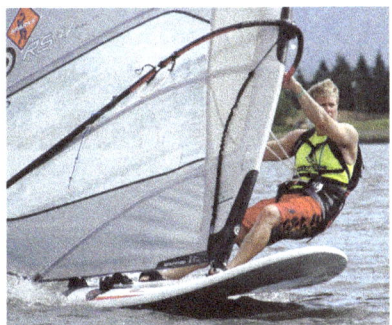
Figure 11.22 Windsurfing[26]

Head injuries remain a problem in sailing. Collegiate and youth sailing teams continue to resist helmets. New England Collegiate Sailing Association has recommended changes in the mast height and composition to reduce the mass of the boom and the likelihood of head trauma, but one of its schools—Massachusetts Institute of Technology (MIT)—has gone a step further. It has required helmets for all team sailors since 2013, and MIT sailors have had no further concussions since 2013. Clearly, the trainers and coaches at MIT realize that every concussion represents a brain injury, and they apparently desire to keep every student athlete's brain in tip-top shape! (That is certainly not the sentiment of some of the "yahoos" who frequent sailing forums and who insist that their children and students learn and practice *situational awareness*.) U.S. Sailing correctly discusses the difference between traumatic brain injury (TBI) and concussion, although it neglects to state that in the United States, at least, the synonym for concussion is mild traumatic brain injury (mTBI).[27] And while acknowledging that there is a brain injury that occurs with concussion, U.S. Sailing only goes so far as saying that concussions "should be taken seriously in scholastic and collegiate sailing." It is true that helmets may or may not protect against every concussion (they are mainly useful for preventing or ameliorating the more serious damage of TBI). However, it is my opinion that for our youth and collegiate sailors, we should do all we can to keep their brains intact and pristine.

At least one Olympic class also saw the light. The new Nacra 17 class rules (effective date March 25, 2019) state the following:

> C.3 PERSONAL EQUIPMENT MANDATORY
>
> (a) When racing each crew member shall wear a personal flotation device to the minimum standard ISO 12402-5 (Level 50), or USCG Type III, or AUS PFD 2, or EN 393 or equivalent. Inflatable buoyancy vests are not permitted.
>
> (b) Each crew member shall wear a helmet that shall be to the minimum standard EN1385, EN1077, EN 966, ASTM 2040, Snell S98 or equivalent with a brightly coloured region of at least 300 square centimetres of the exterior surface that can be seen from above the water with crew lying face down or face up.

The issue has become very heated lately and reminds me of the controversy concerning helmets for motorcycle usage. I am writing this from Pennsylvania, a state which *repealed* its mandatory helmet law in 2003. Currently, you must wear a helmet only until the age of twenty-one; then it is optional. Head injury deaths from motorcycle accidents increased 66 percent from 2003 through 2008, according to a study by the University of Pittsburgh.

I certainly understand the position of those who relish personal freedom of choice when it does not endanger other citizens (and besides, as a society, we *need* organ donors—harsh but true), but let's not confuse the issue. *We are not talking about recreational boating.* We are discussing children, students, and young adults who are engaged in competitive sports. They are our responsibility. Their brains are still maturing, and I would remind you that final brain maturation does not occur until approximately twenty-five years of age. America's Cup crew wear helmets and amateur high-performance dinghy and catamaran classes are *beginning* to adopt helmets. As more and more boats are traveling faster and becoming more difficult to control (especially with foiling), the need for helmets will only increase.

Notes

1. M. M. Cohen, *Dr. Cohen's Healthy Sailor Book* (Camden, ME: International Marine Publishing, 1983).

2. J. J. Brownfain, "When Is an Accident Not an Accident," *Journal of the American Society of Safety Engineers* (September 1962): 20.

3. L. Evans, "Medical Accidents: No Such Thing?" *British Medical Journal* 307 (1993):1438-1439.

4. U.S. Coast Guard, 2017 Recreational Boating Statistics (Washington, DC: Office of Auxiliary and Boating Safety, 2018), https://www.uscgboating.org/library/accident-statistics/Recreational-Boating-Statistics-2017.pdf.

5. D.L. Goetsch, Occupational Safety and Health, Seventh Edition (Boston: Prentice Hall, 2011), pp. 32-50

6. B. Brown et al., "United States Sailing Association Independent Review Panel Review of the Fatal Accident Involving Aegean During the 2012 Newport to Ensenada Yacht Race on April 28, 2012," https://www.ussailing.org/wp-content/uploads/2018/03/Ensenada-Report-FINAL.pdf; "Navy Promised Changes After Deadly Accidents, but Many Within Doubt It's Delivering on Them," ProPublica, https://www.propublica.org/article/navy-accident-changes-fitgerald-mccain-davidson; J. Rousmaniere, "Sailing Accidents: Lessons Learned," Sail, August 2, 2017, https://www.sailmagazine.com/cruising/sailing-accidents-lessons-learned; "Lessons Learned from Sailing Incidents 2011-2015," Sailing Leadership Forum 2016, U.S. Sailing.

7. O. Schaefer, "Injuries in Dinghy Sailing: An Analysis of Accidents among Beginners," *Sportverletz Sportschafen* 14, no. 1 (2000): 25–39.

8. V. Neville and J. P. Folland, "The Epidemiology and Aetiology of Injuries in Sailing," *Sports Medicine* 39, no. 2 (2009): 129–145.

9. A. T. Nathanson, J. Baird, and M. Mello, "Sailing Injury and Illness: Results of an Online Survey," *Wilderness and Environmental Medicine* 21 (2010).

10. A. T. Nathanson, "Sailing Injuries: A Review of the Literature," *Rhode Island Medical Journal Archives* (February 2019): 23-27.

11. J-L. Rouvillain, F. Mercky, and D. Lethuillier, "Injuries on Offshore Cruising Sailboats: Analysis for Means of Prevention," *British Journal of Sports Medicine* 42 (2008): 202-206, doi:10.1136/bjsm.2006.033175.

12. E. G. Fischer, "Fatal Head Injuries in Sailing," *Seahorse International Sailing* (2001): 251.

13. J.B. Allen and M. R. De Jong, "Sailing and Sports Medicine: A Literature Review," *British Journal of Sports Medicine* 40 (2006): 587–593.

14. J. B. Allen et al., "Sports Medicine Injuries in the America's Cup 2000," *New Zealand Sports Medicine* (2006).

15. J. B. Allen,. "Sports Medicine Injuries in the America's Cup 2000," in *Human Performance in Sailing Conference Proceedings: Incorporating the Fourth European Conference on Sailing Sports Science and Sports Medicine and the Third Australian Sailing Science Conference*, ed. S. J. Legg (Auckland, New Zealand: Massey University, 2003), 45–46.

16. V. Neville, J. Molloy, D. Speedy Allen, "The Pain of PIN," in *Human Performance in Sailing Conference Proceedings: Incorporating the Fourth European Conference on Sailing Sports Science and Sports Medicine and the Third Australian Sailing Science Conference*, ed. S. J. Legg (Auckland, New Zealand: Massey University, 2003), 65-66.

17. V. Neville, J. Molloy, and J. Brooks. "Epidemiology of Injuries and Illnesses in America's Cup Yacht Racing," *British Journal of Sports Medicine* 40 (2006): 304–311.

18. C. Price et al., "Patterns of Illness and Injury Encountered in Amateur Ocean Yacht Racing: An Analysis of the British Telecom Round the World Yacht Race 1996-1997," *British*

Journal of Sports Medicine 36 (2002): 457–462; T. Spalding et al., "Analysis of Medical Problems during the 2001-2002 Volvo Ocean Race," in *Human Performance in Sailing Conference Proceedings: Incorporating the Fourth European Conference on Sailing Sports Science and Sports Medicine and the Third Australian Sailing Science Conference*, ed. S. J. Legg (Auckland, New Zealand: Massey University, 2003), 47-50.

19. Michael Blackburn, *Sailing Fitness & Training*, 3rd ed. (2010). Kindle. This book is the bible for small boat sailing. Dr. Blackburn was one of the pioneers in scientifically studying small boat sailing on the water.

20. Wikipedia Laser Radial sailor Roberto Briffa, 2013-02-22 Debono662.

21. D. Leong et al., "Injury and Illness Patterns in Competitive Sailors of the 43rd ISAF Youth: Sailing World Championship—a 12-month Retrospective Study," *British Journal of Sports Medicine* 48 (2014): 625, doi:10.1136/bjsports-2014-093494.177.

22. Tan et al., "Injury and Illness Surveillance at the International Sailing Federation Sailing World Championships 2014," *British Journal of Sports Medicine* 50 (2016): 673–681, doi:10.1136/bjsports-2015-095748.

23. H. Skarp, "Sailor for life, Injuries for Life? A Study about Sailing-Related Injuries among Dinghy Sailors in Sweden," The School of Sport, Unitec, New Zealand, and The Swedish School of Sport and Health Science, Sweden.

24. https://commons.wikimedia.org/wiki/File:Flying Dutchman_NY_2008_trapeze_2.jpg.

25. R. Dyson, M. Buchanan, T. Hale, "Incidence of Sports Injuries in Elite Competitive and Recreational Windsurfers," *British Journal of Sports Medicine* 40 (2006): 346–350; W. Petersen et al., "Injuries and Injury Mechanism during Windsurfing," *Sports Injury Sports Damage* 17, no. 3 (2003): 118–122.

26. https://en.wikipedia.org/wiki/Windsurfing#/media/File:Bry.jpg.

27. "Safety at Sea Resources: Helmet Use," U.S. Sailing, https://www.ussailing.org/ education /adult/safety-at-sea-courses/safety-at-sea-resources/helmet-use.

Chapter 12

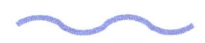

Sleep at Sea

> "Sleep that knits up the ravell'd sleave of care,
> The death of each day's life, sore labour's bath,
> Balm of hurt minds, great nature's second course,
> Chief nourisher of life's feast."
> —*William Shakespeare,* Macbeth, *1606*

> "It's been a hard day's night,
> I should be sleeping like a log."
> —*The Beatles, "A Hard Day's Night," 1964*

Sleep has always been highly prized at sea. The problem of obtaining enough of it arises from the unique marine environment, with its around-the-clock watch duties, extended time offshore, and limited supply of manpower.

For the U.S. Navy's Seventh Fleet, 2017 was a particularly conspicuous year for sleep loss. More than a wake-up call, it was a nightmare. On June 17, 2017, the *USS Fitzgerald*, a $1.8 billion destroyer, collided with a cargo ship off the coast of Japan. Seven sailors died in their sleeping quarters, the deadliest naval disaster in decades. Just two months later, the *USS John S. McCain* turned directly in front of an oil tanker, killing ten additional sailors. An extensive investigation revealed numerous problems, but mission-wide, chronic sleep deprivation was determined to be a major cause for the collisions.

But it's not only the Navy that needs to be concerned with sleep loss. Sleep loss affects the performance of commercial sailors, recreational sailors and power boaters, small boat competitive sailors, day sailors and boaters, and even landlubbers.

How about sleep and the performance of professional athletes? Consider the remarks of Joe Girardi, manager for the New York Yankees, during 2016's spring training: "We start at 11:30. Don't think if I see you here at 7:30 I'm going to be impressed. It's not going to impress me. Sleep! I'm giving you an opportunity to sleep. Sleep!"

In fact, in the years 2013-2018, the National Hockey League, the National Basketball Association, and Major League Baseball all made changes in their union contracts expressly to promote sleep. In basketball and baseball, it actually resulted in an increase in the length of the season![1]

Despite the explosion of knowledge regarding sleep in the last few decades, it is likely that your level of knowledge is roughly that of your grandmother! That is about to change and none too soon.

The trouble is that we have all performed various tasks on borrowed time—that is, late into the night when we should have been asleep. And we generally get away with such behavior—until we don't. Sleep loss presents the same level of risk (or worse) as drunk driving or drug intoxication. And it endangers the entire crew of both the smallest and largest vessels. So, listen up—this may be the most important chapter in the book!

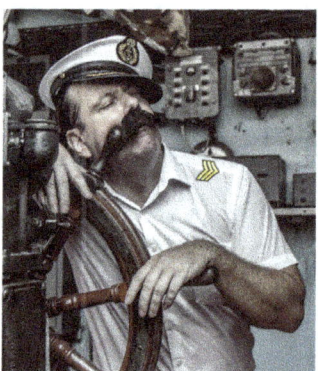

Figure 12.1 Asleep at the wheel—serious humor

Why Do We Sleep?

When I initially wrote this chapter thirty-five years ago, sleep research was in its relative infancy. Since then, it has become an important field of study in human (and animal) physiology and a recognized subspecialty in medicine.

Before we look "under the covers" at some of the newer aspects of sleep science, it is important to ask the fundamental question—why do we sleep? In other words, what is the *function* of sleep? It must have an important function or functions since all mammals and birds engage in sleep that is very similar to our own. Although this is still being investigated, it appears that sleep satisfies the following functions:

(1) Recharge: Sleep allows the body and especially the brain cells to recharge after a long day of physical and mental activity. The importance of sleep restoration always

made intuitive sense—sleep must be critical to survival on an evolutionary basis. Why would nature take the brain and body off-line for hours at a time and allow us to be vulnerable to predators otherwise?

(2) Detoxify: Sleep has recently been discovered to allow the brain to detoxify (see the newly discovered glymphatic system, which drains toxins from the brain and works best if you sleep on your side rather than your back or stomach—no kidding.)

(3) Learn and create: Sleep is extremely important in memory consolidation (memory strengthening). This applies to both procedural memory, such as learning to ride a bicycle or tie a bowline, as well as declarative memory, which is memory for specific information (e.g., book knowledge or autobiographical events in your life). Yes, you learn during waking hours, but memory of all kinds is consolidated while you sleep. Also, during sleep, information in different forms (vision, hearing, smell, etc.) is bound together into a single memory "thing." If you think of a specific meal that you enjoyed, it has been stored in your brain as a collection of information that is bound together in a complex memory that includes taste, color, smell, the setting, the people you were with, and so forth. The binding together of all this information and consolidating it into a single, multifaceted memory trace occurs during sleep. Sleep also seems to be important for creativity.

Circadian Rhythm

The *circadian rhythm* (in Latin, *circa dies* means "about a day") is a complex human timekeeping system that cycles about every twenty-four hours. Sleep is only one part of this large, complex system. Other body functions that normally synchronize to this twenty-four-hour circadian system include body temperature, hormone secretion, salt and water balance, and even some measures of human performance. The advantage of having such a "biological clock" is that it enables the body to predict and prepare for those environmental changes that occur regularly every day. Adaptive responses, which in some cases take several hours to activate, can then be initiated in advance.

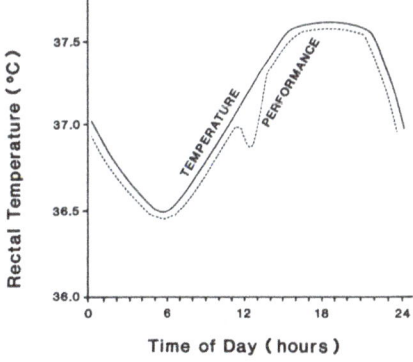

Figure 12.2 Original circadian rhythm and performance illustration circa 1983

Figure 12.2 is an original illustration from the first edition of this book, published in 1983 and is still roughly correct, although we now understand that only some individuals have an afternoon decline in performance and that it has nothing to do with eating lunch. The circadian system is much more complicated than simply the relationship of sleep, temperature, and performance. Figure 12.3 demonstrates how, on average, various functions cycle through the day. Distributing functions throughout the day presumably allows the body to function more efficiently. However, these are just averages—your individual times may vary. For example, some people are morning types (so-called "larks") and some people (and all adolescents) are evening types (so-called "owls"). These personal differences are referred to as our *chronotype*.

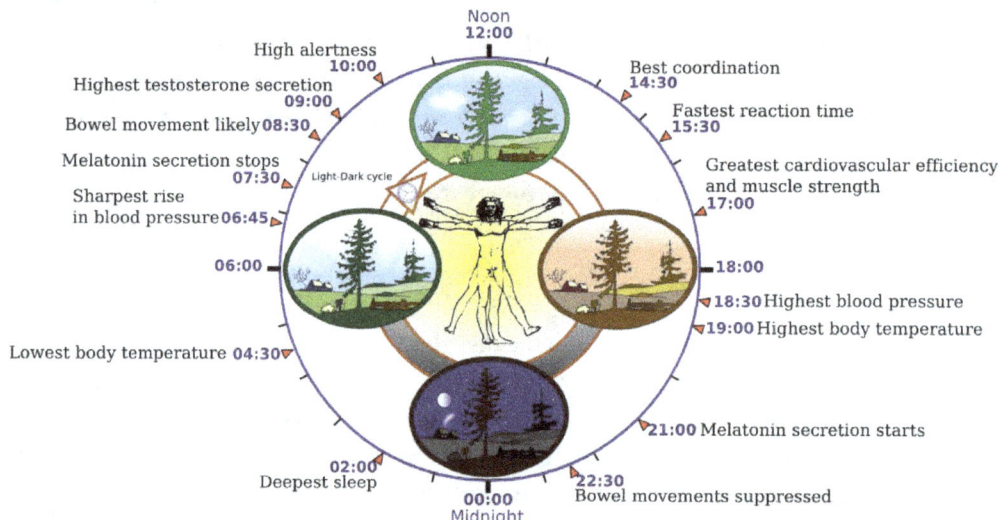

Figure 12.3 Circadian clocks[2]

Secretion of melatonin—a hormone that the brain produces to signal that it is time for sleep—starts in the evening and stops in the morning. Its blood concentration curve would be very different from the temperature and performance curve depicted in Figure 12.2 and would look more like Figure 12.4. Therefore, it is best to think of multiple body functions as a kind of symphony with various instruments playing their role at different times throughout the day and night.

Sleep at Sea

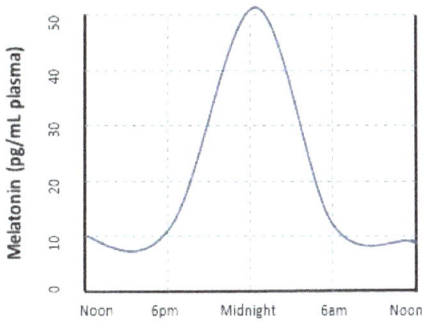

Figure 12.4 Melatonin levels throughout the day[3]

The Two-Step Model (Formerly One Step!)

During the twentieth century, life was rather straightforward: the circadian rhythm paradigm governed how we thought about sleep. It turns out it is a bit more complicated. The current model of sleep consists of two steps or competing processes—*the two-step model*.

Let's deal with the first step. The first step is the circadian rhythm for arousal designated *Process C* (for circadian). This is the daily "call to arms" by an area of the brain—the hypothalamus—which when turned on gives marching orders to multiple other areas of the brain to secrete brain chemicals (neurotransmitters) that wake up most of the nerve cells in the brain.

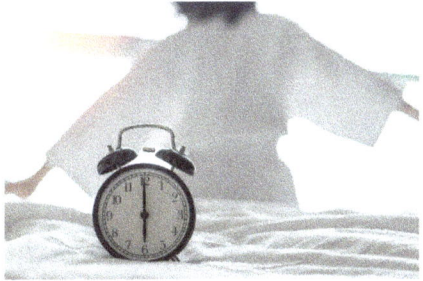

Figure 12.5 Waking up is hard to do

You may be familiar with some of these neurotransmitters: serotonin, norepinephrine, dopamine, and acetylcholine. What turns on the system? It possesses its own clock that keeps pretty good time over twenty-four hours. The internal clock is synchronized with external time by several environmental cues or *zeitgebers* (*time givers* in German), which help the internal clock structure the daily, twenty-four-hour routine. Zeitgebers include light and darkness (the most influential), activity and rest, meal routines, personal interactions, and other social rituals. All of these influence circadian rhythm.

Doe the internal clock in the hypothalamus and the external zeitgebers ever get out of sync? (Yes—see the section titled "Circadian Rhythm Disturbances.")

To review so far, we have the circadian rhythm, or Process C, turning on in the morning, keeping us aroused and active during the day, slowing in the evening, and turning off at night when the sun goes down, allowing us to sleep. What more do you need? Nothing really. The system could work with just the circadian rhythm. What it wouldn't account for is the *time* and *activity* since our last sleep. For example, if we sleep in until the afternoon on Sunday, we can expect to have difficulty falling asleep Sunday night. The one-step model with Process C doesn't account for that. To understand the second part of the two-step model, we need to discuss one other aspect of basic physiology and chemistry.

The second process in our two-step model is *Process S* (for sleep drive). This sleep drive or sleep pressure is a function of the amount of time that has elapsed since the last episode of restorative sleep. That is, the longer we have been awake, the stronger the pressure for sleep becomes, and conversely during sleep, this pressure dissipates (see Figure 12.6).

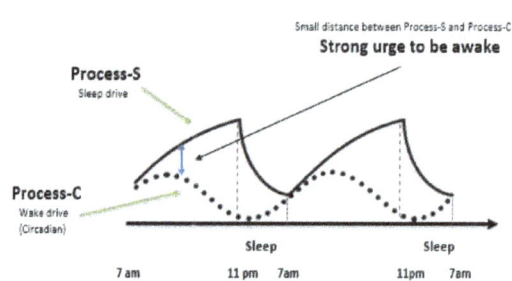

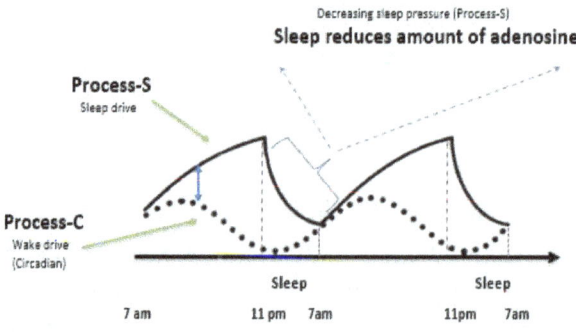

Figure 12.6 How sleep-wake homeostasis (Process S) and the circadian rhythm (Process C) work throughout the day[4]

The longest distance between the sleep drive (Process S) and circadian rhythm (Process C) is when we are most tired and sleepy around 11 p.m.; the shortest distance is when we are most alert at 7 a.m. Note, however, that this curve is just an average and may be shifted one to two hours either way, depending on our personal "chronotype"—this is, if we are a lark or an owl.

The "nuts and bolts" of how Process S operates is still being elucidated, but it appears that the heart of the issue has to do with energy expenditure and the buildup of *adenosine*. As we perform activity during the day, we use energy, become increasingly tired, and eventually fall asleep. The primary source of energy in the body is *adenosine triphosphate* (ATP—If you are unsure of this, review Chapter 9 "Sailing Nutrition," and see Figure 9.12). The triphosphate refers to the three phosphate bonds. There is energy stored in these phosphate bonds. The body uses the energy in these bonds (especially in the third bond to the left) to power cells and muscle activity, by turning ATP into adenosine diphosphate (ADP). Eventually, some of the ADP is turned into adenosine monophosphate (AMP), which in turn is enzymatically turned into plain adenosine, with all phosphate bonds removed.

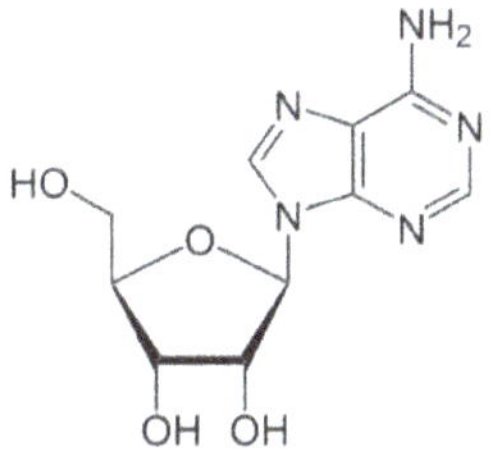

Figure 12.7 Adenosine

As the level of adenosine increases in the brain (from all the hard work you have been doing), the adenosine activates specific brain receptors that cause an increased pressure to sleep—Process S. During waking hours while working, you are using energy (ATP) and generating increasing amounts of adenosine; the buildup of adenosine pressures you to fall asleep. During sleep, the body removes adenosine (much of it used to make more ATP), the adenosine level falls, and by morning the pressure to sleep is low—just in time for the circadian arousal system to activate.

This is where coffee comes into the picture. Caffeine blocks the adenosine receptor in the brain and, in so doing, blocks Process S, which allows you to wake up (Figure 12.8).

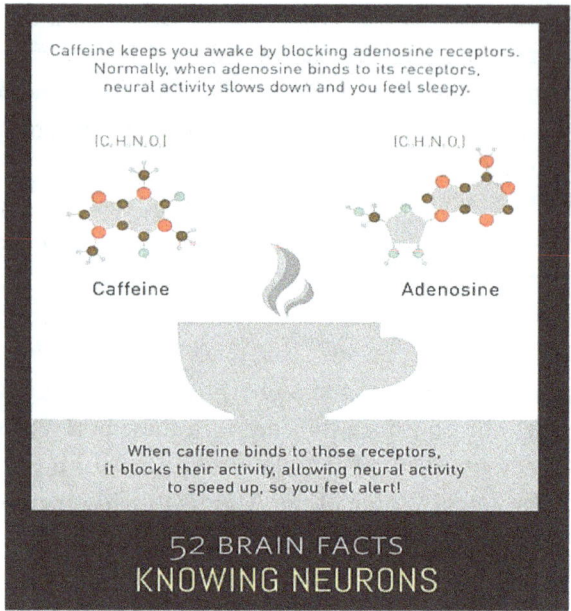

Figure 12.8 Caffeine and adenosine[5]

What Happens When We Fall Asleep?

A normal night's sleep consists of five cycles, each lasting about ninety minutes (Figure 12.9).

Each cycle consists of rapid eye movement (REM) sleep and non-REM sleep. REM sleep is characterized by rapid eye movements that can be seen beneath the closed eyelids and associated with vivid dreaming. Although the person is dreaming and their eyes are moving side to side, the other muscles of the body are entirely paralyzed. Non-REM sleep consists of several stages, including stage 1, which is relatively light sleep; stage 2, which is important in memory consolidation; and the deeper sleep of stages 3 and 4, known as slow-wave sleep.

During each cycle, we spend time in all four stages of non-REM sleep and end each cycle with a period of REM sleep.

It is still unknown why sleep is arranged this way, but it does seem as though non-REM sleep is primary and REM sleep in some way complements and is dependent upon non-REM sleep. Most of the recharging of the brain's energy occurs in non-REM sleep, as does detoxification. Basic memory consolidation also occurs in non-REM sleep. So, what is left for REM sleep to do? REM sleep, which contains most—but not all—of our dreaming, appears to be important in making and solidifying memory connections between different parts of the brain. It is during REM sleep when we experience weird surrealistic dreams. Making these connections may be a time of great creativity while we are asleep. It is also important for emotional memories.

Why should we care? Because something important *must* be going on as evolution has kept this system with only minor changes in virtually all mammals and birds!

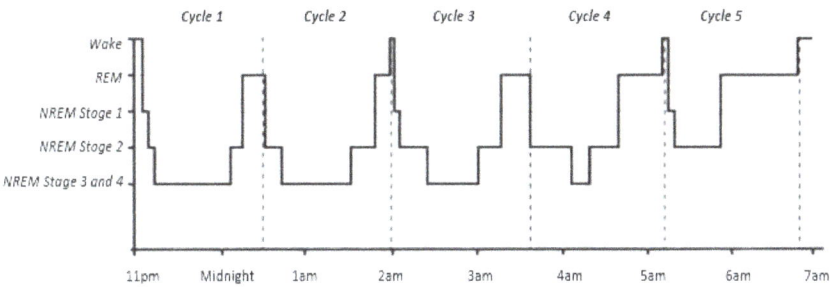

Figure 12.9 Sleep cycles through the night[6]

Now that we understand what sleep is all about, we can address the consequences of insufficient sleep and disrupted sleep, problems related to Process S (acute or chronic sleep loss), and problems related to Process C (disturbances of the circadian rhythm). Let's first address Process C.

Circadian Rhythm Disturbances (Process C)

In order to appreciate the degree to which the circadian sleep-wake cycle can be modified, let us examine two situations that all of us face from time to time: jet lag and the "Monday morning blues."

Refer back to the discussion of zeitgebers, or the environmental cues that help to synchronize internal time with external time. Sometimes, though, internal and external time get out of sync. For example, if you leave New York at 7 p.m. on a flight to London, you will arrive in London at, say, 8 a.m. local time. But due to the five-hour time difference, it will be 3 a.m. New York time. Nevertheless, you may be expected to function straightaway at a high level of performance even though if you were back in New York you would be in the midst of your normal sleep. If, by 11 p.m. London time, you decide to go to sleep, this will correspond to a late afternoon (6 p.m.) nap in New York time. And on awakening the next morning at 7 a.m. London time, you will probably feel as though it were 2 a.m. New York time—and for good reason! Although the sleep-wake cycle begins to resynchronize in a couple of days, it takes approximately seven to ten days for the entire circadian system to resynchronize under optimal circumstances, that is, when time shifts only once and all of the zeitgebers stay in concert. *As a rough guide, it takes about one day to recover for each time zone you have crossed.*

Symptoms of jet lag include:

(1) Disturbed sleep—obviously
(2) Daytime fatigue
(3) Mood changes
(4) A general sense of not feeling well
(5) Difficulty concentrating
(6) Nausea and other gastrointestinal problems (your gastrointestinal tract has a clock too, see Figure 12.3)

The jet-lag syndrome has many practical consequences. It is now common practice to fly all or part of the crew to a vessel that may be on the other side of the globe. These crew members are often expected to participate immediately in the watchkeeping system of the ship. This is usual procedure on merchant vessels and larger private vessels, which may sail with a "bare-bones" crew and must fly in replacements. If the crew member, who is still disoriented from jet lag, is now subjected to a continually changing watchkeeping schedule, it is easy to imagine that his or her circadian rhythm may not straighten itself out for weeks!

Or, consider the sailing athlete who may fly to Europe, the Middle East, or Asia to compete in a sailing event. Might the symptoms of jet lag interfere with performance? Absolutely.

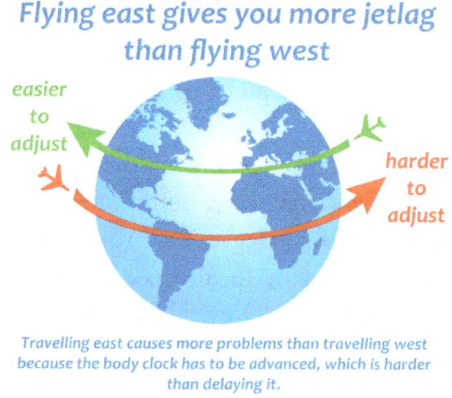

Figure 12.10 Jet lag

Eastward travel (advancing the sleep cycle) tends to cause more symptoms than westward travel (Figure 12.10). You may want to remember the expression "west is best, and east is least." If possible, sailors should gradually shift their sleep-wake cycle to their destination. After arriving, they should maximize exposure to bright daylight in the morning during the day and maximize exposure to darkness before bedtime. Modafinil (and related armodafinil), a medication that is useful for sleep disorders, may be helpful in the morning after arrival. As with all medication, discuss with your physician.

Another common example of the synchronization is the Monday morning blues. During the week, we normally sleep from 11 p.m. to 7 a.m. What happens if we stay out late on Saturday night and don't retire until 2 a.m.? We temporarily phase delay our sleep cycle so that we do not arise on Sunday until 10 or 11 a.m. This usually does not present a significant social problem since Sunday is an "off" day. The difficulty begins Sunday night when we try to phase advance our sleep cycle (i.e., go to sleep earlier), find ourselves unable to, and suffer insomnia. Sleep may not be possible until, say, 1 a.m.

Even worse, on arising Monday morning at the usual 7 a.m., it feels like the middle of the night. No wonder Monday morning is often such a dreadful time of the week. Occasionally, this phase delay can be used to an advantage. For example, what if the sailor needs to stay awake for one night for an overnight race or cruise. Simply staying up late the night before and sleeping late the morning of the race or cruise will phase delay the cycle. The boater doubtless finds the subsequent night watch more tolerable.

Sleep Pressure Disturbances (Process S) and Sleep Loss

Remember, the longer we are awake the greater the pressure to go to sleep. But despite the tiredness and the urge to go to sleep, what happens when we don't get enough sleep?

There are two types of sleep loss: *sleep deprivation*, in which the individual is deprived of sleep and remains awake for an extended period (mainly a problem for long-distance solo sailors), and *sleep restriction*, in which the individual restricts his or her sleep by a few hours each day over a period of days, weeks, months, or years!

On the water, boaters and sailors are primarily concerned with sleep restriction.

The average adult should get approximately seven to eight hours of continuous sleep per day to maintain high levels of attention and cognition (thinking). As we will see below, many of the watchkeeping systems do not allow sufficient quantity, quality, or continuity of sleep—as any midshipman will attest and as the U.S. Navy is trying to remedy.

It turns out that sleep loss is cumulative and results in sleep *debt*—like monetary debt and almost as difficult to pay off! And it takes significantly longer than most individuals imagine and is more than hour for hour, not unlike interest on your monetary debt. For example, the boater who works during the week and sleeps only six hours per night from Monday through Friday cannot possibly make up the sleep debt on the weekend. Even if the number of hours can be roughly repaid, the sleep debt requires much longer time than a two-day weekend will allow. *Therefore, every boater who is sleep deprived during the week will function at an impaired level while boating on the weekend!*

And after seven to ten days of six hours per night sleep, his or her performance is similar to that of someone who has been awake for twenty-four hours. If that didn't grab your attention, consider this: *Performance after sleep restriction for only nineteen hours is equivalent to being legally intoxicated at .08 blood alcohol concentration.*[7]

In general, *the greater the sleep debt, the greater the loss of vigilance and attention*. Vigilance is simply the state of being awake and alert. Attention is the ability to attend to something: the compass, the radar screen, a gauge—whatever is important at the time. It is the lack of attention that is responsible for many accidents at sea. In addition to performance being impaired by the lack of attention to the task at hand, there is another phenomenon that occurs when the pressure of sleep continues, and that is termed *microsleeps*. For brief periods of time, the individual actually falls asleep; however, time spent sleeping is so brief that the person may not even realize that he or she was asleep at the wheel, so to speak. This can be catastrophic and worse than sailing (or driving) drunk. A person who drives a car while *legally intoxicated* has impaired reaction time; it may take longer to brake, for example. A person who drives while *sleep deprived* may be worse off because in addition to impaired reaction time, there may be periods of *microsleeping*, and during the microsleeps, he or she may not brake at all! The same problem can occur on the water—just substitute avoiding an impediment or collision with another ship.

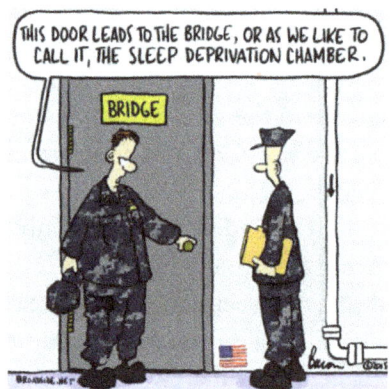

Figure 12.11 Sleep deprivation chamber[8]

To make matters worse, the person who is sleep deprived is often unaware that he or she is sleep deprived. Just like an intoxicated individual who says, "Give me the keys, I'm fine to drive," a sleep-deprived individual may feel that he or she is fine as well. But at least with the intoxicated individual, it is likely the person was seen drinking by others. Sleep deprivation is more insidious because most crew members will keep the knowledge of their restricted sleep to themselves.

One final point about alcohol and sleep. The impairment of attention when sleep deprivation and alcohol intoxication are combined is beyond additive—it is multiplicative!

Choosing a Watchkeeping System

The number of possible watchkeeping systems is virtually limitless. The major determinants are the tasks that need to be performed and the crew that is available. These two variables determine the number of watches that can be set. If possible, the captain should not be assigned a set watch, since he or she is already expected (unrealistically) to be at peak efficiency on an around-the-clock basis. See Appendix G for additional watchkeeping schedules and sleep information.

One Watch

The most serious limitation in having only one watch is that inevitably, there are periods when there is no one watching! This is one of the accepted hazards of singlehanded sailing. In the 1972 Original Single-Handed Transatlantic Race (OSTAR), information on the sleep routine of twenty-one sailors was made available after the race. Five woke hourly, or more often than hourly, all the time, or nearly all the time. One of them managed to wake himself every half hour, day and night, for thirty-eight days. Four sailors established a schedule in which they woke less often than every hour. Twelve did not establish a sleep-wake schedule, but slept at irregular intervals. Unfortunately, the numbers were too small (and there were too many other variables) to establish whether sleep-wake routine had a recognizable effect on sailing efficiency.

Two Watches

There are several two-watch schedules shown in Figures 12.12 through 12.15. Probably the most traditional, which dates to at least the eighteenth century, is the traditional "watch and watch" or "four on, four off" (see Figure 12.12). It can be used with or without the "dogged watch," depending on the need for rotation. Many sailors will recognize the continuity of their nautical heritage in the passage from John Masefield's *Sea Life in Nelson's Time* in endnote 9.[9]

Name	Time	Day 1	Day 2	Day 3
First watch	2000–0000	Team 1	Team 2	Team 1
Middle watch	0000–0400	Team 2	Team 1	Team 2
Morning watch	0400–0800	Team 1	Team 2	Team 1
Forenoon watch	0800–1200	Team 2	Team 1	Team 2
Afternoon watch	1200–1600	Team 1	Team 2	Team 1
First dog watch	1600–1800	Team 2	Team 1	Team 2
Second dog watch	1800–2000	Team 1	Team 2	Team 1

Figure 12.12 Four on, four off[10]

Three and Four Watches

The Dreaded Five and Dime

> A former surface warfare officer still cringes thinking about the deployment where she stood the Navy's notorious "five and dime" watches: five hours on, ten off, then repeat—no matter what time of day or night. "The hardest part is being awake at some point every night and still doing a job all day. It is hard on a body and hard on the mind."

3 five-hour watch sections

	Day 1	Day 2	Day 3
2200–0200	Team 1	Team 3	Team 2
0200–0700	Team 2	Team 1	Team 3
0700–1200	Team 3	Team 2	Team 1
1200–1700	Team 1	Team 3	Team 2
1700–2200	Team 2	Team 1	Team 3

Figure 12.13 A "noncircadian" watchbill: The dreaded "five and dime"[11]

It should be obvious why sailors dread the "five and dime" (Figure 12.13). The watches are five hours in length except for the 2200-0200 four-hour block at night. This schedule leads to a circadian monstrosity—a nineteen-hour day! And the rotations are constantly switching so no one ever adjusts. Why was this perpetuated? In a word, tradition. Speaking of tradition, in Navy speak "port and starboard watch" refers to schedules where one stands six (or four or eight) hours on, has the same amount of time off, then goes back to the same amount of time back on. It has been referred to as "port and stupid."[12]

As you will see in Figures 12.14 and 12.15 below, if the tasks and crew permit the addition of extra watches, it becomes possible to create a more physiologic watchkeeping system.

To design an optimal watchkeeping system, you should optimize both Process C (circadian system) and Process S (sleep pressure). You should now appreciate how difficult that will be. The watchkeeping system (known as the "watchbill" by the U.S. Navy) depends on a number of factors, including the manpower, the teams, the conditions, and so forth. Most boaters will not have the luxury of having sufficient manpower to utilize many of the naval watchbills. Even the U.S. Navy has had this same difficulty—explaining at least in part the referenced accidents at the opening of this chapter. However, analyzing the thought process of the Naval Postgraduate School is instructive, and will help the rest of us design the best watchbill for our limited crew.

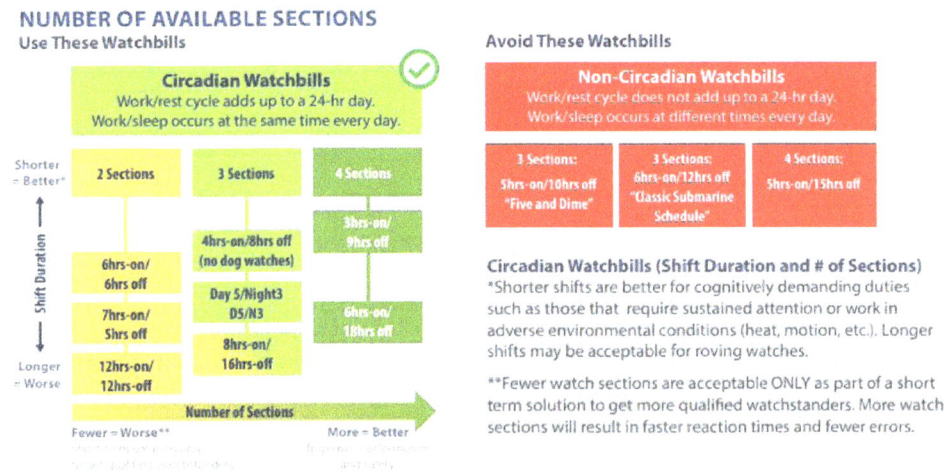

Figure 12.14 Designing a circadian watchbill

One priority would be to design a "circadian watchbill" (Figure 12.14) satisfying Process C. In these watchkeeping systems, the work/rest cycle mimics a twenty-four-hour day. It is also helpful if work and sleep occur at the same time each day, so the sailor can accommodate to the schedule. A second priority would be to satisfy Process S: obtaining seven to eight hours of sleep per day, preferably continuous quality sleep.

The current U.S. Navy's "ideal" systems have greater manpower requirements and are somewhat more complicated, but they do maximize Process C and Process S. Figure 12.15 shows the "3/9 Circadian Watch Rotation."

Yes, it is complicated, and undoubtedly that is one of the reasons the Navy has had difficulty implementing it. It is also a four-man watch system, so that any function that needs watch keeping—Officer of the Day, Engine Officer, and so forth—requires four men. That is a lot of personnel. But it is a circadian system (Process C), it is nonrotating (typically changes are made on the weekend every three weeks or so), and it provides for protected sleep every day (Process S).

The Navy has other watchbills for other crew configurations. See Appendix E.

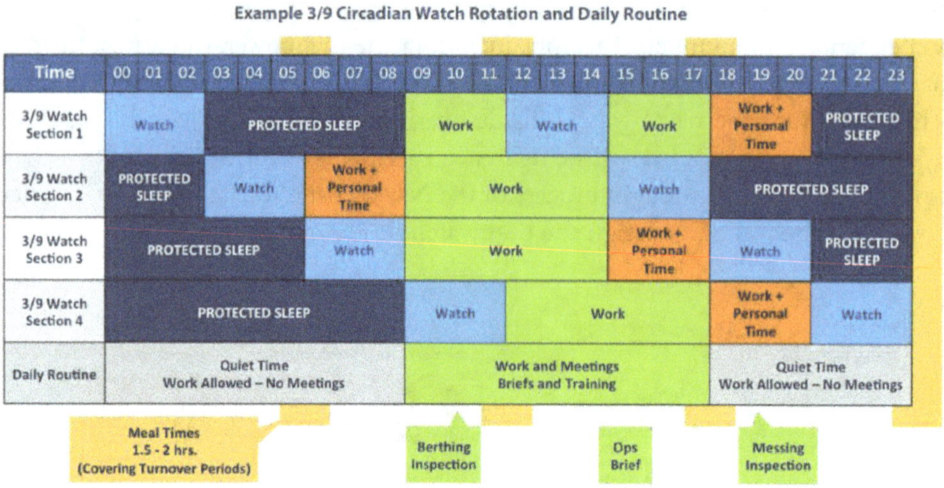

Healthy Boating & Sailing

Example 3/9 Circadian Watch Rotation and Daily Routine

Figure 12.15 U.S. Navy 3/9 Circadian Watch Rotation

Waking up After a Sleep Period—Sleep Inertia

Despite the best designed watch-keeping system, crew members are going to have problems sleeping on board. That's not surprising, since many of the crew members will bring their insomnia with them from shore. Before we look at the problem of insomnia on the water—especially the problem of falling and staying asleep—let's look at the other end of the sleep process, waking up. The difficulty of awakening after sleep is referred to as *sleep inertia*. That is, there is a period of fifteen to sixty minutes during which there is drowsiness and some disorientation associated with impaired sensory and motor acuity, impaired attentiveness and mental ability, and subjective fatigue. This sleep inertia occurs in the absence of sleep deprivation.

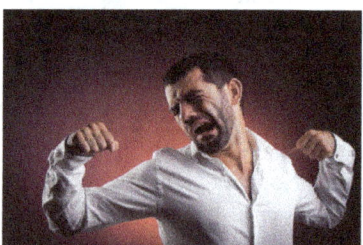

Figure 12.16 Sleep inertia

What if the crew member has some accumulated sleep deprivation? With sleep deprivation, there is a compensatory increase in the time spent in stage 3, slow wave non-REM deep sleep, rather than stages 1, 2, or REM sleep. Awakening during stage 3, slow wave sleep, is associated with even greater sleep inertia.

What can be done? Recognizing sleep inertia and allowing the crew member to awaken fully before requiring critical tasks—like keeping watch, making decisions, or performing other safety-critical tasks—is a good start. Keep in mind that there may be impaired reaction time, reduced motor dexterity, and deficits in spatial memory because of sleep inertia. Bright blue light and of course that cup of Joe will help shorten sleep inertia.

"Measure Twice, Cut Once" (Old English Proverb)

Are there any tools available to document a sleep disorder or sleep debt in your crew or yourself?

One simple approach that can be very instructive is to complete a two-week sleep diary (Appendix E). This can be helpful in differentiating a true sleep disorder from self-inflicted sleep debt! Additionally, if you suspect that you have an actual sleep disorder, this can be very valuable when given to a sleep specialist. It would not be necessarily appropriate to ask your crew to keep such a diary, unless perhaps they are also a relative!

Alternatively, if there is any chance that you or a crew member has chronic insomnia, you may consider completing the Insomnia Severity Index, a seven-question index that will provide a rapid assessment as to whether you have a sleep disorder, and, if so, an estimate of the severity (Appendix E).

Evaluating and quantifying sleepiness would be extremely valuable prior to embarkation. There are a number of tools available worldwide. One of the most frequently used in clinical practice in the United States is the Epworth Sleepiness Scale. As the name implies, it is a subjective measure of someone's sleepiness at one point in time. It is self-rated and based on a score of zero to twenty-four. You can analyze your own score or that of a crew member. Is it intrusive to ask crew members to complete this simple tool? Yes, perhaps, but anyone who stands watch has by definition other people's lives dependent upon their vigilance and attention (Appendix E).

If, on the other hand, your goal is to follow a crew member or members over a period of time, then it may be useful to turn to one of the simple analog scales, such as the Karolinska Sleepiness Scale, which goes from one to nine:

(1) Extremely alert
(2) Very alert
(3) Alert
(4) Rather alert
(5) Neither alert nor sleepy
(6) Some signs of sleepiness
(7) Sleepy, but no difficulty remaining awake
(8) Sleepy, some effort to keep alert
(9) Extremely sleepy, fighting sleep

Treatment Strategies for Insomnia

Most adults have experienced insomnia at some point in their lifetime. An estimated 30 percent to 50 percent have intermittent insomnia, and 10 percent have chronic insomnia. That ensures that some of your crew or you yourself will have some level of insomnia before embarkation. What is the best strategy to deal with insomnia?

The American Academy of Sleep Medicine recently published clinical guidelines, and they are eye-opening.[13] In looking at virtually all of the commonly prescribed medications for insomnia, the authors performed meta-analyses (combining studies focused on the same outcome in order to enlarge the number of subjects and improve the reliability of the results). From the evidence, researchers concluded that proof of efficacy for all medications studied was *weak*. The researchers looked at the following:

- Sleep onset (how long it took to fall asleep)
- Total sleep time
- Wake after sleep onset
- Sleep efficiency (percentage of time in bed during which sleep occurs)
- Number of awakenings

Results of this study don't mean that all sleeping pills are ineffective or inappropriate; to the contrary, the academy does discuss specific recommendations, and the fact that different medications may affect different aspects of sleep (e.g., some reduce sleep latency, others improve total sleep time, etc.). It's just that all the studies, which were funded by the pharmaceutical industry and only compared with a placebo, were scientifically weak! Despite the shaky scientific evidence, either you or your crew may be relying on certain pills to get to sleep, or to stay asleep. It is worth knowing what to expect. Does the crew member have difficulty falling asleep, but once asleep, is able to sleep through? Or is it mainly a problem of sleep maintenance? In short, pinpointing the exact nature of the issue will increase the likelihood of finding an effective sleep medication.

What is missing from the study are some of the most commonly used medications for sleep, including alprazolam (Xanax), lorazepam (Ativan), and diazepam (Valium). One reason is that these medications were developed for other purposes, and are being used (frequently) "off-label." Therefore, there are a paucity of well-controlled studies of these drugs even though they are among the most commonly used in clinical practice. In general, they tend to be short acting and may help with sleep onset but not sleep maintenance.

The seldom-discussed problem is that virtually all of the older—and even some of the newer—sleeping pills "sedate" you rather than assist you into sleep. Sleeping pills act by interfering with the higher regions of the brain (like alcohol does) and do not produce "natural" sleep. For example, EEG brain wave recordings of people on sleeping pills reveal that the normal "architecture" of sleep, as shown in Figure 12.9, is disrupted. Sleeping pills help with sleep—but not normal, natural sleep. In addition, there are many

Recommended for treating Sleep Onset Insomnia
Eszopiclone (Lunesta)
Ramelteon (Rozerem)
Temazepam (Restoril)
Triazolam (Halcion)
Zalepon (Sonata)
Zolpidem (Ambien)
Recommended for treating Sleep Maintenance Insomnia
Doxepin
Eszopiclone (Lunesta)
Temazepam (Restoril)
Suvorexant (Belsomra)
Zolpidem (Ambien)
Not Recommended for treating either Sleep Onset or Maintenance
Diphenhydramine (Benadryl) 50mg size
Melatonin 2mgs
Trazadone
L-tryptophan
Valerian

Table 12.1 Medication recommendations from the American Academy of Sleep Medicine

unwanted side effects, including grogginess, prolonged sleep inertia, daytime forgetfulness, and impaired reaction times.

The only possible exception may be melatonin.[14] Melatonin is a naturally occurring brain chemical that "sets the table" for sleep, but does not really put you to sleep. Recent information from the 2019 American Academy of Neurology Annual Meeting says that the dose of melatonin should be low—no more than 1 to 2 milligrams—and it should be given three hours, not thirty minutes, before sleep. Since it is not a "medication," the dose on the bottle may or may not reflect active ingredients. Finally, you should be aware that diphenhydramine (Benadryl) at a strength of 25 milligrams is the active ingredient in many of the over-the-counter sleeping medications, at least in the United States.

In place of medication, *first-line insomnia treatment should be behavioral in nature*. Cognitive behavioral therapy (CBT) is becoming standard. The variation used specifically for insomnia is often referred to as CBT-I (for insomnia). It is basically short-term, problem-focused therapy, usually conducted by psychologists or psychiatrists, that attempts to change your behavior and eliminate the "issues" that interfere with sleep. It is very practical and usually requires only a limited number of sessions. Rather than addressing the "root cause"—your mother probably did prefer your sister over you—the therapy focusses on shutting down any intrusive thoughts, so that you can get to sleep. The problem with CBT (less so with CBT-I) is price and availability of practitioners.

Another approach is mindfulness meditation. Rather than recognizing and shutting off the "issues" as with CBT techniques, mindfulness meditation teaches you to focus on something else—breathing for example. Mindfulness meditation should be practiced during the day or evening, but is also useful in awakenings during the night to get back to sleep. I admit to using mindfulness meditation daily and at night. There are mindfulness meditation apps for your phone (and there are apps for CBT-I as well), although, traditionally, CBT requires some face-to-face interaction. In Appendix E, I have included the four-seven-eight breathing pattern, which is worth a try.

A major advantage of these nonmedication approaches is that the gains made during treatment are more durable, whereas the gains with medication dissipate as soon as the medication is withdrawn.

Finally, here are some basic recommendations from the Naval Postgraduate School for good sleep hygiene at sea.

Basic rules of healthy work and sleep patterns:

- Obtain eight hours of uninterrupted sleep per twenty-four-hour period, preferably at the same time each day
- Compensate for any sleep loss with naps; if possible, allow yourself thirty minutes or two hours for napping with less sleep inertia
- If possible, use bright light to improve alertness at your workplace
- Avoid light (especially blue light) exposure before bedtime
- Exercise, but no later than two to three hours before your bedtime
- Avoid large meals and beverages, especially caffeinated and alcoholic beverages, before bedtime
- To the extent possible, use the twenty-four-hour circadian rhythm to set the foundation for your work and rest periods
- Build a stable daily work schedule, including the watchbill that maximizes rest opportunities
- Minimize rotating shift changes to allow your circadian clock to adjust to your work schedule
- Use caffeine during the first part of your shift to promote alertness; caffeine may prevent sleep so time its use wisely
- Learn and understand the effects of good sleep practices
- Get supporting analysis before you make a final decision to change the work and rest schedules of your crew

Notes

1. Both this data and the above quote from Joe Girardi are from a lecture by Scott Kutscher, a neurologist from Stanford. He delivered "Sleep for Resiliency, Recovery and Performance: Sleep and Athletic Performance" at the American Academy of Neurology meeting in Philadelphia in 2019.

2. https://commons.wikimedia.org/wiki/File:10_caffeine_knowing-neurons.jpg#filelinks.

3. Matthew Walker, *Why We Sleep: Unlocking the Power of Sleep and Dreams* (New York: Scribner, 2017). This is an excellent up-to-date exploration of all aspects of sleep. Highly recommended.

4. Redrawn image from Walker, *Why We Sleep*. The following illustration is from "Sleep-Wake Homeostasis" at howsleepworks.com. It nicely demonstrates just Process S and how it may be altered by both sleep loss and inappropriate napping.

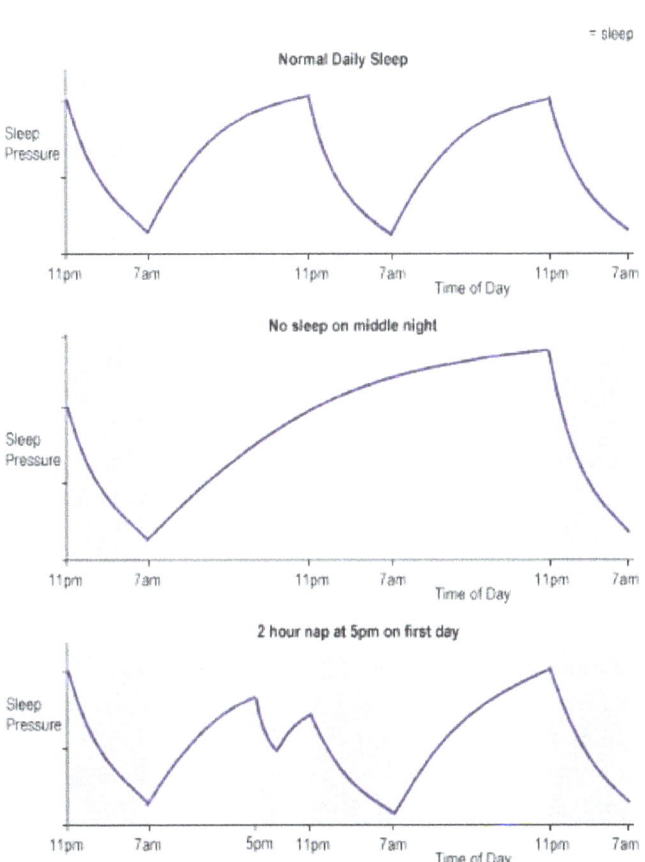

The upper graph demonstrates that sleep pressure increases from 7 a.m. until 11 p.m. and then decreases during sleep to begin the process all over again the next day. So, sleep pressure is relieved by sleep. That makes sense. In the middle graph, sleep pressure continues to build because of the "all-nighter" until the following night when it dissipates. The lower graph demonstrates that the two-hour nap at 5 p.m. will decrease the sleep pressure that evening (and may make it more difficult to fall asleep).

5. https://en.wikipedia.org/wiki/Adenosine_receptor#/media/File:10_caffeine_knowing-neurons.jpg.

6. Redrawn after Walker, *Why We Sleep*.

7. A. M. Williamson and A. Feyer, "Moderate Sleep Deprivation Produces Impairments in Cognitive and Motor Performance Equivalent to Legally Prescribed Levels of Alcohol Intoxication," *Occupational Environmental Medicine* 65 (2000): 649-655.

8. Crew Endurance Handbook: A Guide to Applying Circadian-Based Watchbills, *United States Navy*, https://my.nps.edu/web/crewendurance/about-crew-endurance.

9. The day of a man-of-war's man began at midnight, or at four in the morning, according to the alternation of the watches. If he had the middle-watch, from 12 A.M. till 4 A.M., he came on deck at midnight and remained there till 4 A.M., doing any duty which appeared necessary. . . . The men had but to trim the sails and be ready for a call. . . . The remainder of the watch were supposed by the Articles of War to keep awake on pain of death. Some captains and lieutenants allowed those not actually on watch as look-out men to sleep during their night-watches, if the weather was very fine. The act of sleeping during a night watch in the tropics was known as "taking a caulk," because by lying on the plank-seams the sailors' jackets were marked with lines of tar. In those ships aboard which the sailors were expected to keep awake, the boatswain's mates walked round with their starters, or kept buckets of water ready to wake anyone who fell asleep. . . .

A few minutes before eight bells, or 4 A.M., the quarter-masters stole down the after-ladders to call the midshipmen, mates, and lieutenant of the other watch. The boatswaill's mates . . . blew the prolonged, shrill call "All Hands" following it up by a shout of "Starboard (or larboard) Watch Ahoy. Rouse Out There, You Sleepers. Hey. Out or Down Here." At this order, the watch below, who were snugly sleeping in their hammocks, turned out at once without waiting till they were properly awake. When they had turned out they put on their clothes (if they had taken them off) and bustled up on deck with the starters after them. . . . The men of the other watch, who had kept the deck since midnight, were then allowed to go below to their hammocks. . . .

Before 5 A.M. the watch took off their trousers to the thigh, rigged the pumps, got out the scrubbers and buckets, and began to wash the ship down. . . . At about half-past seven the boatswain's mates went below to the berth-deck and piped "All Hands. Up Hammocks," a pipe which brought up the sleepers and filled the deck with scurrying figures. . . . By 8 A.M. at a word from the captain the boatswain piped to breakfast, eight bells was struck upon the ship's bell, and nearly every man except the helmsman, lookout men, and officers on duty, slipped down to breakfast. Half-an-hour was allowed for this meal on weekdays. At half-past eight the watch was called, and those who had slept from 4 till 7:30 A.M. came upon deck . . . employed in the work of the ship, in the rigging, or about the guns, doing the never-finished duties of sailormen. . . .

Dinner generally took about half-an-hour, from twelve till half-past. It was a merry meal, eaten cheerily, with a great buzz of talk all along the gun deck. At half-past twelve there came a great clink of cans and banging of tin plates on the tables. The fifer took his flute to the main or upper deck, where the master's mate stood by the tub to dispense sea ambrosia to the ship's company. . . . Grog time was the one happy hour of the day. With grog and an occasional battle, a sailor was often almost contented. At half-past one o'clock, when the last oozings of the blackjack had been drained, the watch on deck was called to duty. The watch below were sometimes allowed to keep below, to sleep if they could. . . . At 4 P.M. the boatswain piped to supper, which lasted half-an-hour, and was made pleasant by the second serving out of grog. Shortly after supper, but before sunset, the drummer beat to quarters. All hands had to repair to their stations. . . .

At eight o'clock the first night-watch was called and set, and the watch below went down to their hammocks until midnight. The lights were extinguished, or covered over, so that they would not show from a distance. . . . The watch and watch system, four hours on and four hours off, with the four hours off constantly broken in upon by the ship's routine, was severe and harassing. It meant that the sailor had but four hours of sleep one night, and a bare seven hours the night following. The little naps they managed to take in the forenoons and afternoons were hardly worth mentioning; they were too uncertain, too liable to interruption. Even in their watches below at night they were liable to be called on deck to tack, to wear, to shorten sail, or to go to their stations. Once a month, at least, they were drummed up to general quarters in the middle of their dreams. John Masefield, *Sea Life in Nelson's Time* (New York: Macmillan, 1925), pp. 185-193

10. https://en.wikipedia.org/wiki/Watchkeeping#Watch_systems.

11. https://en.wikipedia.org/wiki/Watchkeeping#cite_note-usni357-6.

12. Jeff Crowell, "A Glossary of Military Terminology, Jargon, and Slang" *Sailor Speak*, May 2013, http://www.combat.ws/S4/SAILOR/INDEX.HTM.

13. "Practice Guidelines," *American Academy of Sleep Medicine*, https://aasm.org/clinical-resources/practice-standards/practice-guidelines/.

14. "Melatonin and Sleep," *National Sleep Foundation*, https://www.sleepfoundation.org/articles/melatonin-and-sleep.

Chapter 13

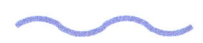

Sailing Psychology 1

> "The sea won't tolerate the inept or pretentious for long. The measure of a man, whether he is an unranked seaman or an ex-admiral of the blue—his hopes and fears, the fiber of his temper, facets of character that might otherwise remain hidden all of his life behind a web of status and sophistication—are soon known on a long small-ship voyage."
> —*Charles A. Borden*, Sea Quest

> "Time and Tide wait for no man."
> —*St. Marher*, 1225

Everyone who goes down to the sea in ships has his or her own set of goals and expectations. For some boaters or sailors, it is the personal challenge of making a successful passage across a bay, or around the world. Others enjoy the organized chaos of sailboat racing. Still others prefer the sense of solitude and withdrawal from the hurly-burly of modern society—Walden Pond on a larger scale.

In addition to goals and expectations, we each carry aboard our own mental and emotional "baggage"; that is, we bring with us our own style of decision making, of dealing with discomfort (on occasion even adversity), of interacting with others, and of simply amusing ourselves. This psychological repertoire, of course, stamps us as individuals.

Since we are all unique, it is difficult to predict how each of us would respond to the variety of stressful situations we can encounter at sea. It would be helpful, for example, if we could predict which sailors are not psychologically "cut out" for long-distance, singlehanded sailing or whether a particular sailor will "fit in" as a crew member. Many of us have doubts about our ability to compete. Nevertheless, although the discipline of psychology cannot yet offer us the means and capacity to make reliable predictions, it has identified patterns of behavior and has redefined the limits of normality in a number of situations. Sometimes the results have been surprising—as in the case of isolation and the singlehanded sailor.

Singlehanded Sailing

The singlehanded sailor must face a staggering array of psychological challenges. Isolation, lack of sleep, physical discomfort, and a multitude of other stresses conspire to reduce an otherwise highly efficient sailor to a dangerously inefficient one. A few sailors—the lone voyagers—appear to thrive on the solitude that most of us would find unbearable. Clearly, they are a rare breed, endowed with an unusual psychological makeup.[1] For the rest of us, long-range single handing is an occasional experience. It may be planned (a solitary cruise or solo race) or unplanned (a lack of crew or shipwreck). In either case, it behooves us to appreciate the psychological hazards that are involved. These hazards are represented by the three S's: *sensory deprivation*, *sleep loss*, and *stress*.

Sensory Deprivation

Although solitude or isolation can be intensely enjoyable at times, it can also be oppressive, and highly dangerous. In a remarkable account of his experience in solitary confinement, Christopher Burney made the following observation: "Variety is not the spice of life; it is the very stuff of it."[2] Although as sailors we are not likely to encounter situations as extreme as solitary confinement, monotony, boredom, and a lack of varied sensory stimuli are important and enduring problems aboard ship.

One of the first shipboard concerns to be addressed systematically was that of boredom and job-related monotony. In studies for the Royal Air Force during World War II, N. H. Mackworth investigated the phenomenon that radar operators on antisubmarine patrol frequently failed to detect as many U-boats as were known to be operating in the area. The radar operators usually worked in isolation, watching a radar screen for hours at a time. Mackworth developed an analogous laboratory model and found that performance in any prolonged vigilance task (such as those a radar operator or lookout performs) begins to decline within twenty minutes. Because of this, and subsequent confirmatory research, the typical tour of duty for such personnel has generally been shortened. An important corollary implication of this study is that if the sailor expects to function at his or her best, the sailor should be exposed to a varied and variable sensory environment.

Following Mackworth's investigations, interest in brainwashing, aroused during the Korean War, motivated psychologists[3] at McGill University (and later elsewhere) to explore the effects of reducing the overall level of sensory stimulation. These studies, collectively known as *sensory-deprivation experiments*, have been conducted in several ways.

First, the absolute number of stimuli that reaches a subject may be reduced, producing true *sensory deprivation*. This was initially accomplished by placing the subject in a totally dark, soundproof room with gloves and arm bandages to reduce the tactile (touch) stimulation. The water-immersion technique popularized in the movie *The Ipcress File* produces the same results. Although this degree of sensory deprivation does not occur at sea, visual deprivation is a common occurrence for anyone (including sailors) who must stare off into the uniform blackness of space for long periods of time. This hazard is well known to long-distance truck drivers and aviators. After many hours, they may begin to experience illusions (misinterpretations of something that is seen, heard, or felt, for example) or hallucinations (images of nonexistent objects) because of the visual deprivation. The nature of the illusions and hallucinations is discussed shortly.

Second, the absolute amount of stimulation may be kept constant, but the variability may be reduced. This is referred to as *perceptual deprivation* and is simulated in the laboratory by special goggles that admit only diffuse, patterned light, and earphones that transmit meaningless sounds. The effects of perceptual deprivation are similar to those of sensory deprivation.

For the boater, the unchanging visual pattern of the sea, the monotonous sound of the wind in the rigging, and the steady noise of the waves ensures that at least some degree of perceptual deprivation can be expected on every blue-water cruise.

There are two additional situations capable of wreaking havoc with the human psyche: *immobilization* and *social isolation*. Immobilization is rarely a problem for the boater, but social isolation certainly is. Every singlehanded sailor must deal in one way or another with social isolation. Its symptoms are virtually identical with those of sensory or perceptual deprivation.

What are the warning symptoms the sailor should keep in mind? Often, there is an early decline in performance, including both fine and gross motor skills. Perception may also be affected, with objects appearing larger or smaller than normal, or straight lines seeming to be curved. Some sailors develop an impaired ability to concentrate and maintain a train of thought. The perception of time passage may be grossly distorted. An alteration in mood is also common, and on occasion an oscillation between irritability and euphoria, which may appear childish. Sensory-deprived subjects are said to be more susceptible to persuasion (brainwashing). The most characteristic symptoms, however, are illusions and hallucinations. Dr. Glin Bennet has written extensively on the psychological phenomena of singlehanded sailors. In his study of the 1972 OSTAR, he examined the type and frequency of perceptual disturbances among the racers. Half of the competitors who completed daily records experienced one or more illusions or hallucinations. Auditory sensations were the most common, followed by visual, olfactory (smell), and spatial (déjà vu). One singlehanded sailor whom Dr. Bennet studied had the following experience after a long stint at the helm:

> He saw his father-in-law at the top of the mast. They were aware of one another's presence, and the experience was in no way alarming. At the top of the mast there is a metal radar reflector, a box-like structure 12 in. (30 cm.) or so across. A short time later the same evening he looked down into the cabin and saw his wife, then his mother, then his daughter lying on the bunk where a sleeping bag was stretched out. Later again he was up at the bow changing a sail and saw in the water by the bow a large flat fish like a ray—very unlikely off the east coast of England—which was probably a misinterpretation of the boat's bow wave . . .

On occasion, the visual hallucinations may be quite complex, as the following case demonstrates:

> The sailor was lying below on his bunk when he heard someone on deck putting the boat about on the other tack. He stirred himself to go up and investigate, but as he went up on deck an unidentified man passed him coming down into the cabin. On deck he found that the boat had indeed been put about properly and that everything was in order. The process was repeated several times. As the sailor went up the man came down; when the sailor came down the man went up. But the man was not recognized.[4]

As the first example demonstrates, it is often difficult to distinguish illusions from hallucinations and even from dreams, daydreams, images, or fantasies. For this reason, psychologists often refer to all these visual experiences as reported visual sensations. Often (but not invariably) illusions precede hallucinations, and less complex hallucinations (dots, lines, patterns) precede more complex hallucinations (such as animals or people). Auditory illusions and hallucinations are even more common than visual ones. During a gale, one of the OSTAR racers felt that voices in the rigging were calling "Bill, Bill," in a high-pitched voice. During the same gale, another sailor reported, "Someone knocked on the side deck as if asking to come in. I was petrified."

Vito Dumas, a veteran singlehanded sailor, once overheard the following conversation coming from the forward locker of his boat while sailing from France to South America:

> "Listen," began a voice with a strong Spanish accent, "I'm going to look for something to eat."
>
> "Shut up; he'll hear you.". . . "No, he won't."[5]

At the time, Dumas was not able to leave the helm, but later, when he had the time to investigate, he realized that no one could possibly be stowed away in his forward locker. Even so, the voices were so lifelike that he assumed that people had been on board and that they must have swum ashore.

Any of the other senses may also be involved in sensory-deprivation experiences. Some sailors have reported the feeling of being touched or struck on the arm, whereas others sensed that another body was beside them in their bunk. Still other sailors have reported the smell of cooking, or freshly brewed coffee—olfactory hallucinations. *Déjà vu phenomena*, the feeling of having been there before, have also been described. One OSTAR racer had "this strong feeling of locality—in this case, for where I have been becalmed for close on 24 hours. I keep thinking of it, as a place I have been to before and can almost picture it." A few days later, "I still have this preoccupation with place, to the extent that if I did not have a compass it would be very easy to become unbalanced about it. It is as though the time and weather conditions constituted a locality."[6]

What can the sailor do to combat the effects of sensory deprivation? Dr. David Lewis has experienced numerous hallucinations on his solo voyages and offers the following suggestion:

> When I was very tired and had spent numerous hours at the helm in winds too light for the vane, sometimes heard voices. . . . Hallucinations seem to occur only when solitude and fatigue are accompanied by monotonous occupations. . . . I would think that varying tasks demanding physical and/or mental effort would be valuable in preserving emotional stability.[7]

Indeed, there is evidence from experimental psychology that physical exercise reduces the effects of sensory deprivation. Mental exercises are not as helpful, and are more difficult to sustain.

Sleep Loss

The consequences of sleep loss have been discussed in Chapter 12. Many of the effects such as mood changes and a decline in performance, are similar to those of sensory deprivation. The illusions and hallucinations that occur with sleep loss are indistinguishable from those due to sensory deprivation. In fact, since both hazards frequently occur simultaneously when singlehanded sailing, it is often difficult to place the blame accurately. A typical example would be the singlehanded sailor who is engaged at the helm for hours on end, attempting to claw off a lee shore. If the sailor begins to hallucinate, is it due to his or her sleep loss? Or is it due to the accumulated solitude of weeks alone at sea? Unlike in the laboratory, it is often impossible to separate the effects of sleep loss from those of sensory deprivation at sea.

Stress

The final "S" with which the sailor must cope is stress, in its 1,001 nautical forms: being becalmed, battling a storm for seventy-two hours, avoiding a lee shore, managing gear failure, and so on. The sailor's underlying personality structure determines, to a great degree, what is stressful to him or her, and how well he or she can deal with each particular stressful situation. (For individual reactions to highly stressful situations, see "The Psychology of Disaster" later in this chapter.)

If the psychological stresses are severe enough and continue long enough, they may produce a full-blown nervous (psychotic) breakdown. There is evidence that these stress-induced breakdowns are more likely to occur in people who have susceptible personalities, especially in those who have suffered nervous breakdowns previously. It seems prudent to suggest that since the psychological stress on the single hander is so intense, anyone who has had a previous breakdown should forgo singlehanded sailing. But even in the absence of a prior psychiatric disorder, severe environmental stress may produce a psychotic reaction. The best-documented case is that of Donald Crowhurst, a contestant in the 1968 *Sunday Times* around-the-world, singlehanded race. N. Tomalin and R. Hall's *The Strange Last Voyage of Donald Crowhurst* is an extraordinary and disturbing account of the unremitting disintegration of a human psyche. The story is unique because of the extensive documentation available, including logbook writings, tape recordings, and even film. There is also a movie (*The Mercy* with Colin Firth and Rachel Weisz) and a documentary (*Crowhurst*).

From the beginning, Crowhurst experienced significant psychological stresses: a failing business, tremendous publicity, serious self-doubt, and an ill-prepared and untested boat that was beset with problems. After only two weeks at sea, Crowhurst realized that the boat would never withstand an around-the-world voyage. At this point, he decided to execute an elaborate deception—a fabricated circumnavigation complete with bogus sightings, phony log entries, and faked messages. All the while, he was waiting off the east coast of South America for the proper moment to "reenter" the race.

The nervous breakdown occurred over a one-week period. The apparent cause of the breakdown was the sinking of his nearest rival. He had no means of escaping the hero's welcome that awaited him, and the attendant public scrutiny. Crowhurst harbored suspicions that his deception might be discovered. Prior to the breakdown, he was able to sail and navigate with adequate precision, but once his grasp on reality began to loosen, he allowed the boat to drift aimlessly.

His writing, now voluminous, became increasingly cosmic and bizarre:

> Mathematicians and engineers used to the techniques of system analysis will skim through my complete work in less than an hour. At the end of that time problems that have beset humanity for thousands of years will have been solved for them. Aspects I have no need to mention will tumble into place, and the distressing struggles of man to reach an understanding of the driving forces between God and Man, and the physical universe [will be over].

He became obsessed with the idea of life as a game:

> During his lifetime, each man plays cosmic chess against the Devil. Each man can decide for himself who has won. The moves of the game are all well-known. It is a difficult game to follow who is winning the game because God is playing with one set of rules, and the Devil with the other exactly opposite set of rules.

On July 1, the day of his death (and the 243rd day of his voyage), he sat down to set the record straight. His last entries were individually timed, and the final two entries were directed to God, since the next "move" was up to him:

> 11 15 00: It is the end of my game the truth has been revealed and it will be done as my family require me to do it.
>
> 11 17 00 : It is the time for your move to begin I have not need to prolong the game It has been a good game that must be ended at the I will play this game when I choose I will resign the game 11 20 40 There is no reason for harmfula[8]

At approximately 11 20 40, Donald Crowhurst walked off the boat to merge with the Atlantic Ocean and the universe. The boat, with all his logs, tape recordings, and home movies, was found ten days later, floating peacefully, undisturbed.

Should the story of Donald Crowhurst cause concern for single handers, or is this a special case? Certainly, it is special in the sense that it is so well documented. Most single handers who perish do not leave behind such a copious record. Little, however, sets Crowhurst apart psychologically. He did not suffer from a prior psychiatric disorder, and he never had a previous psychotic breakdown.[9] In modern psychologic and psychiatric parlance, it would be characterized as a (brief) psychotic disorder with an obvious stressor. Moreover, his symptoms, are entirely unlike those of sensory deprivation or sleep loss, al-though it is possible that either may have been contributory. We are forced to conclude that Crowhurst suffered a stress-induced psychosis.

Sailing Crews and Small-Group Behavior

It is logical to assume that there are fewer psychological hazards for the small, isolated group, such as a nautical crew, then for the singlehanded sailor. Indeed, the presence of at least one other person does significantly "enrich" the environment. Crew members, for example, experience far fewer episodes of hallucinations, illusions, and other grossly abnormal sensations than do isolated individuals.

But small groups are not without their own stresses. Laboratory experiments, studies, and accounts of groups in isolation, isolated duty stations in polar regions, sea voyages and disasters, submarine service, people in space, and people beneath the sea all provide examples. Some of the problems of crew behavior can be anticipated and avoided, whereas others can often be successfully defused. First one must recognize the stresses that the crew are likely to experience.

There are three major stresses: (1) when confined, even the most enriched environment tends to become boring and monotonous; (2) many of the usual sources of gratification and release are no longer available to the crew; and (3) crew members are forced to interact socially in crowded and otherwise unfavorable conditions. The interdependence of crew members blocks many overt means of expressing frustration. After all, a crew member can ill afford to alienate the remainder of the crew.

The degree of stress also depends on the size of the group, its composition, and its organization. Two-person "groups" can be devastating unless the individuals are known to be well suited. Admiral Byrd has graphically detailed the potential difficulties with two people in isolation (in this case, at an advance base in the Antarctic):

> It doesn't take two men long to find each other out. And, inevitably, this is what they do, whether they will it or not, if only because once the simple tasks of the day are finished there is little else to do but take each other's measure. Not deliberately. Not maliciously. But the time comes when one has nothing left to reveal to the other; when even his unformed thoughts can be anticipated, his pet ideas become meaningless drool, and the way he blows out a pressure lamp or drops his boots on the floor or eats his food becomes a rasping annoyance. And this could happen between the best of friends.[10]

With larger crews, a variety of individual reactions may be observed. Within days or weeks there are often signs of interpersonal frictions, such as irritability, uncooperativeness, minor acts of rudeness, and even hostility. At this point, some crew members begin to withdraw from group involvement, a process sometimes referred to as cocooning. Many crew members are surprised to discover how lonely they feel, even though they are surrounded by others sharing the same experience. This phenomenon has been aptly dubbed "the lonely crowd."

As communication and other social interactions become reduced to a minimum, territoriality and privacy needs assume prominence. The claiming of objects and areas is a feature of all isolated groups. A poignant example is the case of two life raft survivors, adrift for a month. One of the two survivors refused to give up his only flashlight, even when he became too weak to use it for signaling. Such instances of territoriality reflect an attempt to maintain some measure of privacy. To quote Admiral Byrd again:

> Even at Little America I knew of bunkmates who quit speaking because each suspected the other of inching his gear into the other's allotted space; and I knew of one who could not eat unless he could find a place in the mess hall out of sight of the Fletcherist who solemnly chewed his food twenty- eight times before swallowing . . . little things like that have the power to drive even disciplined men to the edge of insanity. During my first winter at Little America I walked for hours with a man who was on the verge of murder or suicide over imaginary persecutions by another man who had been his devoted friend. For there was no escape anywhere. You are hemmed in on every side by your own inadequacies and the crowding pressures of your associates. The ones who survive with a measure of happiness are those who can live profoundly off their intellectual resources.[11]

With so many stresses and so few opportunities for expression and release, it is not surprising that psychosomatic symptoms are common. Difficulties with sleep are widely cited, as are headaches and episodes of nausea. Irritability and depression are frequent. Occasionally there are near-psychotic episodes that create a tense atmosphere for the remainder of the crew. What is more common, and almost as stressful, is the tendency for people to resort to compulsive behavior. Compulsive acts (which in other circumstances would be dismissed as minor eccentricities) may be magnified into major annoyances for the remainder of the group.

The Psychology of Stress and Disaster

Contrary to popular mythology and culture, most individuals confronted with disaster do not panic, act hysterically, or become frozen with fear. In fact, the majority of disaster victims are able to contribute at least something to their own welfare and that of their companions.

It should not surprise us, however, that individuals do react somewhat differently to the tremendous stress of disaster. Survivors' immediate reactions to trauma are complicated and due in part to the underlying personality of each victim, their cultural background, their coping and life skills and those of their immediate family, and the specific nature of the disaster. Although reactions vary quite a bit, they are not necessarily a sign of psychopathology. Coping styles vary from very emotional to very reticent, and from a take-charge approach to one that is more reflective. Anyone responsible for the lives of others—and every captain of a vessel certainly is—should be able to recognize some of the various characteristic responses to tragedy and disaster. Clinically, a response style is much less important than the degree to which the coping efforts allow one to successfully continue his or her activities, maintain and enjoy interpersonal contacts, and regulate emotions. *Initial reactions* to trauma can include the following:

- Anxiety
- Sadness and depression
- Confusion
- Exhaustion
- Numbness
- Agitation
- Dissociation
- Blunted affect
- Physical arousal[12]

Indicators of a more severe reaction would include severe dissociation symptoms, intensive intrusive recollections of the disaster, and continuous distress without rest.

Delayed responses include:

- Sleep disorders and nightmares
- Anxiety focused on flashbacks
- Depression
- Persistent fatigue
- Irritability or hostility
- Mood swings and instability
- Emotional detachment with feelings of vulnerability

In *Two Against Cape Horn*, Hal Roth provides one of the best descriptions of severe dissociation and continuous stress. During a storm at night off Cape Horn, the Roths' anchor fouled and their boat was driven ashore. They were accompanied on this leg of their journey by a photographer and his wife (referred to as Adam and Eve). The Roths had never sailed with the photographer, and they had only spent a few days sailing with his wife. Both were novices aboard ship. The following account reminds us that the psychological reaction to disaster is no respecter of either size or sex.

I had been so busy thinking about the wreck that I hadn't paid much attention to Adam. Now, when I looked closely at him, my heart sank. He was shaking in his boots. His eyes had become slits and he was almost crying. Instead of looking at me when he spoke, Adam looked at the ground. During World War II and the Korean War, I had seen what fear could do to a man.

"The yacht is finished," he said. "We don't even have a radio. How much food is there? I want an inventory of the food right away. We must count the cans."

"Water?" said Adam nervously. "How much is there? How many days will it last? How much can we have each day? Let's sound the tanks right away."

I tried to reassure him. "I think we can get the yacht off," I said. "We may have to work in the water a little. I have a thick rubber wet suit . . . "

"Work in the water?"

I saw that Adam was horrified. It was clear that he wanted nothing more to do with the yacht. . . .

Then, while I worked inside to expose the hull damage, I asked Adam to take the dinghy and row out an anchor. The wind had dropped, and the job was easy. I told him exactly what I wanted, but when I looked out later, I saw he had put the anchor out to the south, not the west. A fifteen-minute job had taken two hours and instead of securing the anchor warp to the port bow cleat to help pull the yacht toward deep water, Adam had put the warp on the starboard stern cleat which meant that he was tying the yacht to land. Maybe on purpose. Poor Adam was wandering about in a daze.

We had thousands of feet of new 16-mm film and two cameras on board. "How about taking some footage of the wreck and what we're doing?" said Margaret to Adam during the afternoon. "After all, a photographer doesn't have this opportunity every day."

"You're entirely right," said Adam in his deep bass voice. . . .

Adam talked eloquently but he took no photographs—then or in the days to follow. Later he climbed into the yacht where I was working. He was looking for something and began to pick up things from the high dry side and let them fall into the water on the low side of the saloon or galley. He took a large plastic jar with all my taps and dies and drills from a tool drawer that I had open. His eyes were searching for something else, so he simply dropped these irreplaceable tools into the salt water. I gasped. I could hardly believe what I had seen. At first I was angry, but as I moved closer to shout at him I saw Adam's eyes were glazed and that he was breathing heavily. He was sick with fear and not in control of himself. . .

He slept at least ten hours a night and spent hours writing furiously in a notebook. We repeatedly asked him to use the movie cameras, but nothing happened.[13]

This is an acute stress disorder. Only after a period of time will certain people develop symptoms of a chronic stress disorder known as posttraumatic stress disorder.

Crew Harmony

But before we discuss some of the issues that can affect small groups, we need to look at the concept of work itself. We are not talking about employment work but rather something closer to the physical-science definition of work where work equals force exerted over a distance (work = force x distance). Work might entail hauling up a sail, cooking in the gallery, or even working at the navigation station, but it is accomplishing something concrete. In small groups, members of the crew tend to be purposefully chosen, and assigned those tasks for which they already have experience and qualifications. One person may have the qualifications to be captain (more on this later), whereas another may have mechanical expertise, and yet another may be an excellent cook. People will tend to sign on knowing implicitly or explicitly what their tasks will likely be. This all sounds reasonable and appropriate, but what if one task does not require as much time and energy as the others? And what if some of the crew want to learn (or at least begin to learn) many of the different types of tasks required to pilot a boat? These types of issues may produce resentment, alienation, and other psychological responses that can easily disrupt the efficiency of the group. What can be done?

There are a number of approaches to achieving harmony, including job rotation (this will depend on the size and experience of the crew), job enlargement (combining multiple tasks that had been separated but are related in some way), job enrichment (the individual crew member can take on vertically integrated tasks), and finally, the establishment of semiautonomous work groups for specific tasks (this is the most difficult route and is only viable with medium- to larger-sized groups). However, if harmony is important in your crew—and when isn't it?— how work is apportioned becomes a critical issue. After all, for most of us, boating or sailing is a way to escape the tedium of our employment work, so the last thing we want is to be assigned an onerous or tedious task for hours or days at a time that feels like "work." One obvious example might be a woman who is blithely assigned to be in the galley when in fact that is the last place she wants to be.

Dr. Michael Stadler, whose book *Psychology of Sailing* forms a major contribution to the sailing literature, has outlined several recommendations to avert crew frustration:

1. Do not withhold information—everyone wants to know what is going on
2. Distribute as many jobs cooperatively as possible
3. Knowledgeable sailors should not think themselves above menial tasks
4. Develop a rotation for the unpopular as well as the popular tasks
5. To encourage motivation, point out interesting and educational aspects
6. Combine unpopular with popular, responsible tasks
7. Avoid assigning very narrow tasks that are meaningless out of context
8. If the crew is large enough, encourage work groups for certain tasks[14]

First, even before discussing assignments, it is important that the goals of the voyage be clear to everyone at the outset. It is a crucial mistake to assume that the goals are either obvious or implicit. Second, it is equally important that all roles be discussed (see above) and that the leadership be formal and defined. The captain will wish to retain decision-making for all matters affecting the safety of the crew and vessel, and this should be clearly stated. In other areas, group decision-making may be appropriate. These areas should also be explicitly defined. Several different variations of communication and decision-making are possible, but the best choice depends in large part on the size of the crew. If the crew is small, then it is most efficient that each of the crew communicates directly with the captain. In larger crews, chains of command will develop—either naturally or, better yet, proactively. The absence of explicit rules for communication and decision-making invariably leads to accusations and recriminations, becoming the bane of many a cruise.

What can a captain do to influence and improve group behavior among the crew? Thoughtful selection of crew members is an important first step. Just as in solitary confinement, various individuals adapt differently to group confinement. The best indicator of future success as a crew member is prior crew experience, and/or other exposure to small groups. In addition, the three factors of work motivation, emotional stability, and social compatibility are helpful in assessing a potential crew member's suitability. Biographic data has not yielded consistent predictors and should not be relied upon. Anyone with inappropriate, personal motivations (e.g., escaping marital conflict) should be scrupulously avoided.

Anything safe that relieves boredom and monotony aboard ship is to be welcomed. Every shipboard confinement contains numerous minor annoyances that are collectively trying, including lack of water for washing up, crowding, extremes of temperature, humidity, noise, and limited toilet facilities. These annoyances are to be expected, but should be minimized as much as possible. In this regard, food is consistently noted as a highly important aspect of confined living, probably because it is one of the few pleasures still available; therefore, provisions are important, and should be kept in mind when planning a long voyage.

An Effective Captain

We have looked at the problems of crew satisfaction, which is critical for a successful voyage, but what about the attributes of an effective captain? After all, the captain not only affects the success of the voyage but also its safety. Professor Stadler again enumerates some of the important behavioral characteristics of a successful captain:

1. The strictest adherents to group standards, e.g. observation of safety precautions, fulfillment of galley duty, no smoking below deck (or at all).

2. They participate fully especially with difficult maneuvers (and don't just sit back and issue orders).

3. They do not take solitary decisions but rather when feasible discuss with the crew the options available allowing them to choose—and if this is not possible explaining why a specific action was taken.

4. They do not undertake themselves all the difficult tasks (such as harbor maneuvers or sail changes) but allow the crew the opportunity to learn and grow in confidence of their boating skills.

5. When the captain issues orders they should be well thought out and not open to misinterpretation or amendment. (U.S. history may have been quite different if on the first day at the Battle of Gettysburg, General Lee's orders to take Culp's Hill had not included the phrase "if practicable"). Orders should be directed at a specific person and that person should not be given too many orders at one time.

6. Finally, a good captain gets to know the strengths, weaknesses, and interests of his crew and makes allowances for them in assigning duties.

7. Finally, a good captain gets to know the strengths, weaknesses, and interests of his crew and makes allowances for them in assigning duties.

Effective Leadership

There is no single set of personality traits that will ensure that one will become successful captain or a successful coach of the sailing team. In *Finding a Way to Win: The Principles of Leadership, Teamwork, and Motivation*, Bill Parcells, a successful professional football coach, enumerates what he believes to be the most important components of effective leadership:

- Integrity—values must be communicated and disseminated
- Flexibility—sometimes rules and traditions need to be broken
- Confidence—instill confidence and support sailors' decision-making
- Accountability—take full responsibility when appropriate
- Candor—speak directly and accurately but appropriate to the individual
- Preparedness—always have a plan B and possibly plan C
- Resourcefulness—refusal to give in even when the outcome appears bleak
- Self-discipline—critical to accomplish any task
- Patience—knowing what changes need to be made and when to make them[15]

Notes

1. Certainly, one of the most prototypic of these lone voyagers would be Bernard Moitessier. His story, documented in *The Long Way*, is that of a veteran sailor participating in the first Golden Globe Race, a solo circumnavigation including rounding Cape Horn. After seven months battling storms, gear failures, numerous knockdowns, and fatigue, he was leading the race near the finish line when he decided to pull out and sail solo for another three months. He ended his 37,000-mile solo adventure in Tahiti. Why? You need to read the book.

2. Woodburn Heron, "The Pathology of Boredom," *Scientific American* 196 (1957): 52-56. Burney's quote was actually a counter quote. The original was from the British poet William Cowper (1731-1800): "Variety's the very spice of life, that gives it all its flavor." Johnny Carson (1925-2005), an American comedian, also had a counter quote: "If variety is the spice of life, marriage is the big can of leftover Spam."

3. Initially, Professor Donald O. Hebb at McGill performed this research. Hebb was and is hugely influential in the fields of psychology and neuroscience. "Cells that fire together, wire together." He was from Nova Scotia and was an avid sailor.

4. Glin Bennet, "Medical and Psychological Problems in the 1972 Singlehanded Transatlantic Yacht Race," *Lancet* 2 (1973): 747-754.

5. Glin Bennet, "The Challenge of the Mind," *Cruising World*, August 1982, A36-41.

6. Bennet, "Medical and Psychological Problems," 12.

7. E. C. B. Lee and K. Lee, *Safety and Survival at Sea* (New York: Norton, 1980), 177.

8. N. Tomalin and R. Hall, *The Strange Last Voyage of Donald Crowhurst* (New York: Stein and Day, 1970), 248, 259, 274.

9. This is not to imply that there is nothing noteworthy about Crowhurst's psychological state. Both his egomania and his attempt at deception suggests some element of personality disorder. However, these personality traits are not by themselves associated with a psychotic breakdown.

10. Seward Smith, "Studies of Small Groups in Confinement," in *Sensory Deprivation: Fifteen Years of Research*, ed. J. P. Zubeck (New York: Appleton-Century-Crofts, 1969), 381.

11. Smith, "Studies of Small Groups in Confinement."

12. Center for Substance Abuse Treatment, "Trauma-Informed Care in Behavioral Health Services," (Rockville, MD: Substance Abuse and Mental Health Services Administration, 2014), www.ncbi.nlm.nih.gov/books/NBK207191.

13. Hal Roth, *Two Against Cape Horn* (New York: Norton, 1978), 187-191.

14. Michael Stadler, *Psychology of Sailing: The Sea's Effects on Mind and Body* (London: Adlard Coles, 1987).

15. Bill Parcells, *Finding a Way to Win: The Principles of Leadership, Teamwork, and Motivation* (New York: Doubleday, 1985).

Chapter 14

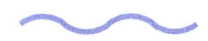

Sailing Psychology 2

"To reach a port, we must sail—Sail, not tie at anchor—Sail, not drift."
—*Franklin D. Roosevelt*, 1882–1945

"Our plans miscarry because they have no aim. When a man does not know what harbor he is making for, no wind is the right wind."
—*Lucius Seneca*, 5 BCE–65 CE

If you just finished Chapter 13, you may be asking yourself, "What? A second chapter on sailing psychology? Is that really necessary?" The answer is yes. The previous chapter can be considered *sailing as conquest*: human against the ocean, a small crew on a day sail, or even a naval encounter with the enemy. Most commonly a personal conquest is directed toward achieving a personal or common goal.

This chapter, on the other hand, deals mainly with *sailing as contest* rather than *conquest*. And most of these are athletic contests. But if you think about it, every conquest can be considered a contest and most contests entail a conquest.

Sport psychology, often referred to as exercise and sport psychology, is a relatively new field. It incorporates the study of human movement (including physiology, kinesiology, and biomechanics) as well as the study of human behavior (psychology). The entire field has evolved over the last thirty years, subsequent to the first edition of this book. And since sport psychology captures both mind and body issues in athletic contests (including sports as "complex" as sailing), it is no wonder that the field is broad. At one end of the spectrum it deals with issues such as goal setting, stress reduction, performance anxiety, confidence, motivation, mental imagery, and teamwork. These are often referred to as *psychological skills training* (PST). At the opposite end of the spectrum are the problems that are classically within the field of psychology—anxiety, emotional and personality issues, depression, and so forth. However, even this aspect of sport psychology has been evolving. Until recently, the dominant treatment was *psychotherapy*, or talking therapy. Psychotherapy attempts to uncover and understand the root cause of the problem (e.g., a difficult childhood, a sense of loss, difficulty with a coworker—anything that can interfere with performance). It is a form of therapy that can be effective, but may last years.

More recently, the emphasis has further changed. More and more practitioners, especially those in the field of sport psychology, have embraced *cognitive behavioral therapy* (CBT). CBT has many variations, but all involve features that are, I believe, more helpful to the sailing athlete. It is based on the idea that our thoughts cause our feelings and behavior rather than external things like events or people. And we can change our thoughts and the way we feel even if the situation does not change. This approach differs from traditional psychotherapy in that it is generally limited to fifteen to twenty sessions. It is structured, and directed toward specific goals, it involves collaborative problem solving, and it includes both education and homework for the client (sailor) to complete.

What does this have to do with the sailing athlete? Dr. Tim Herzog, a lifelong sailor and now a psychologist and counselor, has documented that sometimes the athlete has typical psychological problems that affect performance and that need to be addressed, sometimes the athlete needs to work on PST, and sometimes the athlete requires both.[1]

It is worth noting that many amateur and professional sports teams in the United States, Great Britain, and around the world have made extensive use of sports psychologists to improve both individual performance and teamwork. This includes numerous Olympic sailing teams as well as the U.S. Navy. The Midshipmen Development Center at the U.S. Naval Academy is certainly "onboard":

> The Midshipmen Development Center provides mental skills training to students who are trying to achieve their optimal performance in athletics and military performances. Mental skills can be used in many areas of your life from performance on the PRT to test taking to athletic competitions. What predicts high achievement in persons with talent is the integrated use of a set of mental and behavioral skills that can be learned. Our goal is to promote learning and personal development that is consistent with the USNA's mission to develop midshipmen "morally, mentally and physically."

Sport psychology is here to stay. The techniques discussed in this chapter are just as applicable to your nonmaritime endeavors as they are to sailing contests. Skip this chapter at your own peril.

Sailing Psychology 2

Psychologic Skills Training

Goal Setting

> "What you get by reaching your goals is not nearly so important as what you become by reaching them."
>
> —Zig Ziglar, 1926-2012 (falsely attributed to Thoreau)

Why is goal setting so important? Because it creates both direction and focus. It helps channel your energy so that you perform at a consistently high level while at the same time identifying specific areas that require additional work and improvement. There are three main types of goals:

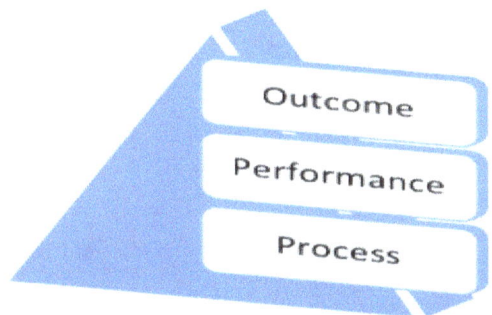

Figure 14.1 Outcome, performance, and process goals

Outcome goals are the most obvious; they are also the most difficult. Winning the next race… Finishing first in your racing class… Beating the best time at your club… and so forth – these are all example of such goals. Outcome goals are useful in setting the direction, but there are inherent problems with them. In any contest, there are always unseen and uncontrollable factors that may make accomplishment (e.g., winning) impossible. You may be very well prepared, but all the other contestants may also be prepared, and although you perform flawlessly, you still may not win. Therefore, outcome goals—perhaps the holy grail of goals—are the least under your absolute control.

Performance goals are more under your control. They consist of improvements relative to previous performances by you or your team and are the performance levels you need to realize if you have any chance of making your outcome goal. Unlike outcome goals, they are measurable. For example, a 100 meter runner may focus on a specific run time. For sailors, it might include the absolute time to sail the course or some other specific event that can be compared to previous performances. Performance goals may be short term or long term, but they must be specific, observable, measurable, and somewhat challenging. Performance goals can be physical, technical, tactical, or mental, but they should be measurable. They represent a benchmark.

Process goals are related to performance; they represent the nuts and bolts of what needs to be focused on while performing a specific skill. They can be thought of as short-term specific skills that are critical to achieving the desired performance, and ultimately the desired outcome. Examples might include:

- Hiking out for a longer time before muscle fatigue and pain set in
- Sailing with a constant heading for extended periods without losing focus
- Sailing close hauled without falling off or heading up
- Sailing well in light air
- Heavy weather reaching
- Heavy weather running
- Gybing
- Mark rounding
- Starting well
- Executing good windward tactics
- Sailing at night

In general, process goals in sailing are going to fall into one of these five categories:

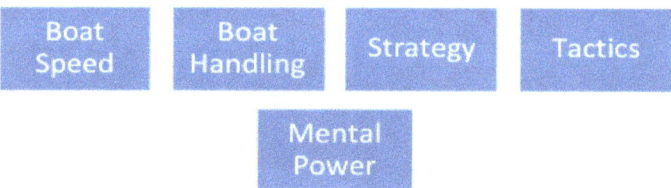

Figure 14.2 The five major boating process goals

Training drills are a good way to work on these process goals. A number of on-water training drills are included in Blackburn's *Sailing Fitness and Training*.[2] Drills like these can help define those skill areas that need the most work—and you will need to prioritize your goals.

SMART Goals

It is useful to think of these goals as a kind of actionable pyramid: concentrating on the specific process goals makes it more likely that you will accomplish your *performance goals*, which in turn increases the likelihood that you will attain your *outcome goal*. There are several principles to assist in formulating effective, *SMART goals*:

Specific—The more clearly defined and specific the goal setting, the more effective they will be. Specific goals leave no room for doubt or confusion. These goals can have physical (strength conditioning), technical (both speed and handling), tactical, psychological, and organizational attributes.

*M*easurable—As we have mentioned, goals should be specific, objective, and measurable. They should have a completion date, and it is also very helpful if the goals are made public. There is now ample research documenting the fact that goals are more likely to be achieved if they are made public, or at least conveyed to someone else.

*A*djustable—The goal may have to be adjusted both in terms of the size of accomplishment, or the time it will take to accomplish the specific goal. You must be flexible.

*R*ealistic—Goals should be realistic but moderately difficult. Goals that are either too difficult or not difficult enough will be either frustrating or trivial. Approach goal setting realistically, and be willing to make changes when necessary.

*T*imely—Short-term goals usually last weeks to a month, intermediate goals last several months, and long-term goals are on the order of one year or longer.

Finally, it is important that goals should be positive rather than negative. After all, goal setting activates our inner reward system, and is the basis for drive and motivation. See Appendix F for a "Goal Setting Worksheet" and supplemental information.

Common Mistakes in Goal Setting

(1) Not writing them down
(2) Failing to set specific goals
(3) Setting unrealistic goals
(4) Setting too many (or too few) goals
(5) Setting negative goals
(6) Not reviewing progress
(7) Failing to adjust goals
(8) Underestimating completion time

Mental Imagery

"Before every shot I go to the movies inside my head. Here is what I see. First, I see the ball where I want it to finish, nice and white and sitting up high on the bright green grass. Then, I see the ball going there; its path and trajectory and even its behavior on landing. The next scene shows me making the kind of swing that will turn the previous image into reality. These home movies are a key to my concentration and to my positive approach to every shot."

—*Jack Nicholas in* Golf My Way, *1974*

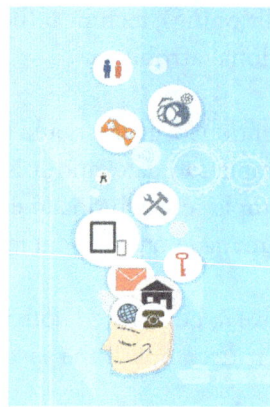

Figure 14.3 Mental imagery

Do you have *aphantasia*? Probably not, because it is relatively uncommon. It describes a condition in which a person is unable to create mental images. That is, he or she is unable to imagine in their "mind's eye" the face of a friend, a picture of their house, or a beautiful sunset over the water. The ability to use mental imagery is absent. This condition is different than *prosopagnosia*, or face blindness, which is the inability to recognize specific faces. Rather, aphantasia is the inability to conjure up in one's mind a pictorial representation of a face, an object, or a situation.

The capacity for mental imagery is extremely important to boaters, sailors, and small boat racers. Let's deal with boaters and sailors first; we'll catch up with the racers shortly.

Imagery is a key tool for problem solving all types of nautical problems. Most of you (those who do not have aphantasia, anyway) use mental imagery often, but don't think about it; it comes naturally. Being at sea in a large boat or ship consists of constantly solving problems, large and small. The problems may involve technical repairs, or something in the environment, such as an unexpected change in the weather. Although we do not think about it this way, we are constantly using mental imagery to solve specific problems. From Galileo and Mozart to Einstein and Hawking, mental imagery has been an important component of problem solving and discovery. Most of us are not solving problems at the genius level, but we are nonetheless, picturing in our mind's eye solutions to common problems or situations that occur on land or on the water. These include:

(1) Jogging your memory (putting a face to a name you have forgotten)
(2) Rehearsing a future encounter (e.g., docking in a storm)
(3) Giving directions (to your house or to your boat)
(4) Solving everyday problems (Where did I leave those boat keys?)
(5) Practicing relaxation or motivation techniques (imagining yourself relaxing on an island somewhere or alternatively working hard to finish a task)
(6) Picturing the mental image of a secluded cove you visited last summer

So, without thinking about it, you are already using mental imagery to preview new experiences all the time *before* they happen, giving you the opportunity to try out different scenarios (like trying out a play in a different city before bringing it to Broadway in New York). These scenarios may include figuring out in advance what works and what does not work, and even experiencing some of the emotions that will occur in your imagery (e.g., anxiety). In this sense, your brain is a time machine allowing you to fast-forward the visual narrative into the future.

But it's not just about visualization. Vision may be the most vivid sensation, but mental imagery may also involve the other senses. Here's a frequently cited definition of imagery:

> An experience that mimics real experience. We can be aware of "seeing" an image, feeling movements as an image, or experiencing an image of smell, tastes, or sounds without actually experiencing the real thing. Sometimes people feel that it helps to close their eyes. It differs from dreams in that we are awake and conscious when we form an image.[3]

As described, mental imagery is multisensory and may include sight, taste, sound, smell, and touch. It is for this reason that the term *visualization* has given way to *imagery*. Although imagery is invariably used in sport (as we will see below), it is widely used by musicians, surgeons, dancers, and military personnel as well. The imagery might include the following:

- Imaging a specific set of skills
- Imaging a specific strategy in competition
- Imaging a goal-oriented response such as winning a race
- Imaging a state of mind, such as confidence or relaxation prior to competition

Types of Imagery

There are two general types of imagery perspective. The first is referred to as *internal imagery*, where you image the performance of a specific skill from your own vantage point. It is as if you had a camera—like a GoPro—mounted on your forehead. You are visualizing the execution of the skill from your own perspective. If, for example, you are hiking out, you imagine the sails, bow of the boat, and water directly in front of you as though you are looking out during competition. Alternatively, you may use *external imagery*, where you view yourself performing a skill from the perspective of an outside observer. It is as though you are watching yourself in a movie. People vary in terms of their preference for internal or external imagery—often switching between the two. Internal imagery appears to make it easier to bring in other senses such as sound, smell, and the kinesthetic sense of body movement. However, your imagery mileage may vary, so to speak.

Developing an Imagery Program—PETTLEP

In 2001, Holmes and Collins proposed the PETTLEP program, which includes the following elements:

Physical—it is helpful to wear the appropriate clothing that is similar to the clothing worn in competition. It is also important to approximate the environment physically as much as possible and to employ physical implements that would be used in competition.

Environment—it is important to use imagery of the environment, such as the lake or river where the competition may be held. When that is not possible, photographs or videos may be a useful substitute for the imagery.

Task—the image of the task should be identical to the actual performance of the task, or as close as possible. After all, what you are trying to do is activate the identical sensorimotor brain networks, in the same sequence that would occur in competition. It is mental practice that simulates as closely as possible the physical practice.

Timing—everything should occur in real time since you are simulating the sequence of skills as closely as possible.

Learning—the sophistication of the imagery will change as the participant/athlete becomes more skillful.

Emotion—it is important to include emotions that normally occur with the skill set.

Perspective— consider internal imagery versus external imagery.[4]

Imagery is useful almost any time but especially during the following situations:

(1) When recovering from an injury
(2) During the off-season
(3) Before (and even after) competition
(4) During breaks in the competition
(5) Before (and after) practice

See Appendix F for a worksheet from the Human Performance Resource Center titled "Create Your Performance Imagery Script."

The key to imagery is the concept of *functional equivalence*—that is, *the same areas of the brain are activated by the actual movement and the imagined movement*. Think about that. Your brain activity looks very similar (with fMRI and/or EEG) when you simply think about hoisting the mainsail, as compared to when you actually hoist the mainsail. In one EMG study of weightlifting, the participants who were imagining they were lifting heavier weight actually became physically stronger without lifting weights—by just imagining the weight was heavier. Functional equivalence extends to the neural activity involved in seeing, hearing, smelling, and so forth. That is why the closer the imagery is to the actual activity, the greater the results will be.[5]

Self-Talk and Performance Routines

Self-talk has been studied off and on in sport psychology since the 1970s. Self-talk is defined as the production of recognizable words that may be expressed internally or out loud and has expressive, interpretive, and self-regulatory functions. It is the voice in your head—although we will often use self-talk to talk out loud. Self-talk may be instructional ("Pull that line tight, now let it out slowly") or motivational ("Come on, don't give up now").

Clinical research on the athlete's spontaneous self-talk has been difficult because it varies over the course of the contest, and athletes may have difficulty recalling what they were thinking and speaking out loud during the contest—and there is currently no simple way to measure self-talk during the event.

In general, it does appear that positive self-talk is helpful, and that negative self-talk should be avoided, but research is ongoing.[6]

In addition to self-talk, many athletes engage in performance routines or rituals. *Performance routines* include:

- *Pre-event routine*—a sequence of actions taken before the event
- *Preperformance routine*—a sequence of thoughts or actions adhered to immediately preceding a skill execution
- *Post-mistake routine*—a sequence that the athlete uses to forget a mistake or missed opportunity

Most of the research interest has been in pre-performance routines. Although the results of studies to date have been inconsistent, evidence tends to favor the advantage of preperformance routines.[7]

Concentration and Focus

> "If you can keep playing tennis when somebody is shooting a gun down the street, that's concentration."
>
> —*Serena Williams*

Most of us can remember when either a parent or teacher said, "Concentrate! Focus on the problem. Don't think about anything else… Focus!" What do we mean by *concentrate*? And how is it different from *focus*? The words are used more or less synonymously, but usually, when we think of focus, we think of narrowing our focus, and that is not always what is needed on the water. In fact, one of the problems for sailors is that (almost

Healthy Boating & Sailing

more than any other sport) we need to constantly shift our attention from a near to a far focus, and go back and forth constantly, sometimes for hours at a time.

The most popular model of attention, concentration, and focus was proposed by Dr. Robert Niedeffer in 1976 and expanded upon in a series of publications.[8] It is referred to as the *theory of attentional and personal style* and is critical for the sailor to understand. He proposed that concentration can be thought as having two dimensions: a *width* (narrow to broad) and a *direction* (internal to external).

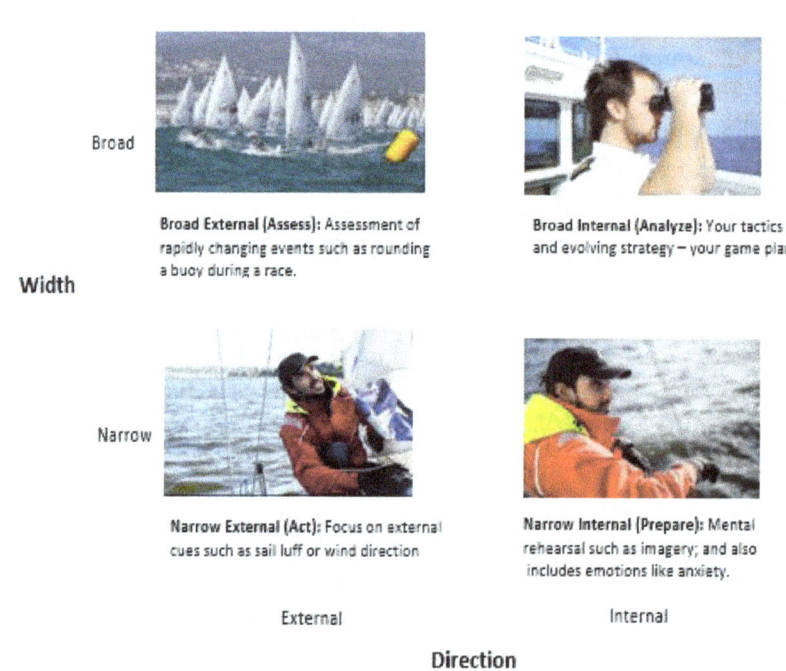

Figure 14.4: Concentration and strategies for controlling it

As sailors, we can think of the following situations:

Narrow internal (prepare)—mentally rehearsing something specific (possibly using mental imagery) like an upcoming tack or gybe. But narrow internal also includes emotions like anxiety, which can impair performance.

Narrow external (act)—focusing on external cues such as the sail luff or change in wind direction (this is where your *process goals* come in).

Broad internal (analyze)—your tactics and evolving strategy; your changing game plan.
Broad External (assess)—assessment of rapidly changing events vis-à-vis the ever-changing situation at the starting line or when rounding a buoy.

So, what does this mean? Well, for starters, let's look at multitasking. For those of you who have been asleep for most of the twenty-first century, multitasking is largely a myth. For the most part, it doesn't exist. Rather, we are constantly shifting attention and concentration (and focus) rapidly from one task to the other so that we think we are doing them simultaneously—but we're not. One second we are looking at the sail trim, while a second later we are approaching the starting line trying to decide whether we can make it on that tack and get across the line without having to tack again, or go over the line early. We have gone from:

> Narrow internal (mentally rehearsing the start, perhaps highly anxious) → narrow external (watching the wind direction, watching the luff of the sail) → broad external (looking over the fleet as you approach the line) → broad internal (analyzing whether you can make it across without being forced to come about).

You get the idea. Improving your concentration has a lot to do with deciding what you should be focusing on. Therefore, concentration is complex, multidimensional, and easily lost.

Distraction is the enemy of concentration. The distraction may be internal or external. Internal distractions would include dysfunctional thoughts, dwelling on previous mistakes, or physiologic symptoms of acute anxiety such as a bounding pulse, rapid breathing, or sweaty palms. External distractions might be a rapid change in the weather, unsportsmanlike conduct, and so forth

Things that can help you stay in the moment, ("mindful" in modern parlance), include:

- *Establishing performance routines*—the more your movements are routinized, the less you need to think about them and the more you can concentrate on other things
- *Establishing performance cues*—it could be a word or a phrase that you can say to yourself to get you back on track (i.e., self-talk)
- *Having well-established process goals*—these can lead you back on track
- *Identifying and avoiding distractors*—these can lead you off track; you should keep a list of things and situations that have been a distraction in the past and be super aware of them

Niedeffer and others have pointed out that some people adopt one of these four attentional focus types as a dominant personality characteristic. That can be problematic. Since, as sailors, we need to constantly refocus our concentration from one category to another, having a dominant personality type makes this more difficult and can get in the way. With a modicum of introspection—and honesty—you should be able to figure this out and make the necessary adjustments. A coach may be able to help. One problem that can take over our internal state—or *narrow internal*—and wreak havoc with our performance is anxiety.

Anxiety

There is no such thing as pure pleasure; some anxiety always goes with it.
—*Ovid, 43 BCE–18 CE*

As discussed by Drs. Weinberg and Gould in their excellent text "Foundations of Sport and Exercise Psychology," it is important to understand and distinguish the terms stress, arousal, and anxiety. Let us deal with stress first.

Stress is defined as "a substantial imbalance between demand (physical and/or psychological) and response capability, under conditions where failure to meet that demand has important consequences."[9] McGrath proposed four stages, as shown in Figure 14.5.

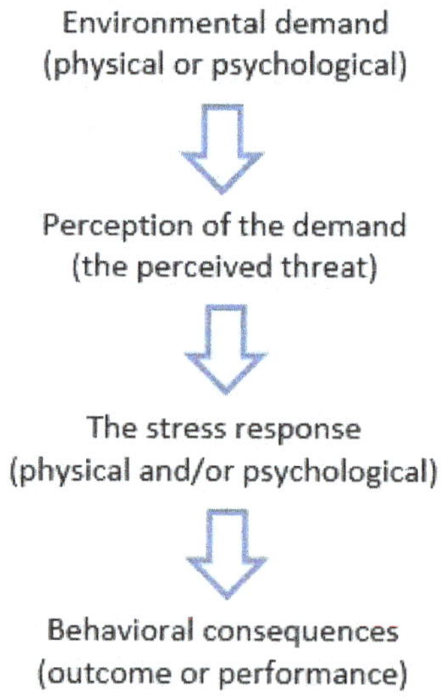

Environmental demand
(physical or psychological)

Perception of the demand
(the perceived threat)

The stress response
(physical and/or psychological)

Behavioral consequences
(outcome or performance)

Figure 14.5 Stress

Do you have stress in your life? If you are alive, the answer is probably yes. It is endemic in Western culture and we must find a productive way to deal with it—on land and at sea.

Arousal is defined as the psychological and physiological activity of the person. Arousal falls on a continuum, ranging from deep sleep to intense excitement or even frenzy. Often arousal is equated with anxiety, but I'm guessing that if you are lucky enough to win the lottery, you will be highly aroused, but not necessarily suffering from high anxiety!

Anxiety, on the other hand, is an emotional state associated with feelings of worry and apprehension, and often, but not always, associated with arousal. Although anxiety is for the most part a negative state, a certain amount of anxiety may not negatively affect performance, and may in fact be beneficial. This is reflected in Figure 14.6, where the level of performance is very low when there is no anxiety (and probably not enough arousal) and rising to a peak with a medium amount of arousal and then falling off as the level of anxiety rises too high.

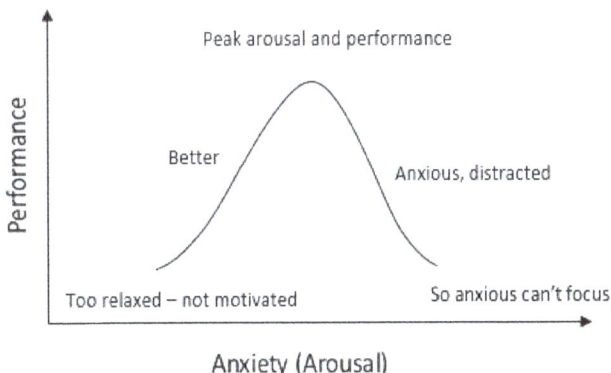

Figure 14.6 Performance versus anxiety[10]

Anxiety produces changes in your brain and body. Adrenaline is released, which causes increased heart rate, perspiration, and increased breathing rate. This is the so-called *fight-or-flight* response. Your sympathetic nervous system is turned way up. The flip side is the *parasympathetic nervous system*, which tends to chill you out. Instead of the fight-or-flight response, the parasympathetic nervous system response produces a state of "rest and digest."

Anxiety is generally broken down into trait anxiety, and state anxiety.

Trait anxiety is a part of the personality structure of an individual. It predisposes the person to respond to a perceived threat that may or may not be real. We all know people who are anxious about anything and everything. That is trait anxiety. It is a trait in their personality.

State anxiety, on the other hand, refers to the anxiety that is generally a temporary feeling of tension and apprehension, associated with a specific condition such as the beginning of a sailboat race, or the anxiety associated with a rapidly developing squall. Obviously, boaters who have a high level of underlying trait anxiety will tend to respond poorly in the face of an unexpected situation causing state anxiety.

Different people have differing *individualized zones of optimal functioning* (IZOF; Figure 14.7). Some athletes thrive in a high state anxiety (for example Athlete C). Others do not. Athlete A functions best in low state anxiety situations whereas Athlete B represents our "Average Joe," whose performance most closely correlates with the inverted U-shaped curve of Figure 14.7.

There are various psychological tools to measure trait and state anxiety. And if the anxiety you experience is severe, you should unquestionably seek the advice of a sports psychologist. However, all of us need to deal with anxiety (some more than others), and there are several techniques that have proven to be helpful.

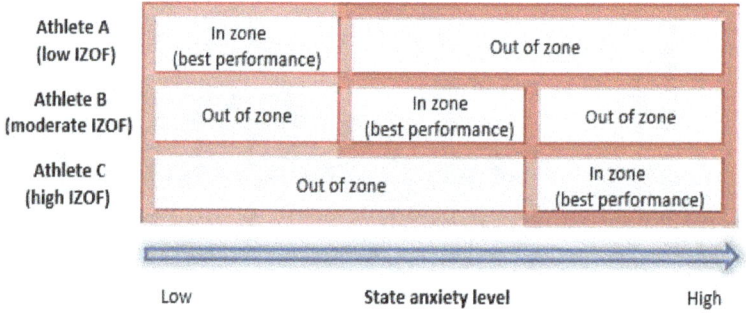

Figure 14.7 IZOF

Emergency Anxiety Relief on the Water

Close your eyes and imagine… You are in the middle of the bay crossing a shipping lane at night. You don't know the area, and you are beginning to become anxious. You feel tense, slightly nauseated, your heart rate is through the roof, and you are breathing rapidly and shallowly—the fight-or-flight response. You are cursing yourself for never following through with the stress reduction program you were planning to begin.

Is there anything you can do? Yes. The body's natural way to relieve stress is to engage the parasympathetic nervous system—rest and digest. How do you do that in the middle of the bay? Deep breathing is the most direct route to the parasympathetic system. Conscious deep rhythmic breathing slows the heart rate and helps quiet your overactive, racing mind. Try deep diaphragmatic (belly) breathing. When you are anxious you breathe rapidly and in a shallow fashion, mainly from the upper chest. Now you want to do the opposite. It means slowly protruding your abdomen as you breathe in (diaphragmatic breathing). Put your hand over your abdomen and feel the intake of breath. Breathe in through your nose and breathe out *slowly* through your mouth through pursed lips as though you are blowing out all of the candles on your birthday cake.

What does a Navy SEAL do to fire up the parasympathetic system? *Box breathing*.[11] Since the life of a Navy SEAL is probably more stressful than yours, I would give this a trial.

(1) Breathe in for four seconds with diaphragmatic and chest breathing
(2) Hold the breath for four seconds without inhaling or exhaling
(3) Exhale for four seconds, slowly as discussed above
(4) Hold lungs empty for four seconds

One cycle equals sixteen seconds (4 x 4). Repeat the above for five to ten minutes or until you are centered without anxiety. It will not make you tired or overanxious—just cool, calm, and collected.

Interested in going further in stress reduction? Next I'll discuss mindfulness meditation.

Mindfulness Meditation

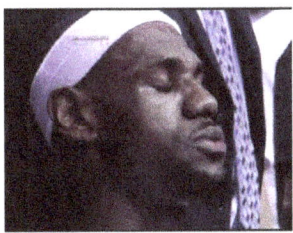

Figure 14.8 Lebron James

The field of sports psychology, as we have seen, is thirty to forty years old. But it is only in the past decade that *mindfulness meditation* has emerged as an important tool for maximizing performance. It became especially influential in the United States after its adoption by marquee athletes in virtually every sport. In basketball, Michael Jordan, Shaquille O'Neal, Kobe Bryant, and Lebron James practiced (or practice) it to prepare for games. Many elite athletes in other sports use it too, including Tiger Woods and Rory McIlroy (golf), Derek Jeter (baseball), Tom Brady (American football), Novak Djokovic (tennis), Carli Lloyd (soccer), and Misty May-Treanor and Kerri Walsh (Olympic beach volleyball).

Meditation has not and will not replace *psychological skills training* (PST). Those techniques have stood the test of time. But PST is not always effective, and mindfulness can be considered a technique to underpin or complement those skills.

In the United States, initial interest in controlled breathing and yoga began in the 1960s and 1970s. Breathing exercises are an integral part of yoga, and except for those who had been practicing it, the importance of breathing was unknown in the West until the landmark work of Harvard cardiologist Dr. Herbert Benson. Benson was studying the relationship between behavior and blood pressure in monkeys when he was approached by people from the *Transcendental Meditation* (TM) movement, who felt they could reduce blood pressure using TM. The result was Benson's book, *The Relaxation Response*, written in 1975 and still in print. The relaxation response combines breathing techniques that engage the parasympathetic system to release internal body stress and psychological stress. But it also addresses relaxing the muscular (motor) system to release stored muscular stress that many of us Westerners carry around, especially in our neck and shoulder muscles. (see Appendix F for an example from *The Relaxation Response*).[12] The emphasis of the relaxation response was and is physical (muscular) relaxation for stress reduction.

Although similar in many respects, and also coming from a Buddhist tradition, mindfulness meditation emphasizes mindful awareness of internal feelings and sensations with no explicit relaxation instructions. Mindfulness meditation was developed and popularized by Dr. Jon Kabat-Zinn, whose work has become extremely influential, especially in sports psychology. Whereas Dr. Benson's approach focused on the stress-related symptoms and signs—especially muscle tension—Kabat-Zinn's emphasis is focusing on the present moment and accepting one's feelings, thoughts, and bodily sensations. (see Appendix F for an example of mindfulness meditation). His original definition is still relevant today:

> Mindfulness means paying attention in a particular way: on purpose, in the present moment, and without judgment.

The idea is that mindfulness models (and there are now many variations) of performance enhancement attempt to change our relationship with internal experiences, as opposed to changing the experience itself. This is in contrast with PST, which tries to create ideal thinking and emotions for performance enhancement.

> The core belief of a mindful approach is that a person performs best when staying with a nonjudgmental moment-to-moment awareness and acceptance of one's internal state, with his or her attention focused on what is essential for performance and a consistent, intentional behavioral effort of actions that support what he or she values most.[13]

Please be sure you understand that preceding paragraph. Whereas traditional PST (goals, imagery, self-talk, etc.) attempts to reduce negative thoughts and emotions and improve self-control, mindfulness practice teaches the individual to recognize the internal state (for example, high state anxiety, disappointment due to a poor start, anger, etc.) but not allow it to interfere with performance. "Accept it and move on . . . you've got a job to do."

Both the relaxation response and mindfulness have been studied in neuroscience. Despite a great deal of overlap in the brain's response, it turns out that there are distinct brain mechanisms. The brain areas that are active in the relaxation response are more involved in muscular control and muscular relaxation (which is the focus of the relaxation response), whereas in mindfulness, the areas of the brain that monitor internal sensations are more active.[14] In one experimental study, after only eight weeks of training, meditators who were learning mindfulness training had an increase in the density of gray matter in the left hippocampus.

With consistent practice of mindfulness, there is an automatic response to behavioral decision making—improved mental efficiency and an ability for the athlete to direct his or her attention to whatever is essential without, needing to reduce or control reactions to potentially distracting sensations or feelings.

> This is different from [a] traditional PST approach. The traditional approach has been to try to reduce or eliminate negative experiences first and then intentionally shift to more positive thoughts and feelings to perform better. Mindfulness and acceptance-based approaches, on the other hand, stress the absence of intentional effort. Through daily mindfulness practice, improved attention becomes automatic, requiring fewer cognitive resources to achieve the desired focus state.
>
> The practice of entering a nonjudgmental, present-moment focus trains the brain to operate this way without needing to consciously or deliberately turn it on under pressure—when we need it the most. Performing under pressure is a hot topic in sport psychology. Some research suggests that reduced anxiety and a narrow focus of attention are both related to optimal athletic results. But these data on mindfulness suggest that reduced anxiety and closed focus may not, after all, be prerequisites for peak performance. Both high functioning athletes and expert meditators seem perfectly capable of demonstrating higher levels of anxious arousal and broader awareness than novices while still maintaining optimal task performance.[15]

Considering these relaxation methods and their use in sports, I have two observations:

1. Although both grew out of the medical mind-body model adapted from the Buddhist tradition, mindfulness meditation (and its various programs), rather than the relaxation response, has become increasingly a part of sports psychology.

Although the relaxation response has been extremely helpful as a medical approach in dealing with mind-body issues such as hypertension, stress, and anxiety, by its nature, mindfulness is more conducive to improved sport performance.
2. Although I have saved mindfulness until the end, it really deserves to precede PST since the techniques of mindfulness will facilitate development of PST. There are a number of programs that feature mindfulness and are appropriate for athletes. Your coach may be able to suggest a local program that would be best for you.

Mindfulness training may be especially important in a sport such as sailing where we need to shift our focus back and forth for thirty to sixty minutes or more—from narrow internal to broad external to broad internal to narrow external (Figure 14.4). Mindfulness allows us to shift our focus rapidly and frequently without being bogged down by errors in judgment that we may have committed or anger or resentment or whatever adverse emotion we may encounter as we shift back and forth. This is what is meant by being nonjudgmental—"Accept it and move on . . . you've got a job to do." And if you can use mindfulness to seamlessly shift your focus and concentrate on the task at hand using whatever PST is appropriate, then you may find yourself "in the zone," also known as flow.

Flow

Flow is basically the same as being "in the zone."[16] Mindfulness meditation can help athletes experience flow, and that is one of the reasons that it is being introduced into more and more training programs.

But flow isn't only for athletes. In 1972, psychologist Mihaly Csikszentmihalyi published a book called *Flow: The Psychology of Optimal Experience*, where he described the experiences that many creative people have, including athletes, musicians, writers, and artists. It can be encapsulated with the concept that a "good life is one that is characterized by complete absorption in what one does." Csikszentmihalyi describes flow as "being completely involved in an activity for its own sake. The ego falls away. Time flies. Every action, movement, and thought follows inevitably from the previous one, like playing jazz. Your whole being is involved and you're using your skill to the utmost."[17]

The major characteristics of the flow state are:

(1) intense and focused concentration on what one is doing in the present moment (mindfulness); a merging of action and awareness
(2) loss of reflective self-consciousness (athletes describe indifference to the crowd; they are focused on what needs to be done at that moment)
(3) distortion of temporal experience (often described as the clock slowing down or stopping)
(4) experience of the activity as intrinsically rewarding

So, people are happiest and most productive when in a state of flow. And that was Csikszentmihalyi's original concern: what is required for a happy life?

It is necessary that perceived challenges stretch existing skills—a sense that one is engaging challenges at a level appropriate to one's capacities. In addition, one needs clear proximal goals and immediate feedback about the progress being made.[18]

Flow is achieved when there is a balance between the challenge of the sport and the knowledge that you have the skills to meet the challenge. The same kind of thing occurs in music when the musician gets lost in improvisation during a jazz solo. It is incredibly rewarding (I have experienced it a few times playing music, but never in sports, and certainly never in sailing as I had neither the challenge, nor the sailing skills. C'est la vie.)

Csikszentmihalyi has put together a checklist of sorts regarding flow, characterized by nine components:

(1) The *challenge-skills balance*: The task cannot be too easy or too difficult, and the person must have the necessary skills. As athletes improve their skills, the challenge increases and they may continue to improve.

(2) The *merging of action and awareness*: The person's performance feels natural and automatic. The mind is completely present in the activity and not distracted by anxiety or pain (mindfulness). Action is almost automatic.

(3) *Clear goals*: These are part and parcel of the sport. They must be understood. (See SMART goals above.)

(4) *Unambiguous feedback*: The feedback may be internal, such as when an athlete flawlessly performs a difficult maneuver. The feedback from his or her own kinesthetic awareness is as important or more important than the feedback from a judge or fans in the crowd.

(5) *Total concentration and focus*: This is where mindfulness comes into play. In order to accomplish a task when the challenge is just at or above the person's skill level, the task requires complete concentration.

(6) *Sense of control*: People never have ultimate control, but when enveloped in a sense of flow, a person feels he or she has more than sufficient control of the outcome.

(7) *Loss of self-consciousness*: A person is no longer worried about being judged by others, and as mindfulness teaches the person, he or she is no longer harshly judging him- or herself.

(8) *Transformation of time*: The person is totally immersed, and time just passes without notice.

(9) *Autotelic experience*: The experience or activity has an end, or purpose in and of itself. A person doesn't perform for any other reason except that it gives him or her pleasure (i.e., not for specific external rewards). It is not until after the flow experience ends that the person experiences joy.

Csikszentmihalyi discussed the history of flow in a TED talk and presented the diagram in Figure 14.9, which relates back to the first point above.[19] The figure compares the degree of challenge with the development of a skill set, and illustrates the sector of flow.

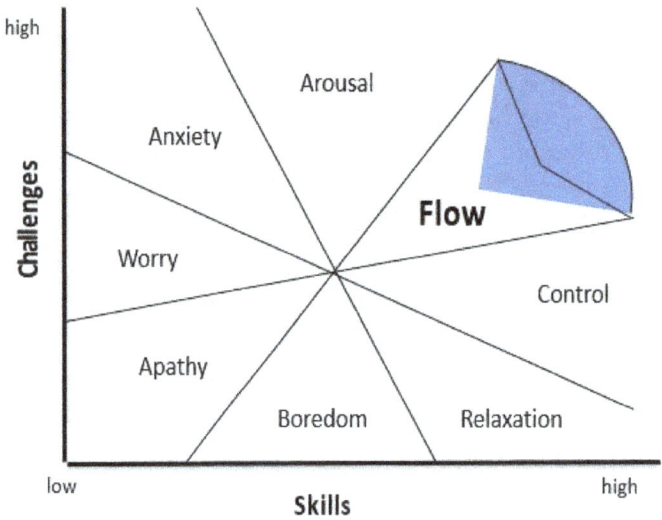

Figure 14.9 Flow: Challenges versus skills

I end with this diagram as it highlights that flow can occur anywhere to any of us; we don't have to be athletes. There were many times in my career that I experienced some element of flow, so I think I understand where Csikszentmihalyi is coming from. And I believe that it also explains what makes some of us humans happy. We are not the only species able to solve problems—not even close. However, to my knowledge, we *are* the only species that experiences enjoyment by setting problems or challenges – beyond what we have previously done – with the express purpose of seeing if we can meet those higher goals, or even beat them! That may be the element that separates the human brain from the primate brain, and the brains of other species: the ability to develop the skills necessary to solve increasingly challenging problems and, at least from time to time, maintaining attention to the degree that we are able to experience flow.

I sincerely hope that this book has given you some of the tools to deal with the challenges of staying healthy on the water. May the flow be with you.

Notes

1. T. Herzog and K. F. Hayes, "Therapist or Mental Skills Coach? How to Decide," *The Sports Psychologist* 26 (2012): 486-499.

2. M. Blackburn, *Sailing Fitness and Training*, 3rd ed. (n.p.: CreateSpace, 2015).

3. White and Hardy, cited in K. J. Munroe-Chandler and M. D. Guerrero, "Psychological Imagery in Sport and Performance," *Oxford Research Encyclopedia of Psychology*, doi: 10.1093/acrefore/9780190236557.013.228.

4. P. Holmes and D. Collins "The PETTLIP Approach to Motor Imagery: A Functional Equivalence Model for Sports Psychologists," *Journal of Applied Sports Psychology* 13 (2001): 60-83.

5. J. Gapin and T. Herzog, "Sailing Video-Imagery: Impact on Imagining Ability," *Journal of Imagery Research in Sport and Physical Activity* (2014): doi 10.1515/jirspa-2012-0002. See also http://thefinalbeat.com/categories/psychology-and-preparation/mental-rehearsal-visualisation-sailing#books

6. J. L. Van Raalte and A. Vincent, "Self-Talk in Sport and Performance," *Oxford Research Encyclopedia of Psychology*, doi: 10.1093/acrefore/9780190236557.013.157.

7. S. Cotterill, "Pre-Performance Routines in Sport: Current Understanding and Future Directions," *International Review of Sport and Exercise Psychology* 3 (2010): 132-153.

8. R. M. Nideffer, *The Inner Athlete* (New York: Crowell, 1986); R. M. Nideffer, "Test of Attentional and Interpersonal Style," *Journal of Personality and Social Psychology* 34: 394-404.

9. J. E. McGrath "Major Methodological Issues," in *Social and Psychologic Factors in Stress*, ed. J. E. McGrath (New York: Holt, Rinehart & Winston, 1970), 19-49.

10. https://www.psychologytools.com/self-help/anxiety/.

11. M. Divine, "The Breathing Technique a Navy SEAL Uses to Stay Calm and Focused," *Time*, May 4, 2016, https://time.com/4316151/breathing-technique-navy%20seal-calm/.

12. Herbert Benson, *The Relaxation Response* (New York: William Morrow, 2000).

13. Eddie O'Connor, "The Psychology of Performance: How to Be Your Best in Life," The Great Courses, https://www.thegreatcourses.com/courses/the-psychology-of-performance-how-to-be-your-best-in-life.html. This is an excellent course in sports psychology reviewing PST, mindfulness meditation, and much more. Highly recommended.

14. G. Sevinc et al., "Common and Dissociable Neural Activity After Mindfulness-Based Stress Reduction and Relaxation Response Programs," *Psychosomatic Medicine* 80 (2018): 439-451.

15. Eddie O'Connor, "The Psychology of Performance."

16. *Flow* is the official term used in sports psychology, whereas "being in the zone" is the more colloquial expression.

17. M. Csikszentmihalyi, *Flow: The Psychology of Optimal Experience* (New York: Harper and Row, 1990).

18. J. Nakamura and M. Csikszentmihalyi. "The Concept of Flow" in *The Oxford Handbook of Positive Psychology*, ed. Snyder and Lopez (New York: Oxford University Press, 2001), 89-105.

19. Mihaly Csikszentmihalyi, "Flow, the Secret to Happiness," *TED*, 2004, https://www.ted.com/talks/mihaly_csikszentmihalyi_on_flow/up-next?language=en.

Appendix A

Motion Sickness Susceptibility Questionnaire Short-Form (MMSQ-Short)

This questionnaire was developed by Professor John Golding mainly for research purposes. It is a modification of a longer questionnaire originally developed by Reason and Brand, the MMSQ. A minimal amount of calculation is required and then you can compare the composite result with the Table of Means and Percentile Conversion Statistics. The fiftieth percentile was 11.3, so a score of 12 and above would place you above the fiftieth percentile and a score of 11 or less below. That should give you or your crew a rough idea of seasickness sensitivity.

The questionnaire is used by permission and is from "J. F. Golding Predicting Individual Differences in Motion Sickness Susceptibility by Questionnaire," *Personality and Individual Differences* 41 (2006): 237-248.

Healthy Boating & Sailing

Motion Sickness Susceptibility Questionnaire Short-form (MSSQ-Short)

1. Please State Your **Age** .... Years.   *2.* Please State Your Sex (tick box) **Male** **Female**
                                                                                         [ ]₁   [ ]₂

This questionnaire is designed to find out how susceptible to motion sickness you are, and what sorts of motion are most effective in causing that sickness. Sickness here means feeling queasy or nauseated or actually vomiting.

Your CHILDHOOD Experience Only (before 12 years of age), for each of the following types of transport or entertainment please indicate:

3. **As a CHILD (before age 12)**, how often you **Felt Sick or Nauseated** (tick boxes):

	Not Applicable - Never Travelled	Never Felt Sick	Rarely Felt Sick	Sometimes Felt Sick	Frequently Felt Sick
Cars					
Buses or Coaches					
Trains					
Aircraft					
Small Boats					
Ships, e.g. Channel Ferries					
Swings in playgrounds					
Roundabouts in playgrounds					
Big Dippers, Funfair Rides					
	1	0	1	2	3

Your Experience over the LAST 10 YEARS (approximately), for each of the following types of transport or entertainment please indicate:

4. **Over the LAST 10 YEARS**, how often you **Felt Sick or Nauseated** (tick boxes):

	Not Applicable - Never Travelled	Never Felt Sick	Rarely Felt Sick	Sometimes Felt Sick	Frequently Felt Sick
Cars					
Buses or Coaches					
Trains					
Aircraft					
Small Boats					
Ships, e.g. Channel Ferries					
Swings in playgrounds					
Roundabouts in playgrounds					
Big Dippers, Funfair Rides					
	1	0	1	2	3

Motion Sickness Susceptibility Questionnaire Short-Form (MMSQ-Short)

Scoring the MSSQ- Short

Section A (Child) (Question 3)

Score the number of types of transportation not experienced (i.e., total the number of ticks in the 't' column, maximum is 9).

Total the sickness scores for each mode of transportation, i.e. the nine types from 'cars' to 'big dippers' (use the 0-3 number score key at bottom, those scores in the 't' column count as zeroes).

MSA = (total sickness score child) x (9) / (9 - number of types not experienced as a child)

Note 1. Where a subject has not experienced any forms of transport a division by zero error occurs. It is not possible to estimate this subject's motion sickness susceptibility in the absence of any relevant motion exposure.
Note 2. The Section A (Child) score can be used as a pre-morbid indicator of motion sickness susceptibility in patients with vestibular disease.

Section B (Adult) (Question 4)

Repeat as for section A but using the data from section B.

MSB = (total sickness score adult) x (9) / (9 - number of types not experienced as an adult)

Raw Score MSSQ-Short

Total the section A (Child) MSA score and the section B (Adult) MSB score to give the MSSQ-Short raw score (possible range from minimum 0 to maximum 54, the maximum being unlikely)

MSSQ raw score = MSA + MSB

Percentile Score MSSQ-Short

The raw to percentile conversions are given below in the Table of Statistics & Figure, use interpolation where necessary.

Alternatively a close approximation is given by the fitted polynomial where y is percentile; x is raw score
$y = a.x + b.x^2 + c.x^3 + d.x^4$
a = 5.1160923   b = -0.055169904
c = -0.00067784495   d = 1.0714752e-005

Table of Means and Percentile Conversion Statistics for the MSSQ-Short (n=257)

Percentiles Conversion	Raw Scores MSSQ-Short		
	Child Section A	Adult Section B	Total A+B
0	0	0	0
10	0	0	.8
20	2.0	1.0	3.0
30	4.0	1.3	7.0
40	5.6	2.6	9.0
50	7.0	3.7	11.3
60	9.0	6.0	14.1
70	11.0	7.0	17.9
80	13.0	9.0	21.6
90	16.0	12.0	25.9
95	20.0	15.0	30.4
100	23.6	21.0	44.6
Mean	7.75	5.11	12.90
Std. Deviation	5.94	4.84	9.90

Table note: numbers are rounded

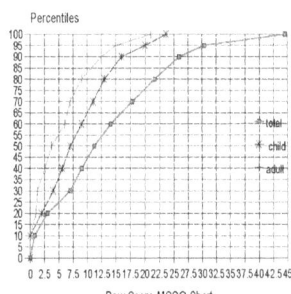

Figure: Cumulative distribution Percentiles of the Raw Scores of the MSSQ-Short (n=257 subjects).

Reference Note

For more background information and references to the original Reason & Brand MSSQ and to its revised version the 'MSSQ-Long', see:
Golding JF. Motion sickness susceptibility questionnaire revised and its relationship to other forms of sickness. **Brain Research Bulletin**, 1998; 47: 507-516.
Golding JF. (2006) Predicting Individual Differences in Motion Sickness Susceptibility by Questionnaire. **Personality and Individual differences, 41:** 237-248.

Behavioral Countermeasures

Behavioral Countermeasure	Comment
Habituation (desensitization)	Effective but stimulus specific. Slow to acquire
Visual horizon	If possible, stay on deck
Avoid reading or visual scanning	Minimize but still need to read monitors and maps
Avoid head movements	If feasible
Lay supine	If feasible, will also reduce head movements
Avoid areas of maximum motion	Avoid the bow of the ship, if feasible
Best to be in control	Pilot / helmsman
Controlled breathing	Reliable and perhaps half as effective as medication
Listening to music	Not proven or reliable but seems to help
Keeping busy (adaptation)	"Toughing it out" (easier to write than to do) does allow for adaptation

After John F. Golding "Motion Sickness Susceptibility and Management at Sea" in *Maritime Psychology: Research in Organizational & Health Behavior at Sea, Springer (Switzerland, 2017).* Professor Golding's chapter is an excellent current review of the overall topic of motion sickness and it's management.

Appendix B

Drugs That Can Interfere with Sweating

1. Cold and Allergy Medications
   - diphenhydramine (Benadryl)
   - hydroxyzine
   - phenylephrine
   - pseudoephedrine
   - triprolidine
   - chlorpheniramine

2. Antidepressants (esp. older)
   - amitriptyline
   - nortriptyline
   - imipramine
   - doxepin

3. Major Tranquilizers
   - clozapine
   - olanzepine
   - risperdal

4. Antianxiety Medications
   - alprazolam
   - diazepam
   - oxazepam
   - flurazepam

5. Other Central Nervous System
   - codeine
   - oxycodone
   - phenobarbital
   - topiramate
   - zonisamide
   - cyclobenzaprine

6. GI Medications
   - atropine
   - cimetidine
   - ranitidine

7. Seasickness and Other Anticholinergics
   - scopolamine
   - meclizine
   - promethazine
   - benztropine
   - dicyclomine
   - solifenacin
   - oxybutynin
   - tolterodine
   - prochlorperazine

8. Diuretics
   - hydrochlorthiazide
   - furosemide
   - bumetanide

9. Respiratory
   - ipratropium
   - tiotropium
   - theophylline

10. Cardiovascular
    - digoxin
    - captopril
    - diltiazem
    - nifedipine
    - triampterene
    - amiodarone

11. Beta-Blockers
    - propranolol
    - atenolol
    - metoprolol
    - nadolol
    - carvedilol
    - labetalol

12. Stimulants and Illegals
    - amphetamines (Adderall)
    - methylphenidate (Ritalin)
    - cocaine
    - methamphetamine
    - MDMA
    - PCP
    - Bath salts

13. Supplements
    - St. John's Wort
    - Gingko

Appendix C

Sweat Rate Calculation

Sweat rate = (A + B) ÷ C

A = Preexercise body weight − post-exercise body weight, recorded in ounces (1 pound = 16 ounces)
B = Fluid consumed during exercise, recorded in ounces (1 cup = 8 ounces; 1 gulp = about 1-1.5 ounces)
C = Exercise duration, recorded in hours (40 minutes = .66 hour)

Example for Mary:

During her regular ninety-minute outdoor run, Mary drank 22 ounces of fluid. Her pre-exercise weight was 125 pounds and her post-exercise weight was 124.5 pounds.

Mary's sweat rate is = (A + B) ÷ C where:
A = Weight change during exercise = 125.0 pounds − 124.5 pounds = 0.5 pounds = 8 ounces
B = Fluid consumed during exercise = 22 ounces
C = Exercise duration = 90 minutes = 1.5 hours

Mary's sweat rate = (8 ounces + 22 ounces) ÷ 1.5 hours = 20 ounces per hour

To meet ACSM hydration recommendations, Mary should plan to drink 20 ounces per hour of exercise, or 30 ounces total for ninety minutes (approximately 5 ounces every fifteen minutes)* when she runs under similar conditions.

*For greatest accuracy, calculate sweat rate under normal workout conditions, weigh without clothing or shoes, and avoid using the restroom prior to post-exercise weigh-in. Otherwise you will need to subtract urine volume—and that may be difficult to calculate! Since factors like outdoor conditions, fitness level, and exercise intensity affect sweat rates, you will need to

recalculate when environmental or fitness levels change, or if you engage in a different type or intensity of activity.

Please note that we are using the word "ounces" with two different meanings: weight and volume. In order to convert to metric, you will need to use two different tables. See Appendix G.

For a simple estimation of your hydration status (if you can't use the above formula), you can modify rehydration based only on weight. If you experience weight loss, hydrate more. If you experience weight gain, hydrate less. Your urine color may be used to confirm.

Appendix D

Various Fitness Tools

(1) Older Sailing Fitness Test

Hiking endurance

Sit with your back flat against a wall with your thighs 90 degrees to your back and your calf 90 degrees to your thighs. Hold for as long as possible.

If you can do two minutes, you're a level I; ten minutes makes you a level V.

Sheeting power

Men: If you can do five to ten pull-ups, congratulations—you are a level I! Thirty makes you a level V.

Women: If you can do ten inverted rows (lie in the floor on your back and pull yourself up to a bar or table top), you are level I. Thirty makes you a level V.

Aerobic fitness

Do a 1.5-mile run, a 3.75-mile bike ride, or a 600-meter swim.

For men, level I time for any of these is thirteen minutes or less; level V is nine minutes or less. For women, level I is fourteen minutes or less and level V is ten minutes or less.

(2) Current Texas A&M University Galveston Sailing Team Personal Fitness Test

Max push-up in ninety seconds: Block placed under chest. Chest must touch the block @ rep.

Max crunches in ninety seconds: Start with shoulder blades touching the ground, flex abdomen until elbows cross your belly button. Arms crossed, hands on shoulders.

Max wall sit: Back on wall, legs at 90 degrees. Hands should remain off knees and thighs.

Max plank: Hold a straight-back position suspended from toes and elbows. Time stops if hips dip or peak.

Max pull-up/inverted row: Hands facing away from the face, pull up until chin clears the bar. Lower to straight-arm position. Women lie in a horizontal position hanging from squat rack and heels supported by chair. No time limit.

Cooper twelve-minute run test (for estimated VO2 max): A simple VO2 Max definition: "V" stands for volume, "O" stands for oxygen, VO2 max refers to the maximum amount or volume of oxygen you can use during intense or maximal exercise within a specific amount of time.

VO2 Max = (Distance covered in twelve min [in meters]) − 504.9 ÷ 44.73

1 mile = 1,609 meters

0.5 miles= 804.5 meters

0.25 miles = 402.25 meters

Maximal oxygen uptake norms for men (ml/kg/min)

rating	Age (years) 18-25	26-35	36-45	46-55	56-65	65+
Excellent	> 60	> 56	> 51	> 45	> 41	> 37
Good	52-60	49-56	43-51	39-45	36-41	33-37
Above Average	47-51	43-48	39-42	36-38	32-35	29-32
Average	42-46	40-42	35-38	32-35	30-31	26-28
Below average	37-41	35-39	31-34	29-31	26-29	22-25
Poor	30-36	30-34	26-30	25-28	22-25	20-21
Very poor	< 30	< 30	< 26	< 25	< 22	< 20

Maximal oxygen uptake norms for women (ml/kg/min)

Rating	Age (years) 18-25	26-35	36-45	46-55	56-65	65+
Excellent	> 56	> 52	> 45	> 40	> 37	> 32
Good	47-56	45-52	38-45	34-40	32-37	28-32
Above average	42-46	39-44	34-37	31-33	28-31	25-27
Average	38-41	35-38	31-33	28-30	25-27	22-24
Below average	33-37	31-34	27-30	25-27	22-24	19-21
Poor	28-32	26-30	22-26	20-24	18-21	17-18
Very poor	< 28	< 26	< 22	< 20	< 18	< 17

(3) Simple Formula to Calculate Twelve-Minute Run Test

Elizabeth Quinn @Verywell Fit November 20, 2018

To calculate estimated VO2 max results (in ml/kg/min), use either of these formulas:

In miles: VO2max = (35.97 x miles) -11.29

In kilometers: VO2max = (22.351 x kilometers) -11.288

(4) Rating of Perceived Exertion (RPE) Scale

This is a relatively simple one to ten scale of perceived exertion. It is relatively easy to use and does not require any specific measurement (e.g., heart rate). It is based on simple physiologic parameters such as breathing, speaking, and sweating.

Healthy Boating & Sailing

RATING OF PERCEIVED EXERTION

10	Maximal Exertion — Cannot push any harder
9	Very Hard Activity
8	Hard Activity — Difficulty breathing, unable to speak
7	Hard Activity — Heavy sweating, difficulty speaking
6	Moderate Activity — Moderate sweating, able to speak
5	Moderate Activity — Speaking is easy, light sweating
4	Light Activity — Breaking a sweat, comfortable speaking
3	Light Activity — Comfortable, slight difficulty breathing
2	Minimum Activity — Barest exertion
1	Resting — No exertion

(5) Borg's RPE

The scale was developed by the Swedish psychologist Gunnar Borg and is known as the Borg Scale, or RPE. It also measures exercise intensity and uses a nonlinear scale from six to twenty, where six indicates no exertion at all and twenty indicates maximum exertion. The advantage of the scale is that if you multiply the Borg RPE by ten you will have a rough estimation of your heart rate. For example, 17 times 10 equals 170, which for you may correlate with the rating of "very hard."

Describe Exertion	Rating	Examples for Most Adults < 65 years of age
None	6	No exertion; reading a book
Very, very light	7-8	Extremely light activity (e.g., tying shoes)
Very light	9-10	Chores with little effort
Fairly light	11-12	Walking with some effort but not enough to effect breathing
Somewhat hard	13-14	Moderate effort, increased breathing and heart rate, not out of breath
Hard	15-16	Bicycling, running, increased heart rate and breathing very fast
Very hard	17-18	Highest level you can sustain
Very, very hard	19-20	Final burst in activity (e.g., end of race)

(6) Knight's Sailing Fitness Toolbox

Knight has a number of test exercises, including the following:

Sit and reach test
Hip flexibility test
Shoulder flexibility test
Squat test
Push-up test
Standing jump test
Cardio test: 1-mile run
Cardio test: O'Neil rowing test
Balance test
Core strength test

Values are broken out for males and females.

(7) Blackburn's Sailing Fitness and Training

Blackburn also has a number of tests to measure your fitness, including the following:

Sit and reach test
Abdominal endurance test
Body weight pull-up test
Wall sit test
Recommendations for the Hike-o-Matic
Aerobic personal time trial

Values are broken out for Club sailor; National level; and International level.

Appendix E

Additional Sleep Information

1. Additional Watchkeeping Schedules

The Brits have their own traditions. Below is the Traditional Royal Navy watch system. There are two watches: starboard or port. It has two "dog watches" of two hours each, which allow (cause) the system to rotate every day. If there are sufficient personnel, it can be divided into four rather than two, but it is still rotating and there are no protected sleep periods.

A 2-section dogged watch

	Day 1	Day 2	Day 3
2000–0000	Team 1	Team 2	Team 1
0000–0400	Team 2	Team 1	Team 2
0400–0800	Team 1	Team 2	Team 1
0800–1200	Team 2	Team 1	Team 2
1200–1600	Team 1	Team 2	Team 1
1600–1800	Team 2	Team 1	Team 2
1800–2000	Team 1	Team 2	Team 1

A 3-section dogged watch

	Day 1	Day 2	Day 3
2000–0000	Team 1	Team 2	Team 3
0000–0400	Team 2	Team 3	Team 1
0400–0800	Team 3	Team 1	Team 2
0800–1200	Team 1	Team 2	Team 3
1200–1600	Team 2	Team 3	Team 1
1600–1800	Team 3	Team 1	Team 2
1800–2000	Team 1	Team 2	Team 3

Figure E.1 2-section and E.2 3-section dogged watch rotations

Variations of the Royal watch rotation include the three team, which produces even more rotation every day, although obviously there is more time off during the day.

Another watchkeeping system is the six-hour watch system, which maximizes rest time:

Various Fitness Tools

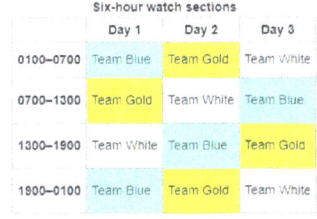

Figure E.3 Six-hour watch rotation

Numerous other systems have been devised, often referred to as a "Swedish" watch-keeping system. There are numerous variations with watches of five, five, five, five, four or six, six, four, four, four. Figure G.4 shows a Swedish system with six, four, two, two, four, six.

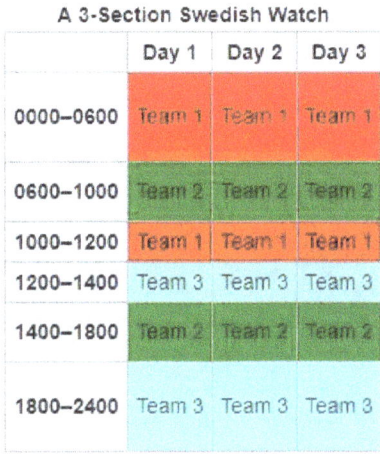

Figure E.4 Swedish watch rotation

The Navy has other watchbills for other crew configurations, including the two watch systems for three-man watchbills shown in Figures G.5 and G.6.

Healthy Boating & Sailing

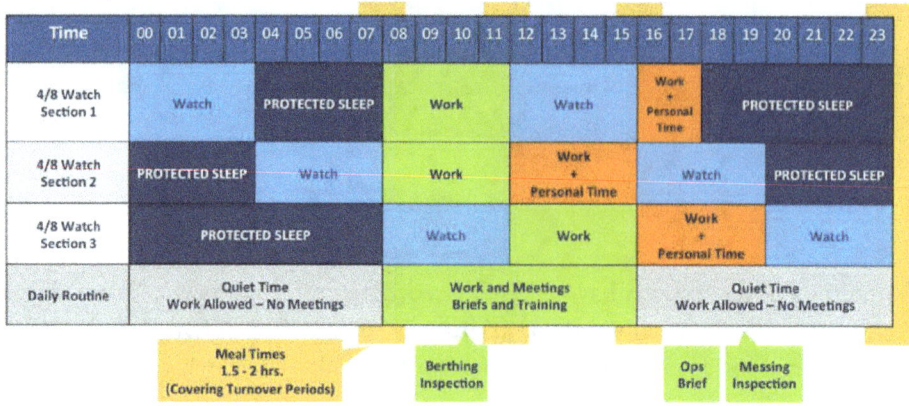

Figure E.5 Four-eight circadian watch rotation and daily routine

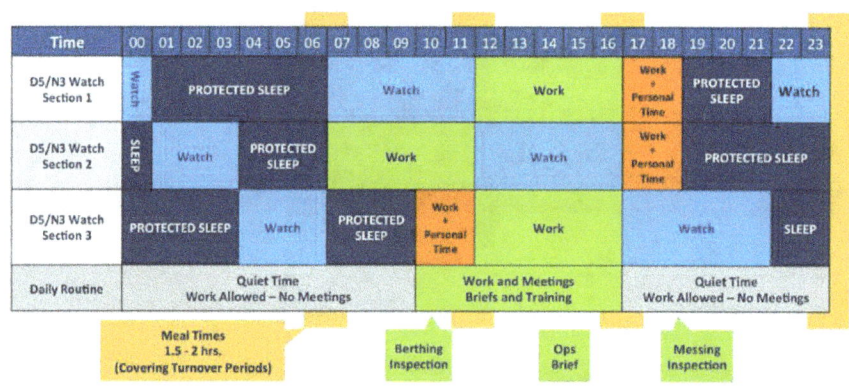

Figure E.6 D5/N3 circadian watch rotation and daily routine

Table E.1 from *Coastal Boating* includes a number of other configurations. Searching the boating literature, you will discover many combinations and permutations depending on number of crew, the social situation, whether or not the captain takes part in the watchkeeping, and so forth. I could spend pages and pages enumerating "favorite" watchkeeping systems. Hopefully you will now be better able to predict which will be best for your situation.

Various Fitness Tools

Some Options for Watchkeeping Schedules		
Crew	**Schedule**	**Benefit**
Single-handed	20 minutes sleep cycle with loud alarms (timer, AIS, radar proximity, radar detector, off course alarm, battery low alarm, etc)	The amount of time to traverse the distance to the horizon seen from the deck of a small vessel. Heave to for longer rest during the day.
Double-handed	6h on/6 h off	Long sleep/relaxation time but also long watch at night
	6h on during the day, 4 h on at night	Both get to see sunrise and sunset on alternating days, and no one gets the midnight shift two days in a row. A loosely defined 6 hours during the day ensures plenty of rest.
	6h on during the day, 3h on at night	Stays on same shift every day so it becomes routine.
	4h on/4h off day and night	Easy to keep track. The main meal would be during the 1600 to 2000 watch which would be shared. The 4 hour watch ties in with the science of sleep – the sleep cycle from light sleep through deep sleep to REM sleep takes 90 – 100 minutes, and the first two such cycles are when most of the good work of renewal is done. So you fit two such cycles neatly into four hours, with enough time to get to sleep, and to rouse yourself for your watch.
	2h on/2h off at night, loose during the day	Least tiring period at night time, long rest periods during the day
Crew of 3	Overlapping 6h or 4h hour intervals. (One crew member changes every 2 or 3 hours)	Fresh crew shares watch with tired crew. Always have 2 people watching each other ready to assist.
	Non-overlapping 4h intervals	Each person has only two 4h watches daily.
Crew of 4	Non-overlapping 3h intervals.	Each person has only two 3h watches daily.
	Two crew paired for watches same as double-handed	Two crew will always have someone watching the other if a problem occurs
Crew of 5	Overlapping 4h intervals	One watch per night per person, but always two people on watch together
Crew of 6	Non-overlapping 4 h intervals	Two watches daily per person, but always two people on watch together

Table F.1 CoastalBoating.net at http://features.coastalboating.net/Editorials/Watchkeeping_Procedures.html

2. Two-Week Sleep Diary

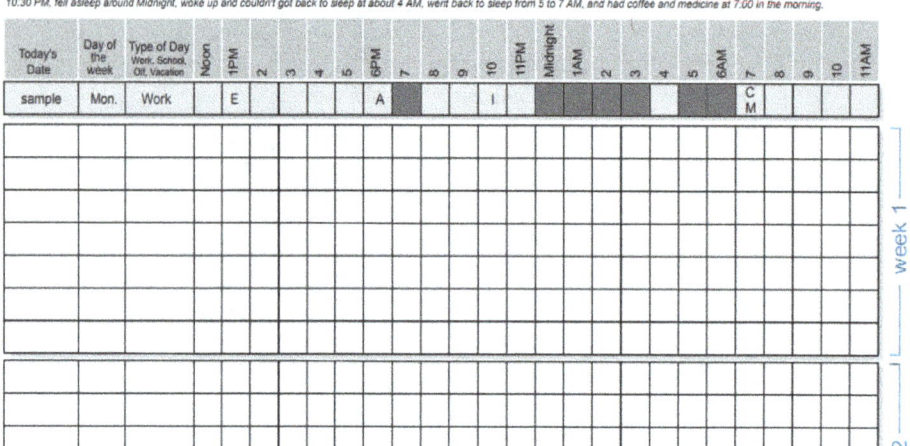

3. Insomnia Severity Index

Insomnia Severity Index

The Insomnia Severity Index has seven questions. The seven answers are added up to get a total score. When you have your total score, look at the 'Guidelines for Scoring/Interpretation' below to see where your sleep difficulty fits.

For each question, please CIRCLE the number that best describes your answer.

Please rate the CURRENT (i.e. LAST 2 WEEKS) SEVERITY of your insomnia problem(s).

Insomnia Problem	None	Mild	Moderate	Severe	Very Severe
1. Difficulty falling asleep	0	1	2	3	4
2. Difficulty staying asleep	0	1	2	3	4
3. Problems waking up too early	0	1	2	3	4

4. How SATISFIED/DISSATISFIED are you with your CURRENT sleep pattern?

Very Satisfied	Satisfied	Moderately Satisfied	Dissatisfied	Very Dissatisfied
0	1	2	3	4

5. How NOTICEABLE to others do you think your sleep problem is in terms of impairing the quality of your life?

Not at all Noticeable	A Little	Somewhat	Much	Very Much Noticeable
0	1	2	3	4

6. How WORRIED/DISTRESSED are you about your current sleep problem?

Not at all Worried	A Little	Somewhat	Much	Very Much Worried
0	1	2	3	4

7. To what extent do you consider your sleep problem to INTERFERE with your daily functioning (e.g. daytime fatigue, mood, ability to function at work/daily chores, concentration, memory, mood, etc.) CURRENTLY?

Not at all Interfering	A Little	Somewhat	Much	Very Much Interfering
0	1	2	3	4

Guidelines for Scoring/Interpretation:

Add the scores for all seven items (questions 1 + 2 + 3 + 4 + 5 +6 + 7) = _____ your total score

Total score categories:
0–7 = No clinically significant insomnia
8–14 = Subthreshold insomnia
15–21 = Clinical insomnia (moderate severity)
22–28 = Clinical insomnia (severe)

Used via courtesy of www.myhealth.va.gov with permission from Charles M. Morin, Ph.D., Université Laval

4. Epworth Sleepiness Score

The Epworth Sleepiness Scale

The Epworth Sleepiness Scale is widely used in the field of sleep medicine as a subjective measure of a patient's sleepiness. The test is a list of eight situations in which you rate your tendency to become sleepy on a scale of 0, no chance of dozing, to 3, high chance of dozing. When you finish the test, add up the values of your responses. Your total score is based on a scale of 0 to 24. The scale estimates whether you are experiencing excessive sleepiness that possibly requires medical attention.

How Sleepy Are You?

How likely are you to doze off or fall asleep in the following situations? You should rate your chances of dozing off, not just feeling tired. Even if you have not done some of these things recently try to determine how they would have affected you. For each situation, decide whether or not you would have:

- No chance of dozing = 0
- Slight chance of dozing = 1
- Moderate chance of dozing = 2
- High chance of dozing = 3

Write down the number corresponding to your choice in the right hand column. Total your score below.

Situation	Chance of Dozing
Sitting and reading	•
Watching TV	•
Sitting inactive in a public place (e.g., a theater or a meeting)	•
As a passenger in a car for an hour without a break	•
Lying down to rest in the afternoon when circumstances permit	•
Sitting and talking to someone	•
Sitting quietly after a lunch without alcohol	•
In a car, while stopped for a few minutes in traffic	•

Total Score = _____

Analyze Your Score

Interpretation:
- 0-7: It is unlikely that you are abnormally sleepy.
- 8-9: You have an average amount of daytime sleepiness.
- 10-15: You may be excessively sleepy depending on the situation. You may want to consider seeking medical attention.
- 16-24: You are excessively sleepy and should consider seeking medical attention.

Reference: Johns MW. A new method for measuring daytime sleepiness: The Epworth Sleepiness Scale. *Sleep* 1991; 14(6):540-5.

5. Four-Seven-Eight Breathing Method

- Part your lips slightly and make a whooshing sound as you exhale through your mouth
- Close your mouth and inhale slowly and silently through your nose to the count of four (in your head)
- Hold your breath for seven seconds
- Exhale with the whooshing sound slowly for eight seconds
- Complete this cycle four times; try to practice without thinking, mindlessly

Appendix F

Psychology Documents

SMART Goals

Your Goal:

S	Specific	What do I want to accomplish? Why? Requirements? Constraints?	
M	Measurable	How will I measure progress? How will I know when I have reached my goal?	
A	Achievable	How can the goal be accomplished? How should I proceed?	
R	Relevant	Is the goal worthwhile and is this the time? Do I possess the resources to accomplish it? Is the goal a long-term objective?	
T	Time Frame	How long will it take to accomplish this goal? When is the due date? When am I going to work on this goal?	

The Relaxation Response

The following is a relaxation response technique from Dr. Herbert Benson's groundbreaking book.

(1) Sit quietly in a comfortable position.
(2) Close your eyes.
(3) Deeply relax all your muscles, beginning at your feet and progressing up to your face. Keep them relaxed. (Relax your tongue—and thoughts will cease.)

(4) Breathe through your nose. Become aware of your breathing. As you breathe out, say the word "one"* silently to yourself. For example, breathe in, and then out, and say "one"*, in and out, and repeat "one."* Breathe easily and naturally.

(5) Continue for 10 to 20 minutes. You may open your eyes to check the time, but do not use an alarm. When you finish, sit quietly for several minutes, at first with your eyes closed and later with your eyes opened. Do not stand up for a few minutes.

(6) Do not worry about whether you are successful in achieving a deep level of relaxation. Maintain a passive attitude and permit relaxation to occur at its own pace. When distracting thoughts occur, try to ignore them by not dwelling upon them and return to repeating "one."*

(7) With practice, the response should come with little effort. Practice the technique once or twice daily, but not within two hours after any meal, since the digestive processes seem to interfere with the elicitation of the relaxation response.

*Choose any soothing, mellifluous sounding word, preferably with no meaning or association, in order to avoid stimulation of unnecessary thoughts.

Mindfulness Meditation

Mindfulness-based stress reduction is like the relaxation response in that both are used to treat the anxiety state directly without undue concern for extended analysis of the "root cause." Whereas the relaxation response focuses on a creating a state of deep rest—the opposite of the "fight or flight" response—mindfulness emphasizes a nonjudgmental approach as a key to stress reduction. Both the relaxation response and mindfulness meditation are based on meditation. Both are highly effective, although they work through different neural mechanisms.

(1) Sit down. Find a place that feels calm and quiet to you.
(2) Set a time limit. Initially, it can help to choose a short time, perhaps five or ten minutes.
(3) Notice your body. You can sit in a chair with your feet on the floor, or you can sit loosely cross-legged in a "lotus posture", or you can kneel—all are fine. Just be certain you feel stable and are in a position you can maintain for a while.
(4) Feel your breath. Follow the sensation of your breath as it goes in and as it goes out.
(5) Notice when your mind has wandered. It will wander. Inevitably, your attention will leave the sensations of your breath and wander to other places. When you notice this—in a few seconds, a minute, five minutes, whatever—simply return your attention to the breath.
(6) Be kind to your wandering mind. Don't judge yourself or obsess over the content of the thoughts you find yourself lost in. Just come back.

Various Fitness Tools

Mental Imagery

Create your own Performance Mental Imagery Script:

CREATED BY THE HUMAN PERFORMANCE RESOURCE CENTER / HPRC-ONLINE.ORG / FROM THE CONSORTIUM OF HEALTH AND MILITARY PERFORMANCE (CHAMP)

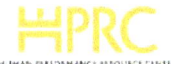 **MENTAL FITNESS**

Create Your Performance Imagery Script

Imagery is a performance psychology skill that involves mentally creating an experience, typically from memory, which imitates a real experience. Good mental imagery incorporates all your senses, and building an imagery script can help boost your confidence while reducing stress and anxiety about an important upcoming performance.

You can generate imagery in your mind for just about any task (for example, taking an exam, performing weapon maintenance in the dark, or having a difficult conversation). Imagery also can help you learn new skills, maintain and improve your current abilities, and take advantage of times when physical practice isn't possible.

To optimize your performance, follow the instructions below to create your own imagery script.

IDENTIFY

Pinpoint what you want to improve through imagery, and specify how you hope it will be helpful.

What task or performance do I want to improve?
Example: Marksmanship, giving a brief, or push-ups…

_____
_____
_____
_____
_____

How will practicing imagery help me?
Example: Learn or improve skills or strategies, increase confidence, or control arousal and anxiety…

_____
_____
_____

INSPIRE

How does this task fit in with your larger goals and what you value? Staying connected to your purpose can help motivate you.

Why does this performance matter to me?

_____
_____
_____

Appendix G

Below are a variety of charts to readily compare metric and English systems. Some day the United States may adopt the metric system that the rest of the world uses—EVEN THE ENGLISH. The only countries which have not adopted the metric system (officially known as the International System of Units (SI):

United States		Liberia		Burma (Myanmar)

Various Fitness Tools

Fahrenheit to Celsius and Celsius to Fahrenheit

Fahrenheit to Celsius and Celsius to Fahrenheit Conversion

°F	°C	°F	°C	°F	°C	°C	°F	°C	°F
-22	-30.0	30	-1.1	82	27.8	-30	-22.0	22	71.6
-21	-29.4	31	-0.6	83	28.3	-29	-20.2	23	73.4
-20	-28.9	32	0.0	84	28.9	-28	-18.4	24	75.2
-19	-28.3	33	0.6	85	29.4	-27	-16.6	25	77.0
-18	-27.8	34	1.1	86	30.0	-26	-14.8	26	78.8
-17	-27.2	35	1.7	87	30.6	-25	-13.0	27	80.6
-16	-26.7	36	2.2	88	31.1	-24	-11.2	28	82.4
-15	-26.1	37	2.8	89	31.7	-23	-9.4	29	84.2
-14	-25.6	38	3.3	90	32.2	-22	-7.6	30	86.0
-13	-25.0	39	3.9	91	32.8	-21	-5.8	31	87.8
-12	-24.4	40	4.4	92	33.3	-20	-4.0	32	89.6
-11	-23.9	41	5.0	93	33.9	-19	-2.2	33	91.4
-10	-23.3	42	5.6	94	34.4	-18	-0.4	34	93.2
-9	-22.8	43	6.1	95	35.0	-17	1.4	35	95.0
-8	-22.2	44	6.7	96	35.6	-16	3.2	36	96.8
-7	-21.7	45	7.2	97	36.1	-15	5.0	37	98.6
-6	-21.1	46	7.8	98	36.7	-14	6.8	38	100.4
-5	-20.6	47	8.3	99	37.2	-13	8.6	39	102.2
-4	-20.0	48	8.9	100	37.8	-12	10.4	40	104.0
-3	-19.4	49	9.4	101	38.3	-11	12.2		
-2	-18.9	50	10.0	102	38.9	-10	14.0		
-1	-18.3	51	10.6	103	39.4	-9	15.8		
0	-17.8	52	11.1	104	40.0	-8	17.6		
1	-17.2	53	11.7			-7	19.4		
2	-16.7	54	12.2			-6	21.2		
3	-16.1	55	12.8			-5	23.0		
4	-15.6	56	13.3			-4	24.8		
5	-15.0	57	13.9			-3	26.6		
6	-14.4	58	14.4			-2	28.4		
7	-13.9	59	15.0			-1	30.2		
8	-13.3	60	15.6			0	32.0		
9	-12.8	61	16.1			1	33.8		
10	-12.2	62	16.7			2	35.6		
11	-11.7	63	17.2			3	37.4		
12	-11.1	64	17.8			4	39.2		
13	-10.6	65	18.3			5	41.0		
14	-10.0	66	18.9			6	42.8		
15	-9.4	67	19.4			7	44.6		
16	-8.9	68	20.0			8	46.4		
17	-8.3	69	20.6			9	48.2		
18	-7.8	70	21.1			10	50.0		
19	-7.2	71	21.7			11	51.8		
20	-6.7	72	22.2			12	53.6		
21	-6.1	73	22.8			13	55.4		
22	-5.6	74	23.3			14	57.2		
23	-5.0	75	23.9			15	59.0		
24	-4.4	76	24.4			16	60.8		
25	-3.9	77	25.0			17	62.6		
26	-3.3	78	25.6			18	64.4		
27	-2.8	79	26.1			19	66.2		
28	-2.2	80	26.7			20	68.0		
29	-1.7	81	27.2			21	69.8		

Length Metric to English and English to Metric

Inch → Centimeter		Centimeter → Inch	
Inch	Centimeter	Centimeter	Inch
1	2.54	1	0.394
2	5.08	2	0.787
3	7.62	3	1.18
4	10.16	4	1.57
5	12.70	5	1.97
6	15.24	6	2.36
7	17.78	7	2.76
8	20.32	8	3.15
9	22.86	9	3.54
10	25.40	10	3.93
20	50.80	20	7.87
30	76.20	30	11.81
40	101.60	40	15.75
50	127.0	50	19.69
60	152.40	60	23.62
70	177.80	70	27.56
80	203.20	80	31.50
90	228.60	90	35.43
100	254.00	100	39.37

Feet → Meters		Meters → Feet	
Feet	Meters	Meters	Feet
1	0.30	1	3.28
2	0.61	2	6.56
3	0.90	3	9.84
4	1.22	4	13.12
5	1.52	5	16.40
6	1.83	6	19.69
7	2.13	7	22.97
8	2.44	8	26.25
9	2.74	9	29.53
10	3.05	10	32.81
20	6.10	20	65.67
30	9.14	30	98.43
40	12.19	40	121.23
50	15.24	50	164.04
60	18.29	60	196.86
70	21.34	70	229.66
80	24.38	80	262.47
90	27.43	90	295.28
100	30.48	100	328.08

Yards → Meters		Meters → Yards	
Yards	Meters	Meters	Yards
1	0.91	1	1.09
2	1.83	2	2.19
3	2.74	3	3.28
4	3.66	4	4.37
5	4.57	5	5.47
6	5.49	6	6.56
7	6.40	7	7.66
8	7.32	8	8.75
9	8.23	9	9.84
10	9.14	10	10.94
20	18.29	20	21.87
30	27.43	30	32.81
40	36.58	40	43.74
50	45.72	50	54.68
60	54.86	60	65.66
70	64.00	70	76.55
80	73.15	80	87.49
90	82.30	90	98.43
100	91.44	100	109.36

Miles → Kilometer		Kilometer → Miles	
Miles	Kilometer	Kilometer	Miles
1	1.61	1	0.62
2	3.22	2	1.24
3	4.83	3	1.86
4	6.44	4	2.49
5	8.05	5	3.11
6	9.66	6	3.73
7	11.27	7	4.35
8	12.87	8	4.97
9	14.48	9	5.59
10	16.09	10	6.21
20	32.19	20	12.43
30	48.28	30	18.64
40	64.37	40	24.85
50	80.47	50	31.07
60	96.56	60	37.28
70	112.65	70	43.50
80	128.75	80	49.71
90	144.84	90	55.92
100	62.14	100	62.14

Various Fitness Tools

Weight Metric to English and English to Metric

Oz. → Grams		Oz. → Grams		Pounds → Kilos		Kilos → Pounds	
Oz.	Grams	Grams	Oz.	Pounds	Kilos	Kilos	Pounds
1	28.375	1	0.035	1	0.454	1	2.20
2	56.8	2	0.07	2	0.91	2	4.41
3	85.1	3	0.11	3	1.36	3	6.61
4	113.5	4	0.14	4	1.82	4	8.82
5	141.9	5	0.18	5	2.27	5	11.02
6	170.3	6	0.21	6	2.72	6	13.22
7	198.6	7	0.25	7	3.18	7	15.43
8	227.0	8	0.28	8	3.63	8	17.63
9	255.4	9	0.32	9	4.09	9	19.84
10	283.8	10	0.35	10	4.54	10	22.04
20	567.5	20	0.70	20	9.80	20	44.08
30	851.3	30	1.06	30	13.62	30	66.12
40	1135.0	40	1.41	40	18.16	40	88.16
50	1418.8	50	1.76	50	22.70	50	110.20
60	1702.5	60	2.11	60	27.24	60	132.24
70	1986.3	70	2.46	70	31.78	70	154.28
80	2270.0	80	2.82	80	36.32	80	176.32
90	2553.8	90	3.17	90	40.86	90	198.36
100	2837.5	100	3.52	100	45.40	100	220.40
200	5675.0	200	7.04	200	90.80	200	440.80
500	14187.5	300	17.60	500	227.0	500	1102.0
1,000	28375.0	1,000	35.20	1,000	454.0	1,0000	2204.0

Volume Metric to English and English to Metric

Quarts → Liters		Liters → Quarts		Gallons → Liters		Liters → Gallons	
Quarts	Liters	Liters	Quarts	Gallons	Liters	Liters	Gallons
1	0.946	1	1.06	1	3.79	1	0.26
2	1.89	2	2.11	2	7.57	2	0.53
3	2.84	3	3.17	3	11.36	3	0.79
4	3.79	4	4.23	4	15.14	4	1.06
5	4.73	5	5.29	5	18.93	5	1.32
6	5.68	6	6.34	6	22.71	6	1.58
7	6.62	7	7.40	7	26.50	7	1.85
8	7.57	8	8.46	8	30.28	8	2.11
9	8.52	9	9.51	9	34.07	9	2.38
10	9.46	10	10.57	10	37.85	10	2.64
20	18.93	20	21.14	20	75.70	20	5.28
30	28.39	30	31.71	30	113.55	30	7.94
40	37.85	40	42.28	40	151.40	40	10.56
50	47.32	50	52.85	50	189.25	50	13.20
60	56.78	60	63.42	60	227.10	60	15.84
70	66.24	70	73.99	70	264.95	70	18.48
80	75.70	80	84.56	80	302.80	80	21.12
90	85.17	90	95.13	90	340.65	90	23.76
100	94.63	100	105.70	100	378.50	100	26.40
200	189.26	200	211.40	200	757.00	200	52.80
500	473.15	300	528.50	500	1892.5	500	132.00
1,000	946.30	1,000	1057.00	1,000	3785.0	1,0000	264.00

Index

Note: Page numbers in *italics* indicate figures; numbers in **bold** refer to tables.

accidents
    alcohol as factor, 254, 255
    Coast Guard Recreational Boating Statistics, *255*
    definition of, 254
    factors contributing to, 255–56
    and human error, 256
    human factors theory, 256, 256–58
    and inappropriate activities, 256
    and inappropriate responses, 256
    in open motorboats, 255
    and the overload factor, 256
    and PFD use, 255, 258
    recent examples, 253, 279
    and sleep deprivation, 256, 258, 279
    and systems theory, 256–58
acetylcholine, 283
actinic damage, 103
active rewarming, 64, 65
acupuncture wristbands, 21
Adderall, 81
adenosine, 285, *285*
adenosine monophosphate (AMP), 285
adenosine triphosphate (ATP), 215–16, *216*, 285
adrenaline, 331
aerobic/cardio exercise, 245–47
aerobic glycolysis, 220–21
aerobic training, 237–40, 248–49
aerodynamic drag, 69
afterdrop, 65

aircraft pilot sickness, 27n21
albacore, 151
alcohol
    and accidents, 254, 255
    and body temperature, 56–57
alprazolam, 296
amberjack, 151
amebic dysentery, 158
American Academy of Sleep Medicine, 296
American College of Sports Medicine, 236
Amitriptyline, 81
amphetamines, 19, 81
anaerobic glycolysis, 220
anaerobic training, 248–49
anchovy, 151
anemia, 209
animals
    seasickness in, 2
    vaccination certificates for, 159–60
    See also marine life
Anson, George A., 208
antibiotics
    for cholera, 160
    for seawater boils, 119
    for stingray injury, 135
    for traveler's diarrhea, 165
anticholinergic drugs, 81
antidepressants, 81
antihistamines, 16, 19, 20, 81, 151
antimigraine medications, 81
antimotility drugs, 165
antiseizure medications, 81
Antivert, 20

anxiety, 330–31
    emergency relief on the water, 332–33
    performance vs., *331*
    state, 332
    trait, 331
arms, keeping warm, 67
arousal, 331
arthritic pain, 261
athletic performance, and thermoregulation, 87–89
Ativan, 296
Australian salmon, 151
autotelic experience, 337
avobenzone, 114

bacillary dysentery, 158
back strength, 250
bacteria
    campylobacter, 161
    E. coli, 161
    marine, 37, 49n7
    in the ocean, 37
    salmonella, 161
    shigella, 161
    staphylococcus, 119
    that produce tetrodotoxin, 150
    vibrio, 161
Bailey, Maralyn, 94
Bailey, Maurice, 94
Baker, Robin, 45
balance training, 243–44
ballistic stretching, 243
balloonfish, 149
barnacle cuts, 124
barracuda, 142
basal metabolic rate (BMR), 210, 211–12
    Mifflin St. Jeor Equation, 211, **212**
Beagle, HMS, 54
Benadryl, 81
Bennet, Glin, 305
Benson, Herbert, 334, 359
beta-blockers, 81
betadine, 162
binoculars, 189
biohacking, ix–xi

biological clock. *See* circadian rhythm
Blackburn, Michael, 248, 250, 269
Blackburn's Sailing Fitness and Training, 351
Blagden, Charles, 79
bleach (sodium hypochlorite), 162, 172n6
blowfish, 149
bluefish, 151
boardsurfing, 274–75
boating accidents. *See* accidents
Boating Basics Online, on sound signals, 31, *32*
boating under the influence (BUI), 254
boats. *See* vessels
body temperature, 73n1
    and immersion hypothermia, *58*
    See also hypothermia
Bombard, Alain, 96
Bonine, 20
bonito, 151
boredom, 304, 315
Borg, Gunnar, 350
Borg Scale of Perceived Exertion, 238–39
Borg's RPE, 350
Bougainville, Louis de, 38
boundary cells, 47
brain
    boundary cells, 47
    caudate nucleus, *46*, 48
    forward-looking cells, 47
    grid cells, 47
    hippocampus, 44–45, *46*, 47
    hypothalamus, 81, 283
    occipital lobe, 49n4
    place cells, 47
    speed cells, 47
breathing
    box, 333
    controlled, 334
    deep rhythmic, 332–33
    diaphragmatic, 333
    four-seven-eight method, 358
bromophenols, 37
bronzers, 121n6

Index

Burney, Christopher, 304
Byrd, Richard E., 310–11

caffeine, 285
calisthenics, 245, 251n9
Callahan, Steven, 93
calories and exercise, 210–13
    basal metabolic rate (BMR), 210
    Dietary Approaches to Stop Hypertension (DASH), 213, *213*
    for endurance athletes, 224n6
    energy sources, *216*
    energy storage, **217**
    exercise activity thermogenesis (EAT), 210–11
    exercise intensity, **212**, *222*
    glycerol/fatty acid structure, *218*
    guidelines for daily carbohydrate intake, **223**
    Mediterranean diet, 213, *214*
    MIND diet, *215*
    non-exercise activity thermogenesis (NEAT), 211
    protein recommendations for athletes, **223**
    thermic effect of food (TEF), 210
    total daily energy expenditure (TDEE), 211–13
    weight-reduction program, 212–13
    See also exercise
camel sickness, 2
campylobacter, 161
canthaxanthin, 121n6
captains
    effective, 316
    influence on group behavior, 315
Caras, Roger A., 145
carbohydrate loading, 224n6
carbohydrates, 204–6, 220
    guidelines for daily intake, **223**
    storage of, 217
cardiopulmonary resuscitation (CPR), 65
carpal tunnel syndrome (CTS), 262, 267–68, *267*
cataracts, 185

caudate nucleus, *46*, 48
CDC Yellow Book, 160
cellulose, 205
Celsius to Fahrenheit, 363
challenge-skills balance, 337, *338*
Chichester, Francis, 84
chloroquine, 171
cholera, 158, 159
    treatment for, 160–61
chronotypes, 282, 285
ciguatera, 146–49, *147*, *148*, 155n34
cinnarizine, 20, 21
circadian rhythm, 281–83, *281*
    circadian clock, *282*
    disturbances in, 287–89
    and sleep drive, 284–85
    and sleep-wake homeostasis, *284*
circuit training, 236, 248
    high-intensity, 236–37, 246
clam-digger's itch, 120
clothing
    for arms, 67
    Army mnemonic, 75n16
    base layer, 75n13
    for cold weather, 66–71, 69–71
    and convection currents, *67*
    for face and head, 68–69
    fishnet underwear, 75n13
    gloves, 60, 112
    hats, 74–75n7
    and hypothermia, 61
    insulating layers, 66–67, 68
    insulation material, 69
    layering, 66–67
    for legs, 67
    shoes, 68
    synthetic, 70
    ultraviolet protection factor (UPF), 117–18, *118*
    ventilation of, 70–71, 72
    wet suits and dry suits, 71
    windbreakers, 68
    woolen, 69, 70
cocaine, 81
cochlea (hearing apparatus), 3–4, 29

coelenterates, 129–30
 feather hydroid, 130
 fire coral, 129
 seawasp, 126–27
 See also jellyfish
cognitive behavioral therapy (CBT), 297, 320
cold shock, 60
cold vasodilation, 60
cold water, 53
 heat escape lessening posture (HELP), 61, *62*
 huddle position, 62, *62*
 immersion hypothermia, *58*
 Rule of Fifties, 61
 strategies for survival in, 60–63
 survival time, 58–59, *58*, *59*
 See also hypothermia
cold weather
 clothing for, 69–71
 keeping warm, 66–69
 natural defenses against, 56–57
 performance in, 72
 tips for staying warm, 72–73
 on/in the water, 53
 wet suits and dry suits, 71
 See also hypothermia
Coles, Adlard, 58
color perception, 189–92, 197n10
 and cones, 190, *190*
 sensitivity by wavelength, *191*
 at twilight, 192
 and water depth, 191–92
compass, internal, 47
compression neuropathy, 261
concentration, 327–30, *328*, 337
concussions, 259, 262, 275–76
conduction, 88
 heat loss through, 55–56
cone snails, 131–33, *132*, 154n12
contact lenses, 181
convection, 88
 heat loss through, 55–56
convection currents, 66–67, *67*
Convention on the International Regulations for Preventing Collisions at Sea, 49n1

Cook, James, 146, 150–51, 208
coral cuts, 124–25
coral polyps, 124
coral reefs, 124–25, 153n1, 153n3
core temperature, 63, 77, 82
Coriolis vestibular reaction, 23–24n7
Creamer, Martin, 39
creatine, 223
crew harmony, 314–16
cross training, 241
Crowhurst, Donald, 308–9, 317n9
crown of thorns, 131
Cryptosporidium parvum, 161
Csikszentmihalyi, Mihaly, 336–38
cumulative trauma disorder, 261
Cunningham, Pete, 247

Dana, R. H., 55
Darwin, Charles, 22, 46, 54
dead man's float, 61
decibel scale, 36, *36*
DEET, 168
dehydration
 and drinking seawater, 95–97
 estimating degree of, 82
 prevention of, 89–91
 progressive, 82
 salt loss in, 83
 and traveler's diarrhea, 163
 urine color as measure of, 89, *90*
 voluntary, 82, 88
 water loss in, 83
depression, 10, 21, 23, 261, 311, 312, 320
depth sounding, 191
desalination, 93–94, *94*
 in open-ocean sailing, 100n16
dextroamphetamine, 17, 18, 19
diarrhea. *See* fluxes
diazepam, 296
dictyopterenes, 37
Dietary Approaches to Stop Hypertension (DASH), 213, *213*
dimenhydrinate, 16, 19, 21, 81
dimethyl sulfide (DMS), 37–38
dimethylsulfoniopropionate (DMSP), 37

diphtheria, 159
diseases
    and international nautical travel, 160–65
    prevention and vaccinations, 165–71
    quarantinable, 158–60
    tropical, 157
    See also *specific diseases by name*
diuretics, 81
dopa, 121n9
dopamine, 283
doxycycline, 160–61, 171
Drake, Francis, 38, 200
Dramamine, 16, 21
drownproofing, 61
drowsiness, 18, 19, 21, 22, 62, 294
drug treatment
    drugs that can interfere with sweating, 345
    effects on body's performance in heat, 81
    for insomnia, 296–97, **297**
    for malaria, 169, 171
    photoallergic reactions, **109**
    photosensitivity, **109**
    phototoxic reactions, **109**
    for seasickness, 16–21, **18**, 27n24
    and skin sensitivity, 108, **109**
    See also antibiotics; sting and bite treatments
dry suits, 71
Dumas, Vito, 306–7
dynamic balance, 244
dynamic stretching, 243

ear protection, 37
Ebola, 159
echolocation, 34, 49n2, 49n4
E. coli, 161
Elavil, 81
electrical fields, ability to sense, 39
electrolytes, 89, 90, 91, 161, 163–64, 209
electromagnetic spectrum, 196n1
endolymph, 3, 5, 24
enema, 64, 82, 94

energy systems
    anaerobic (glocolysis), 218
    ATP-TC (phosphogen system), 218, 219
Entamoeba histolytica, 161
enteroviruses, 161
entrapment neuropathy, 261–62
ephedrine, 19, 81
epicondylitis, 268
Epworth Sleepiness Scale, 295, 358
Ergospirometry, *239*
evaporation, 88
    and heat, 79–83
    and heat exhaustion, 85
    heat loss through, 55–56
exercise
    abs and core, 248
    aerobic/cardio, 245–47
    aerobic training, 237–40, 248–49
    anaerobic training, 248–49
    balance training, 243–44
    for big boat racing, 247–48
    and the Borg Scale of Perceived Exertion, 238–39
    and burnout, 261
    calisthenics, 245, 251n9
    cardio training, 247
    circuit training, 236, 248
    cross training, 241
    and the cruising sailor, 244–47
    and Ergospirometry, *239*
    FITT principle, 229
    flexibility training, 242–43
    and heart rate maximum (HR max), 249
    for heat gain, 54, 57
    (exercise)
    high-intensity circuit training (HICT), 236–37, 246
    high-intensity interval training (HIIT), 241, 246
    and lactate threshold (LT), 240, *240*
    and maximum heart rate (MHR), 238
    muscles used in small boat sailing and sailboarding, *270*
    overload, 230
    and overtraining syndrome, 260–61

recovery, 230
reversibility, 231
at sea, 244–47
slow twitch/fast twitch muscle types, 231–32, *232*
for small boat and Olympic class sailing, 248–50
specificity, 230–31
and strength training, 233–36
variation in training, 234
and VO2 max, 239–40, 249
weight training, 247
with resistance bands, 244–45
See also calories and exercise
exercise activity thermogenesis (EAT), 210–11
exercise and sport psychology. *See* sport psychology
eye disorders
cataracts, 185
keratitis (corneal sunburn), 184
macular degeneration, 184
ocular inflammation, 184
photokeratitis, 184
pinguecula, 184–85
pterygium, 185
eyelid cancers, 186
eye protection, 73
See also sunglasses

Fahrenheit to Celsius, 363
fats, 206–7
white/brown, 73–74n2, *74*
feather hydroid, 130
fevers, 130, 157–58
typhoid fever, 158
typhus, 158
See also malaria; yellow fever
fiber, 205
fight-or-flight response, 331
fire coral, 129
fish juice, 95, 96, 98
fish poisoning
ciguatera, 146–49, *147, 148*
paralytic shellfish poisoning, 151–52
pufferfish, 149–51
scombroid poisoning, 151
fish tapeworm, 153
fitness. *See* exercise
fitness tools, 348–51
FITT (frequency, intensity, time, type) principle, 229
flexibility training, 242–43
flow, 336–38
flukes, 120
flu vaccines, 166
fluxes, 158
amebic dysentery, 158
bacillary dysentery, 158
cholera, 160–61
salmonella, 152, 158, 161
staphylococcal food poisoning, 158
traveler's diarrhea (TD), 161–65
viral enteritis, 158
focus, 327–28, 337
attentional, 328–30
broad external, 329
broad internal, 329
narrow external, 328–29
narrow internal, 328–30
food poisoning, 152
staphylococcal, 158
food pyramid, 202, *202, 213, 214*
forward-looking cells, 47
fugu (pufferfish), 149–51

Gahlinger, Paul, 20
Gatty, Harold, 36, 38, 43, 45, 48
giant grouper, 144
giant tridacna clam, 145
giardia, 161
glare, 175–76, 197n12
Global Positioning System (GPS), 48
globefish, 149
gloves, 60, 112
glucose
blood, 217
and dehydration, 88
and exercise, 204, 206, 220, 221–23

and glycogen, 204, *204*, 217, 221
and insulin, 205
lactate converted to, 240
replenishing, 206
in sports drinks, 163
glycemic index (GI), 205–6
glycogen storage, 204, 217
glycogen supercompensation, 224n6
glycolytic curve, *219*, 220
goals
clear, 337
common mistakes in setting, 323
outcome, 321
performance, 321
process, 322, 328, 329
SMART, 322–23, 337, 359
Golding, John, 341
Gooley, Tristan, 39
grid cells, 47
Griffith, Bob, 119
Guzmán, Alonso Pérez, 2

hair cells, 3, 5
hair jellyfish, 126
See also jellyfish
Hall, R., 308
hallucinations, 305–7
Hatha yoga, 246
hats, 68–69
Hawkins, Richard, 92–93, 207
health, risk factors, **228**
hearing, at sea, 29–37
heat, and hypertension, 87
heat cramps, 84
heat escape lessening posture (HELP), 61, *62*
heat exhaustion, 84–85, *85*
treatment for, 85
heat exposure, 77–99
heat gain, and metabolism, **54**
heat-induced disorders, 84–87
heat cramps, 84
heat exhaustion, 84–85, 85
heatstroke, 86–87
heat syncope, 84

heat loss, **54**, *55*
through sweating, 70
through the head, 68–69, 74–75n7
and water temperature, *58*
heatstroke, 77–78, 81, *85*, 86–87
heat syncope, 84
Heinrich, Herbert, 256
helmets, 275–76
helmsman's rear end, 119
Hepatitis A vaccine, 166
herring, 151
Herzog, Tim, 320
high blood pressure, 87
high-intensity circuit training (HICT), 236–37, 246
high-intensity interval training (HIIT), 241, 246
hiking, 248, 250, 268–69, *269*, 272–73, 274
5 angles of, *273*
hippocampus, 44–45, *46*, 47, 48
huddle position, 62, *62*
human error, 256–57
human factors theory, 256
Human Performance Resource Center, 89
humidity, and thermoregulation, 88
hydration, and athletic performance, 88
hydrofoiling, 273
hydrogen sulfide, 37
hyoscine, 17–18, 19, 81
hypernatremia, 96
hypertension, 87
hypertonic liquids, 96
hypothalamus, 81
hypothermia, 53, *63*
and core temperature, 63
immersion, 58–63
mild, 63–64
moderate, 64
revival of victims, 63
severe, 64
survival time, *59*
symptoms of, 62–63, 72
three stages of, 63–64
treatment of, 64–65
hypotonic liquids, 96

ice melts, 45
image displacement, 183, *183*
imagery
    developing a program, 326–27
    external, 325–26
    internal, 325
    mental, 323–25, 361
    types of, 325–26
immersion hypothermia, 58–63
    See also hypothermia
immobilization, 305
individualized zones of optimal functioning (IZOF), 332
influenza, 159
injuries, 259
    arthritic pain, 261
    in big boat racing, 264–67
    carpal tunnel syndrome (CTS), 267–68, *267*
    on cruising sailboats, 263–64
    entrapment neuropathy, 261–62
    epicondylitis, 268
    (injuries)
    fractures, 263
    as function of crew position, **265**
    to hands and fingers, 263
    to the head, 264, 275–76
    at ISAF Youth Sailing World Championship, 273
    lacerations and contusions, 262
    neck and spine, 266, *266*
    nerve entrapment, 268
    in Olympic class boats, 267–76
    overtraining, 260–61
    overuse injury, 261, 264, 268, 274
    parts of dinghy associated with, *263*
    posterior interosseous nerve (PIN) entrapment, 265, 266–67, *267*
    in recreational boating and cruising, 262–64
    rotator cuff, 265, *266*
    at Sailing Federation World Championship, 273
    to the shoulder and spine, 264–65
    by site, *274*

    soft tissue, 264
    sprains (torn ligaments), 261
    strains, 259, 261
    and trauma, 259, 268
    traumatic brain injury (TBI), 275–76
    while windsurfing, 274–75
inner ear, 3
insect repellents, 167–168, 169
insomnia, 296–98
insomnia severity index, 357
insulating layers, 72
insulin, 205
Interaural Level Difference (ILD), 31
Interaural Time Difference (ITD), 31
intermittent fasting (IF), 225n14
International Certificate of Vaccination, 159
International Maritime Conference (1889), 29–30, *30*
International System of Units (SI), 362
interval training, high-intensity, 241, 246
iodine, 172n6
IR3535, 168
iron depletion, 209, 223
irukandji jellyfish, 128, 129
Irwin, Steve, 154n17
isokinetic training, 235–36
isometric stretching, 242
isometric training, 235
isotonic liquids, 96
isotonic training, 234
jellyfish, 123, 125–26, 128–29
    irukandji jellyfish, 128, 129
    treatment of stings, 128–29
jet lag, 288–89, *288*
job-related monotony, 304
Jordan, Chris, 236

Kabat-Zinn, Jon, 334
kahawai, 151
Kahneman, Daniel, 171
Karolinska Sleepiness Scale, 295
Keppel, H.M.S., 59
keratinocytes, 111
keratitis (corneal sunburn), 184
ketogenic diet (keto diet), 225n14

killer clams, 145
Klika, Brett, 236
Knight, Katherine, 246, 250
Knight's Sailing Fitness Toolbox, 351

lactate threshold (LT), 240, *240*
Lancaster, James, 208
leadership, effective, 316–17
legs, keeping warm, 67
Leonard, Beth, 20
light rays
    absorption, 182–83, *183*
    bending, 181–83
    and image displacement, 183, *183*
    reflected, 196–97n5
    reflection, 182–83, *183*
    refraction, 182–83, *183*
Lind, James, 208
lionfish, 136, 137–38
liver flukes, 153
lorazepam, 296
luminous range, 196

mackerel, 151
Mackworth, N. H., 304
macular degeneration, 184
Maguire, Eleanor, 47
mahi-mahi, 151
malaria, 158, 168–71
    in Africa and Asia, *170*
    in Central and South America, *170*
    medication for prophylaxis, 169, 171
malarone, 171
mammalian diving reflex, 64
manta (giant devil) ray, 143–44, *143*
maps
    mental, 46, 47
    navigation using, 44–45
marine life, 123
    barracuda, 142
    ciguatera, 146–49
    cone snails, 131–33, *132*, 154n12
    coral reef, 124–25
    crown of thorns, 131
    feather hydroid, 130

    fire coral, 129
    giant grouper, 144
    giant tridacna clam, 145
    irukandji jellyfish, 128
    jellyfish, 123, 125–26, 128–29
    manta (giant devil) ray, 143–44, *143*
    moray eel, 142–43, *143*
    needlefish, 144
    octopus, 133–34, *133*
    orcas (killer whales), 144–45
    other coelenterates, 129–30
    Portuguese man-of-war, 127
    pufferfish, 149–51
    rockfish, 138
    scorpionfish, 136–38
    sea anemones, 130
    sea snakes, 135–36, *136*
    sea urchins, 130–31, *131*
    sea wasp, 126–27
    sharks, 138–42, 154n23, 154–55n24
    starfish, 131, *131*
    stingray, 134–35, *135*, 154n17
    stonefish, 136–37, *136*
    weeverfish, 138
    zebrafish, 136
marine signals, 30
Masefield, John, 291
measles, mumps, rubella vaccine (MMR), 165
meclizine, 19–20, 21
meditation. *See* mindfulness meditation
Mediterranean diet, 213, *214*
mefloquine, 171
melanin, 105, 111, *111*, 121n9
melanocytes, 111, 121n9
melanoma, 186
melatonin, 282, 297
memory function
    and the hippocampus, 46, 48
    and navigation, 44–45
    purpose of, 50–51n22
Meniere's disease, 11
mental imagery. *See* imagery
metabolism
    of fat, 223

of food, 78–79, 92, 95
and hypothermia, 54, 64
increasing, 81
of protein, 96
method of loci, 50–51n22
methylphenidate, 81
metric system conversions, 362–66
Mexoryl SX and XL, 114, *115*
microsleeping, 290
Midshipmen Development Center (U.S. Naval Academy), 320
miliaria (prickly heat), 118
MIND diet, *215*
mindfulness meditation, 297–98, 333–36, 360
minerals, 209
minimal erythema dose (MED), 106, *107*, 112–13
Moitessier, Bernard, 317n1
monotony, 315
moon jellyfish, 126
See also jellyfish
moray eel, 142–43, *143*
mosquito repellents, 168, 169
mosquitos
and malaria, 168–69
and yellow fever, 166–67
motion sickness, 2
adaptation schedules, 27n21
in animals, 2, 22n2
current theory of, 6–11
and the motion analyzer, 6–7, *7*
psychological, 13
World War II medications, 26n17
See also seasickness
Motion Sickness Susceptibility Questionnaire Short-Form (MMSQ-Short), 341–44
MRI scans, *46*, 47
muscles
abdominal, *271*
deep multifidi, *272*
iliopsoas, *271*
low back, *272*
quadriceps, 270–71
quasi-isometric contractions, 273
tendons of the knee, *270*
tibialis anterior, *272*
used in small boat sailing and sailboarding, *270*

National Institute for Occupational Safety and Health, 37
nausea, 10
See also seasickness
navigation
Aborigine, 44
celestial, 39
by color, 43
eyeball, 191–92
Inuit, 44–45
by maps, 44–45
by memory, 44–45, 50–51n22
natural, 39–40, 44
Polynesian, 41–43
response system, 46, 48–49
by sea birds, 43–44
and the senses, 38–48
by sight, 38, 49n2
by smell, 38
in snow, 45
by sound, 40
spatial strategy, 46–47, 48
stick chart, 43
by sun and stars, 39–42
by taste, 40
thermometrical, 43
unnatural, 48
using ocean swells and waves, 42–43
using "sixth sense," 45–46
Viking, 40–41, *41*
by wind, 43
needlefish, 144, 151
Nelson, Horatio, 2, 13, 26n19
nematocyst, 125, 153n3
nervous breakdown, 308–9
neurotransmitters, 283
non-exercise activity thermogenesis (NEAT), 211
nonshivering thermogenesis, 54
norepinephrine, 283

norovirus, 161
Norwalk virus, 161
nutrition
    and aerobic glycolysis, 220–23
    and anaerobic glycolysis, 220
    "Basic 4" food groups, *201*
    "Basic 7" food groups, *201*
    calories and exercise, 210–13
    carbohydrates, 204–6
    fats, 206–7
    food pyramid, 202, *202, 213, 214*
    healthy diets, 213–14
    intermittent fasting (IF), 225n14
    ketogenic diet (keto diet), 225n14
    minerals, 209
    MyPlate, 202–3, *202*
    nautical, 199–203
    and our energy systems, 215–19
    protein, 203–4
    and the sailing athlete, 214–15
    USDA guidelines, 201–3
    vitamins, 207–9

ocean
    bacteria in, 37
    smell of, 37–38
ocean sunfish, 149
O'Connor, M. R., 44
octinoxate, *116*
octopus, 133–34, *133*
ocular inflammation, 184
oil of lemon eucalyptus (OLE or PMD)
oral rehydration therapy, 163–65
orcas (killer whales), 144–45
O'Sullivan, H. Barry, 58–60
O'Sullivan, Mrs. H. B., 58–60
overload factor, 256
oxybenzone, 114
oxygen uptake norms, 349
ozone layer, 102, 103

pandemics, 159
para-aminobenzoic acid (PABA), 121n10
paralytic shellfish poisoning, 151–52
parasympathetic nervous system, 331, 332–33

Parcells, Bill, 316
Parry, William, 45
passive rewarming, 64
patellofemoral syndrome, *271*
performance routines, 327, 329
permethrin, 167
persistent pigment darkening test (PPD), 114
personal flotation devices (PFDs), 60, 255, 258, 276
Phenergan. *See* promethazine
phosphogen system, 218, 219
photoallergic reactions, 108, **109**, *110*
photokeratitis, 184
photosensitivity, **109**
phototoxic reactions, 108, **109**, *110*
physical examination, 228
phytoplankton, 37
Picaridin, 168
Pilates, 246–47
pinguecula, 184–85
place cells, 47
plague, 159
pneumococcal vaccines, 166
polarized light, 175, *175*
Polynesian Triangle, *42*
porcupine fish, 149
Portuguese man-of-war, 127
posterior interosseous nerve (PIN) entrapment, 265, 266–67, *267*
posttraumatic stress disorder, 314
potassium supplements, 83
prehydration, 89–90
pressure immobilization technique (PIT), *133*
prickly heat (miliaria), 81, 118, *119*
prismatics, 181
proguanil, 171
promethazine, 18–19, 27n24
    suppositories, 20
proprioception, 39
proprioceptive neuromuscular facilitation (PNF) stretching, 243
protein, 203–4, 217–18
    daily consumption, 223
    recommendations for athletes, **223**
protein complementarity, 203

protozoa, 161
psychological skills training (PST), 319–20, 334–36
    anxiety, 330–32
    attentional focus, 328–30
    concentration and focus, 327–28
    emergency anxiety relief on the water, 332–33
    flow, 336–38
    goal setting, 321–22
    mental imagery, 323–27
    mindfulness meditation, 333–36
    self-talk and performance routines, 327
    SMART goals, 322–23
psychology
    of the effective captain, 316
    of effective leadership, 316–17
    of sailing crew and small-group behavior, 310–16
    of singlehanded sailing, 304–9
psychosis, stress-induced, 309
pterygium, 185
pufferfish, 149–51

quadriceps, 270–71
quarantine, 158–60

radiation, 88
    heat loss through, 55
rainwater, 94
rash, 81, 118
Rasmussen, Knud, 45
rating of perceived exertion (RPE) scale, 349–50
red snapper, 146
red tide, 151
rehydration
    after exercise, 89
    during exercise, 89–90
relaxation response, 334–35, 359–60
repetitive strain injury, 261
resistance bands, 244–45
retention enema. *See* enema
reverse osmosis, 92

rewarming, active/passive, 64–65
risk, 158, 171
Ritalin, 81
Robertson, Dougal, 94, 97
rotator cuff injuries, 265, *266*
rotavirus, 161
Roth, Hal, 312
Rundstrom, Robert, 45

sailboarding, 250
sailing, in cold weather, 53–73
sailing accidents. *See* accidents
sailing crews
    and crew harmony, 314–16
    and small-group behavior, 310–16
sailing fitness test, 348
sailing rules, 31
sailors
    big boat racing, 247–48, 264–67
    competitive, 224n6, 227–28
    cruising, 244–47
    Olympic class, 248–50, 267–76
    Polynesian, 38–39, 40, 41–44, 47
    recreational, 262–64
    singlehanded, 304–9
    small boat, 248–50
    Viking, 40
sailor's skin, 101
salinity, 96
    estimation of, 98
salmonella, 152–53, 158, 161
salt intake, 87
salt tablets, 83, 99n3
sardines, 151
sciatica, 261, *261*
scombroid poisoning, 151
scopolamine, 17–18, 19, 81
    transdermal, 19, 21
scorpionfish, 136–38
scurvy, 157, 207–9
sea anemones, 130
sea birds, 43–44
sea nettles, 126
    See also jellyfish

seasickness, 1–27
    and anxiety, 13
    cause of, 2
    contributing factors, 12–13
    "to do" list, 16
    drug treatment, 16–21, **18**, 27n24
    effects on world history, 2
    exacerbating factors, 12–13
    gut symptoms, **9**
    head symptoms, **9**
    individual variability and sensitivity, 11–12
    prevention of, 13–15
    sensory conflict in the brain, 6–9
    Sopite syndrome, 21–22
    stages of, 8–9
    and the stomach, 12
    symptoms and signs, 9–11
    and the vestibular balance system, 3–5
    and vision, 6
sea snakes, 135–36, *136*
sea urchins, 130–31, *131*
sea wasps, 126–27, 153n3, 153n8
seawater, controversy over drinking, 95–97
seawater boils, 119
seaweed, 37
self-talk, 327, 329
semicircular canals, 3–5, *4*, 6, *6*, 20, 29
sensory conflict theory, 6–9, 24–25n8
sensory deprivation, 304
serotonin, 283
72 COLREGS, 49n1
severe acute respiratory syndrome, 159
Shackleton, Ernest, 22n2
shark repellents, 142
sharks, 98–99, 138–42, 154n23, 154–55n24
shellfish poisoning
    bacterial, 152
        erythematous, 152
        paralytic, 151–52
shigella, 161
shigellosis, 158
shingles vaccine (Shingrix), 166

shivering, 54, 73–74n2, *74*
    and hypothermia, 63
Shlim, David R., 171
shoes
    for cold weather, 67
    wearing in cold water, 60
shoulder stabilization, 250
sight, navigation by, 38
simulator sickness, 2
skin cancer, 101, 103, 110
skin disorders
    actinic damage, 103
    coral cuts, 124–25
    heat-related, 81
    miliaria (prickly heat), 118
    photoallergic reactions, 108, **109**, *110*
    phototoxic reactions, 108, **109**, *110*
    prickly heat (miliaria), *119*
    sailor's skin, 101
    seawater boils, 119
    skin cancer, 101, 103, 110
    sunburn, 103, 105–8
    swimmer's itch, 120
skipjack, 151
sky radiation, 104
sleep
    and alcohol, 290
    choosing a watchkeeping system, 290–94
    circadian rhythm, 281–83
    circadian rhythm disturbances, 287–89
    cycles of, 286–87, *287*
    documenting sleep disorders, 295
    and jet lag, 288–89
    and microsleeping, 290
    and the Monday morning blues, 289
    non-rapid eye movement (non-REM), 286, 294
    process described, 286–87
    rapid eye movement (REM), 286, 294
    reasons for, 280–81
    recommendations for healthy patterns, 298

sleep inertia, 294–95
sleep pressure disturbances and sleep loss, 289–90
treatment for insomnia, 296–98
two-step model, 283–86
sleep debt, 289–90
sleep deprivation, 256, 258, 289–90, 294
accidents caused by, 279–80
sleep diary, 295, *356*
sleep disorders, 295
sleep inertia, 294–95
sleep loss, and singlehanded sailing, 307
sleep pressure, 299–300n4
disturbances in, 289–90
sleep restriction, 289
small-group behavior, 310–16
smallpox, 159
SMART goals, 322–23, 337, 359
smell
navigation by, 38
of the sea, 37–38
social isolation, 305
sodium hypochlorite (bleach), 162, 172n6
solar still, 92, 93
Sopite syndrome, 21–22
sound
in foggy weather, 31, 33
head tilting to disambiguate the vertical, *34*
head turning to disambiguate location, *33*
and Interaural Level Difference (ILD), 31, *33*
and Interaural Time Difference (ITD), 31
judging distance of, 35
localization of, 33–34
navigation by, 34, 40
noise and decibel level, 36, *36*
at sea, 29–37
sound waves over water vs. over land, 35, *35*
Vertical Interaural Difference, *34*
sound signals, 30–31
in foggy weather, 31

spacecraft sickness, 2, 23n6, 27n21
speed cells, 47
sport psychology, 319–20
sprains (torn ligaments), 260, 261
Stadler, Michael, 314
stand-up paddling (SUP), 245, *246*
star compass, 41–42, *42*
starfish, 131, *131*
static balance, 243–44
static stretching, 242
steering rules, 31
stimulants, 81
sting and bite treatments
cone snail envenomation, 133
jellyfish, 128–29
lionfish, 137–38
octopus bites, 134
pressure immobilization technique (PIT), 133, *133*, 136
rockfish, 138
sea snakes, 136
sea urchins, 131
stingray, 134–35
stonefish, 136–37
stingrays, 134–35, *135*, 154n17
stonefish, 136–37, *136*
strains, 259, 261
strength training, 233–36
isokinetic, 235–36
isometric, 235
isotonic, 234
stress
four stages of, *330*
psychology of, 311–12
reduction of, 334
and singlehanded sailing, 308–9
stretching
active versus passive static, 242
ballistic, 243
dynamic, 243
isometric, 242
proprioceptive neuromuscular facilitation (PNF), 243
static, 242
Stugeron, 20

Index

sulfur, atmospheric, 37–38
Summer Olympics
    sailing classes, 249
    training for, 248–49
sunburn, 103, 105–8
sun damage, 101
sunglasses, 176–77
    antireflective coating, 180
    and contact lenses, 181
    how sunglasses work, *176*
    lens material, 180
    lens prescription, 181
    lens shape and frame style, 180–81
    light transmission factor (LTF) and lens color, 177, *178*
    photochromatic lenses, 179
    polarizing lenses, 178–79, *179*, 196n4
    and prismatics, 181
    reflecting or mirror lenses, 177–78
    scratch resistant, 180
    and UV radiation, 180
sunscreens, 104, 112, 113–17
    common chemical and mineral agents, **113**
    Japanese UVA grading system, *115*, 121–22n11
    labeling, *115*, *116*
    penetration of UVA and UVB, *108*
    sun protection factor (SPF), 112–13
    tips for staying safe in the sun, 117
survival, and water loss, 91–99
survival suits, 74–75n7
swamp itch, 120
sweat glands, 80, *80*

sweating
    avoiding, 70
    calculating rate of, 91
    drugs that can interfere with sweating, 345
    and heat, 92
    sweat rate calculation, 346–47
swellfish, 149
swimmer's itch, 120, *120*
sympathetic nervous system, 331
systems theory, 256

Tai Chi, 244, 246
tanning, 105, 110–13
temperature regulation, 88
    See also cold water; cold weather; hypothermia; heat-induced disorders; heat loss
tetanus, diphtheria, pertussis (Tdap or Td) vaccine, 166
tetraodontiformes, 149
Texas A&M University Galveston Sailing Team Personal Fitness Test, 348–49
thermal balance, 54–63
thermic effect of food (TEF), 210
thermogenesis, 73–74n2, *74*
    non-exercise activity (NEAT), 211
    nonshivering, 54
thermoneutral zone, 79
thermoregulation, and athletic performance, 87–89
threshold of hearing (TOH), 36–37
Tinetti Assessment Tool for Balance, 244, 250n8
Tinosorb M and S, 114
Titanic, RMS, 53
titanium, *116*
toadfish, 149
Tomalin, N., 308
topiramate, 81
torn ligaments, 261
tranquilizers, 81
Transcendental Meditation (TM), 334
Transderm Scop, 19, 20, 21
trapezing, 250, 268, 274, *275*
trapped nerves, 261
trauma, acute, 259
traveler's diarrhea (TD), 161–65
    bacterial causes, 161
    levels of risk, 161
    minimizing risk, 161–62
    prevention/prophylaxis, 163
    protozoan causes, 161
    signs and symptoms of dehydration, 163
    signs of adequate rehydration, 163
    treatment for, 163–65
    viral causes, 161

triglycerides, 217
tuberculosis, 159
tub immersion, for hypothermia, 65
turkeyfish, 136, 137–38
twelve-minute run test, 349
2-undecanone, 168
typhoid fever, 158
typhus, 158

ultraviolet (UV) radiation, 102, 120n1, 174
   direct vs. oblique light, 103, *103*
   electromagnetic wave from visible light and UV spectrum, *174*
   exposure to, 102–4
   sensitivity to, 105
   and the skin, *106*
   UVA, 107, *108*
   UVB, 107, *108*
   See also sunburn; tanning
ultraviolet protection factor (UPF) clothing, 117–18, *118*
United States Light List, 196
urine, 89, *90*, 92, 95, 96, 128, 131, 163, 207, 346, 347
utricle and saccule (U&S), 3–5, *4*, 29
UV exposure, 102–4
   and cataracts, 185
   and polarizing lenses, 179–80

vaccinations, 165–71
   flu and pneumococcal vaccines, 166
   Hepatitis A, 166
   measles, mumps, rubella vaccine (MMR), 165
   rabies, 159–60
   shingles (Shingrix), 166
   tetanus, diphtheria, pertussis (Tdap or Td), 166
   yellow fever, 167–68
Valium, 296
Van Dorn, W.G., 145
vasoconstriction, 60
vegetarians, 223

vessels
   lights carried by, 31
   six motions of, 7–8, *8*, *14*
   steering and sailing rules, 31
vestibular balance system, 3–5, *4*, 6–8, 23n5, 29, 39
vibrio, 161
viral enteritis, 158
viral hemorrhagic fevers, 159
virtual reality sickness, 2
viruses, marine, 37, 49n7
vision
   bending light rays, 181–84
   binoculars and other nautical instruments, 189
   blind spot, 193, *194*
   and color perception, 189–92
   contact lenses, 181
   and glare, 175–76
   and the grand spectrum, 174–75
   and luminous range, 196
   nighttime, 193–96
   ophthalmic conditions, 184–86
   rods and cones, 190, 192, 193–95, 197–98n15
   and sailing acuity, 173, 186–89
   and sunglasses technology, 176–81
   at twilight, 192, 197n13
   visual acuity, 186–88
   See also eye disorders; visual acuity
visual acuity, 186–87, *188*, 197n9
   and celestial acuity, 187–88, *188*
   at night, 194
   structure of the retina, *187*
visualization, 325
   See also imagery
vitamin C, 207–9
vitamin D, 110
vitamins, 207–9
vomiting, 10
   See also seasickness

wahoo, 151
Walters, J.D., 98

watchkeeping systems, 290–94
    3/9 Circadian Watch Rotation, 293, *294*
    additional schedules, 352–55, *352–55*
    circadian, 293, *293*
    five and dime, 292–93, *292*
    on a man-of-war, 300–301n9
    one watch, 291
    two watches, 291, *291*
water
    chemical desalination of, 93–94
    depth of, 191–92
    in food, 78–79
    intake of, 78
    in marine life, 94–95
    output of, 78
    rainwater, 94
    requirements for survival, 92
    sources of, 92–93, *98*
    See also cold water; water loss
water loss
    insensible, 79
    and survival, 91–92
    through the kidneys, 79
watermakers, 162–63, 172n7

waypoints, 48
weeverfish, 138
wet suits, 71
windsurfing, 274–75, *275*

Xanax, 296
X-ray exposure, 120n2

yacht racing, 99n6
yellow fever, 158, 159, 166–68
    in Brazil, *168*
    in Sub-Saharan Africa, *167*
    vaccine for, 167–68
yellowfin tuna, 151
yoga, 246–47, *246*, 334

zebrafish, 136, 137–38
zeitgebers, 283–84
zinc, *116*
zinc oxide, 115–16
zone, being in the, 336
zonisamide, 81
zooplankton, 37

www.ingramcontent.com/pod-product-compliance
Lightning Source LLC
Chambersburg PA
CBHW081103080526
44587CB00021B/3432